The Musculoskeletal System

SYSTEMS OF THE BODY
The Musculoskeletal System
BASIC SCIENCE AND CLINICAL CONDITIONS
THIRD EDITION

Sean O'Neill BMED PhD FRACP
Associate Professor
Rheumatology
Sydney Musculoskeletal Health Flagship
University of Sydney Northern Clinical School
Rheumatologist
Royal North Shore Hospital
St Leonards, NSW, Australia

Lyn March MSc MBBS PhD FRACP
FAFPHM
Liggins Professor of Rheumatology and Musculoskeletal
Epidemiology,
University of Sydney
Professorial Rheumatology Department
Royal North Shore Hospital
St Leonards, NSW, Australia

Leslie Schrieber MBBS MD
FRACP
Hon Associate Professor
Rheumatology
Royal North Shore Hospital
St Leonards, NSW, Australia

Terence Rae Moopanar MBBS FRACS FAOrthA PhD
Visiting Orthopaedic Surgeon
Royal North Shore Hospital
Sydney, Australia

William Walter MBBS FRACS
FAOrthA PhD
Department of Orthopaedic Surgery
Royal North Shore Hospital
The Kolling Institute
University of Sydney, NSW, Australia

Series Editor
Stephen Hughes BSc, MSc,
MBBS, FRCSEd, FRCEM, FHEA
Consultant in Emergency Medicine, Broomfield Hospital
Senior Lecturer in Medicine, School of Medicine, Anglia
Ruskin University
Chelmsford, UK

For additional online content visit ExpertConsult.com

ELSEVIER

First edition 2003
Second edition 2010

Notices

Practitioners and researchers must always rely on their own experience and knowledge in evaluating and using any information, methods, compounds or experiments described herein. Because of rapid advances in the medical sciences, in particular, independent verification of diagnoses and drug dosages should be made. To the fullest extent of the law, no responsibility is assumed by Elsevier, authors, editors or contributors for any injury and/or damage to persons or property as a matter of products liability, negligence or otherwise, or from any use or operation of any methods, products, instructions, or ideas contained in the material herein.

ISBN: 978-0-7020-8380-8

Publisher: Jeremy Bowes
Content Project Manager: Fariha Nadeem
Design: Margaret Reid
Illustration Manager: Anitha Rajarathnam
Marketing Manager: Deborah Watkins

Copyedited by Editage, a unit of Cactus Communications Services Pte. Ltd.

Typeset by TNQ Technologies Pvt. Ltd.

Printed in Scotland

Last digit is the print number: 9   8   7   6   5   4   3   2   1

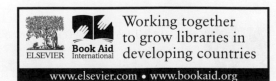

Chapter 1 Rheumatoid arthritis and the hand
Leslie Schrieber MBBS MD FRACP
Hon Associate Professor, Rheumatology, Royal North Shore Hospital, St Leonards, NSW, Australia

and

Nicholas Manolios MBBS (HONS) PhD MD FRACP FRCPA
Professor of Rheumatology, Faculty of Medicine and Health, University of Sydney
Director of Rheumatology, Westmead Hospital, Sydney, Australia

Chapter 2 Soft tissue rheumatic disease involving the shoulder and elbow
Terence Rae Moopanar MBBS FRACS FAOrthA PhD
Visiting Orthopaedic Surgeon, Royal North Shore Hospital, Sydney, Australia

Chapter 3 Nerve compression syndromes
David Stewart MBCHB FRACS (PLAST)
Visiting Hand Surgeon, Royal North Shore Hospital, Sydney, Australia

Chapter 4 Lower back pain
Christopher Needs MBBS MMed BPharm MA FRACP
Senior Clinical Lecturer, University of Sydney
Senior Staff Specialist Rheumatology, Royal Prince Alfred Hospital, Camperdown, NSW, Australia

and

Manuela Ferreira PhD
Professor, The University of Sydney, Faculty of Medicine and Health, The Back Pain Research Team, Institute of Bone and Joint Research, The Kolling Institute, Royal North Shore Hospital, St Leonards, NSW, Australia

Chapter 5 Bone structure and function in normal and disease states
Lyn March MSc MBBS PhD FRACP FAFPHM
Liggins Professor of Rheumatology and Musculoskeletal Epidemiology, University of Sydney Professorial Rheumatology Department, Royal North Shore Hospital, St Leonards, NSW, Australia

and

Roderick Clifton-Bligh BSc (Med) MBBS FRACP PhD FFSc (RCPA)
Associate Professor, Medicine, Northern Clinical School, Kolling Institute, University of Sydney. Head of Department of Endocrinology Royal North Shore Hospital, Sydney, Australia

and

Andrew Ellis OAM MBBS FRACS(Orth) FAOrthA
Visiting Orthopaedic Surgeon, Royal North Shore Hospital, Sydney, Australia
COL Royal Australian Army Medical Corps

Chapter 6 The synovial joint in health and disease: osteoarthritis
Christopher B. Little BVMS MSc PhD DACVS FRSN
Director, Raymond Purves Bone and Joint Research Laboratories Professor, Faculty of Medicine and Health, The University of Sydney Northern Clinical School, Kolling Institute, Institute of Bone and Joint Research, Northern Sydney Local Health District, Royal North Shore Hospital, St Leonards, NSW, Australia

and

David J. Hunter MBBS MSc (Clin Epi) M SpMeD PhD FRACP
Florance and Cope Chair of Rheumatology, Professor of Medicine, Co-Director Sydney Musculoskeletal Health Flagship, University of Sydney, Rheumatologist, Royal North Shore Hospital, St Leonards, NSW, Australia

and

Lyn March MSc MBBS PhD FRACP FAFPHM
Liggins Professor of Rheumatology and Musculoskeletal Epidemiology, University of Sydney Professorial Rheumatology Department, Royal North Shore Hospital, St Leonards, NSW, Australia

Chapter 7 Crystal arthropathies and the ankle
Neil McGill MBBS BSc(Med) FRACP
Visiting Rheumatologist, Royal Prince Alfred Hospital, Sydney, Australia

Chapter 8 Skeletal muscle and its disorders
Matthew J.S. Parker MBChB MRCP FRACP
Staff Specialist Rheumatologist, Royal Prince Alfred Hospital, Sydney, Australia

Chapter 9 Autoimmunity and the musculoskeletal system
Sean O'Neill BMed PhD FRACP
Associate Professor, Rheumatology, Sydney Musculoskeletal Health Flagship, University of Sydney Northern Clinical School, Rheumatologist, Royal North Shore Hospital, St Leonards, NSW, Australia

Chapter 10 Trauma and the musculoskeletal system
Terence Rae Moopanar MBBS FRACS FAOrthA PhD
Visiting Orthopaedic Surgeon, Royal North Shore Hospital, Sydney, Australia

and

Andrew Ellis OAM MBBS FRACS(Orth) FAOrthA
Visiting Orthopaedic Surgeon, Royal North Shore Hospital, Sydney, Australia
COL Royal Australian Army Medical Corps

Chapter 11 Infection and the musculoskeletal system
William Walter MBBS FRACS FAOrthA PhD
Department of Orthopaedic Surgery, Royal North Shore Hospital, The Kolling Institute, University of Sydney, NSW, Australia

Most students now study medicine through a form of integrated curriculum. These courses blend basic science with exposure to clinical medicine from an early stage. These students have the good fortune to be left in no doubt, from the outset, why they are studying medicine. I teach in a medical school that delivers a fully integrated curriculum and I can compare it with the traditional model according to which I received my early medical education. That comparison is very favourable.

Unlike many other texts, the *Systems of the Body* series has been designed very specifically to support an integrated approach to learning medicine. Our carefully selected panel of authors drawn from across the English-speaking world have combined basic science with clinical application. Links to clinical skills, clinical investigation and therapeutics are made clear throughout.

The aim is to offer highly accessible guidance for all student types and stages. It will be invaluable to those who are approaching the subject for the first time or who may have found a topic challenging when using other more traditionally configured resources – as well as greatly assist all students wishing to excel as their course progresses. The clear layout and writing style, together with detail that informs without overwhelming, go a long way to supporting students. It may also provide welcome reminders to postgraduates facing their own examinations.

Whatever curriculum you follow, wherever you are in the world, and whichever stage you are at, we know that the *Systems of the Body* volumes will serve as great places to start when learning something new and enable you to effectively piece together the essential components of each major body system, in a modern clinical context.

Good luck!

Stephen Hughes, MSc MBBS FRCSEd FRCEM FHEA
Senior Lecturer in Medicine
Consultant, Emergency Medicine
Anglia Ruskin University
and
Broomfield Hospital
Chelmsford, UK
Chelmsford, UK

The burden of musculoskeletal disease is high across the world, significantly limiting mobility and dexterity. The World Health Organization points to musculoskeletal conditions as the leading contributor to disability worldwide. Because of ageing and population growth, the number affected is rapidly increasing.

The editors and chapter authors are excited to introduce the third edition of *The Musculoskeletal System* (Basic Science and Clinical Conditions). The aim of this introductory text book is to build on a long-standing enthusiasm for health science education, which arose from passionate clinical teachers within the Department of Rheumatology and the Department of Orthopaedic and Traumatic Surgery at Royal North Shore Hospital and the University of Sydney. We are indebted to and remember in this edition the lives of our dear friends who as Professors and Chairs of these departments commenced the project in 1999, and 20 years ago saw the release of the first edition. We thus acknowledge Professor Phillip Sambrook OAM and Professor Thomas Taylor who gathered the editors and chapter authors together for the task. They recognized the partnership of the two disciplines leading towards success in understanding the nature and treatment of disorders of the musculoskeletal system.

Science underpins knowledgeable treatment, and much has progressed and is incorporated in this new edition. Each chapter introduces the relevant basic science of the various elements of the musculoskeletal system and of the subsequent pathophysiology of their disorders. The superb illustrations, tables and graphics serve to reinforce the key points and aid understanding of structures and functions of musculoskeletal tissues and of immune and metabolic pathways.

Although primarily aimed to support the learning of medical students, there is much in the book of interest to other professionals involved in the care of the arthritic or injured patient. Physiotherapists, occupational therapists, nurses, psychologists, pharmacists and orthotists all contribute a great deal to the comprehensive care of patients with musculoskeletal problems. This book provides a clear explanation of the basic science and clinical conditions of the musculoskeletal system with great utility to many health professionals. It provides an introductory platform that the curious clinician can build on according to their interest and needs.

Using a problem-based format that has proved so successful in previous editions, the reader is led through practical examples of the condition under discussion. A format has been chosen that integrates explanations about anatomy and basic science at the beginning of each chapter. The latter then expands on the clinical disorders and conditions and their treatment with links to further learning at each chapter's end.

Let the authors journey with you, the reader, as foundation knowledge and understanding is built on this critical area of healthcare.

The authors gratefully acknowledge the contributions of the chapter authors of the previous (second) edition of The Musculoskeletal System – Basic Science and Clinical Conditions: David Sonnabend (Chapter 2), Michael Tonkin (Chapter 3), Les Barnsley (Chapter 4), Philip Sambrook (Chapter 5), Rodger Laurent (Chapter 8), Nicholas Manolios (Chapter 9), Andrew Ellis and Thomas Taylor (Chapter 10), and Sydney Nade (Chapter 11).

CONTENTS

AUTOIMMUNITY AND THE MUSCULOSKELETAL SYSTEM 137

TRAUMA AND THE MUSCULOSKELETAL SYSTEM 153

INFECTION AND THE MUSCULOSKELETAL SYSTEM 167

RHEUMATOID ARTHRITIS AND THE HAND

Leslie Schrieber and Nicholas Manolios

Chapter objectives

After studying this chapter you should be able to:

1. Explain the structure and function of synovial joints.

2. Understand the relevant anatomy of the hand and wrist joints.

3. Discuss the basic function of the immune system.

4. Understand the aetiopathogenesis of rheumatoid arthritis.

5. Describe the pathological changes that occur in inflammatory arthritis.

6. Recognize the common clinical presentations and features of rheumatoid arthritis and their pathophysiological basis.

7. Develop an approach to the differential diagnosis of inflammatory arthritis.

8. Describe extra-articular manifestations of rheumatoid arthritis and explain their pathophysiological basis.

9. Understand the principles that govern the team approach to the management of rheumatoid arthritis.

10. Describe the clinical pharmacology and use of non-steroidal anti-inflammatory drugs, corticosteroids, disease-modifying anti-rheumatic drugs and biological therapies in the treatment of rheumatoid arthritis.

11. Discuss the place of orthopaedic surgery in the treatment of rheumatoid arthritis.

12. Appreciate the long-term prognosis of rheumatoid arthritis.

Introduction

Synovial joints, the most mobile type of joints in the body, are susceptible to inflammatory injury leading to arthritis. The synovium is a common target of a variety of insults including direct microbial infection, crystal deposition and autoimmune attack such as seen in rheumatoid arthritis (RA). This chapter will review normal synovial joint structure and function, describe the processes that lead to inflammatory arthritis, outline an approach to differential diagnosis and describe the principles of treatment of RA. The topic and discussion will be illustrated by a patient with inflammatory arthritis found to have RA, the commonest chronic inflammatory rheumatic disease, affecting 1%–2% of the population. RA not only produces extensive morbidity, but also is associated with a reduction in life expectancy.

Essential anatomy and physiology

Synovial joint anatomy

There are three types of joints in the body: synarthroses, amphiarthroses and diarthroses (synovial joints). Synarthroses are joints that have an interlocking suture line between adjacent bones (e.g. skull bones) – this provides a very strong bond. The synarthrosis expands during maturation of the developing brain and is eventually replaced by bony union between the adjacent bones at the end of brain growth. Amphiarthroses are joints that have fibrocartilage between adjacent bones – this results in limited flexibility and strength. They are found in

the rib cage, the sacroiliac joint, symphysis pubis and between vertebral bodies – the intervertebral discs.

Diarthroses, or synovial joints, are the commonest type of joint and are the most flexible. They possess a synovial membrane, have a cavity that contains synovial fluid, and are subclassified into ball and socket (e.g. hip), hinge (e.g. interphalangeal) and saddle (e.g. first carpometacarpal) types. These joints (see Fig. 1.1A, B) allow the cartilaginous surfaces of the joint ends to move efficiently and smoothly, with low-frictional resistance. Different designs allow for different movements, including flexion (bending), extension (straightening), abduction (movement

Case 1.1 Rheumatoid arthritis: 1

Case history

Mrs Gale is a 43-year-old woman who, together with her husband, runs a domestic cleaning company. She presents with a 9-month history of painful hands and wrists. Her symptoms started with occasional early-morning stiffness and swelling in her right knee, followed shortly afterwards by similar symptoms in her hands and wrists. Mrs Gale says she is no longer able to help her husband in the cleaning business. The pain is getting worse. Physical examination reveals symmetrical soft tissue swelling in all the proximal interphalangeal and metacarpophalangeal joints of both hands and wrists. Her right knee joint is swollen and has an effusion. The metatarsophalangeal joints are tender to palpation.

A provisional diagnosis of an inflammatory arthritis, probably rheumatoid arthritis, is made. Interpretation of this presentation requires knowledge of synovial joint structure in general and the hands in particular as well as knowledge of the immune system in health and disease.

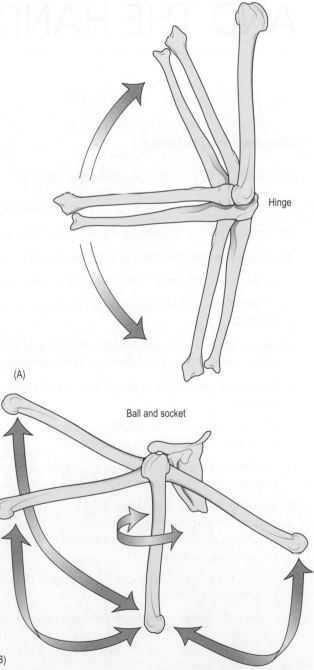

Hinge

(A)

Ball and socket

(B)

Fig. 1.1 Types of synovial joint: (A) hinge joint; (B) ball and socket joint.

away from midline), adduction (movement towards midline), and rotation. Synovial joints are more susceptible to inflammatory injury than are other types of joints.

Synovial joints are surrounded by a capsule that defines the boundary between articular and periarticular structures (Fig. 1.2). Reinforcing the capsule are ligaments and muscular tendons, which act across the joint.

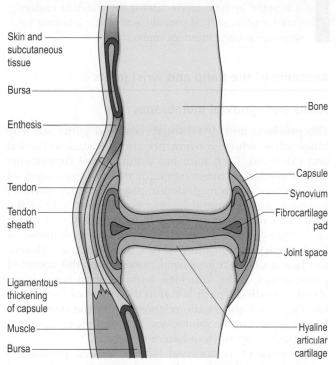

Fig. 1.2 Structure of a synovial joint.

Skin and subcutaneous tissue

Bursa

Enthesis

Tendon

Tendon sheath

Ligamentous thickening of capsule

Muscle

Bursa

Bone

Capsule

Synovium

Fibrocartilage pad

Joint space

Hyaline articular cartilage

The joint capsule, ligaments and tendons are composed principally of type I collagen fibres – type I collagen is the major fibrous protein of connective tissue.

The synovium has a lining layer that consists of special cells called synoviocytes that are normally one to three cells thick. There is no basement membrane separating the synoviocyte layer from the subintima (Fig. 1.3). There are at least two different types of synoviocytes: type A and type B. Type A are of bone marrow-derived macrophage (phagocyte or 'hungry cell') lineage and type B are fibroblast-like synovial (FLS) cells of mesenchymal origin. Other cell types in this layer include dendritic cells – antigen-processing cells involved in generating an immune response. The synoviocytes lie in a stroma composed of collagen fibrils and proteoglycans, a diverse group of glycosylated proteins that are abundant in the extracellular matrix of connective tissues, which is continuous with the subintima. The latter may be fibrous, full of fat or areolar containing loose connective tissue. The subintima contains a dense network of fenestrated capillaries (small blood vessels) that facilitate the exchange of nutrients and other molecules between the circulation and the synovium. The vessels are derived from branches of the arterial plexus that supply the joint capsule and juxta-articular bone. There is also a lymphatic drainage system that is involved in removing large molecules and interstitial fluid from the synovium. The synovium is innervated and pain sensitive, particularly during inflammation.

Synovial joint physiology

Normal synovial joints are highly effective in allowing low-friction movement between articulating surfaces.

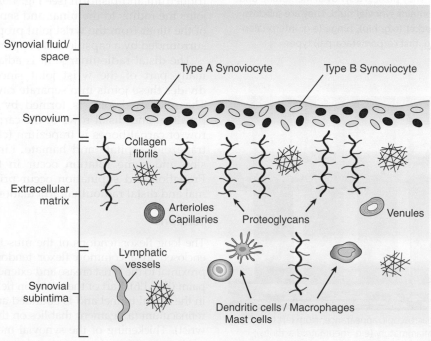

Synovial fluid/ space

Synovium

Collagen fibrils

Extracellular matrix

Lymphatic vessels

Synovial subintima

Type A Synoviocyte

Type B Synoviocyte

Arterioles Capillaries

Proteoglycans

Venules

Dendritic cells / Macrophages Mast cells

Fig. 1.3 Histology of a normal synovial joint.

Articular cartilage is elastic, fluid-holding, analogous to a sponge, attached to a relatively impervious layer of calcified cartilage and bone. Load-induced compression of cartilage forces interstitial fluid to flow laterally out of the cartilage and into the surrounding tissue or joint space. This 'shock-absorbing' effect decreases the pressure load on the joints and assists in protecting the cartilage against mechanical injury.

Synovial fluid (Fig. 1.4) is present in small quantities in normal synovial joints. It is a yellowish coloured, relatively acellular, viscous fluid within the joint that bathes the surface of the synovium and cartilage. Synovial fluid is an ultrafiltrate of blood to which hyaluronic acid is added. Hyaluronic acid is secreted by synoviocytes and is the molecule responsible for synovial fluid viscosity, acting as a lubricant for synovial–cartilage interaction. Synovial fluid provides trophic factors to the cartilage that is avascular and allows for exchange of nutrients and metabolic by-products between plasma, synovial membrane and cartilage. The synovial cavity can be used to advantage as a site at which therapeutic agents can be introduced, for example, intra-articular corticosteroids to treat inflamed synovium, as well as for diagnostic aspiration.

Normal synovial fluid contains only small quantities of low molecular weight proteins compared with plasma. The barrier to the entry of proteins probably resides within the synovial microvascular endothelium.

Interesting facts

Anatomy of synovial joints

Synovial joints are the commonest and most mobile type of joint in the body. They possess a synovial membrane and have a cavity that contains synovial fluid. They are subclassified into ball and socket (e.g. hip), hinge (e.g. interphalangeal) and saddle (e.g. first carpometacarpal) types.

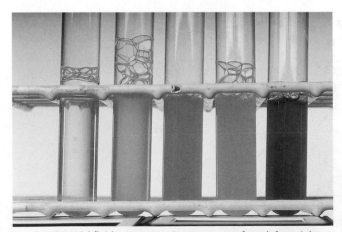

Fig. 1.4 Synovial fluid – macroscopic appearance, from left to right: normal or osteoarthritis; inflammatory (e.g. rheumatoid arthritis); gout; septic; and haemarthrosis (blood).

Interesting facts

Synovial fluid

Synovial fluid, present in small quantities in normal synovial joints, is a clear, yellowish, relatively acellular, viscous fluid that covers the surface of synovium and provides trophic factors to the cartilage. It is an ultrafiltrate of blood to which hyaluronic acid is added. Hyaluronic acid is secreted by synoviocytes and is the molecule responsible for synovial fluid viscosity, acting as a lubricant for synovial–cartilage interface contact.

Anatomy of the hand and wrist joints

Joints and synovial membranes

The proximal and distal interphalangeal joints are true hinge joints whose movements are restricted to flexion and extension. Each joint has a thin dorsal (upper surface) capsular ligament strengthened by expansion of the extensor tendon, a dense palmar (under surface) ligament, and collateral ligaments on either side of the joint. The metacarpophalangeal joints are also considered hinge joints and their ligaments resemble those of the interphalangeal joints. When the fingers are flexed, the heads of the metacarpal bones form the rounded prominences of the knuckles, with the joint space lying about 1 cm distal (peripheral) to the apices of the knuckles. Figure 1.5 shows the relationship of the dorsal and lateral aspects of the joint space, synovial membrane and the articular capsule to adjacent structures.

The wrist or radiocarpal joint is formed proximally by the distal end of the radius and the articular disc, and distally by a row of carpal bones, the scaphoid, lunate, triquetrum and pisiform (see Fig. 1.5A). The articular disc joins the radius to the ulnar and separates the distal end of the ulnar from the wrist joint proper. The wrist joint is surrounded by a capsule and supported by ligaments.

The distal radioulnar joint is adjacent to but not normally part of the wrist joint since the articular disc divides these joints into separate cavities (see Fig. 1.5A). The midcarpal joint is formed by the junction of the proximal and distal rows of the carpal bones. The distal row of carpal bones is trapezium (closest to the thumb), trapezoid, capitate and hamate. Limited flexion, extension and some rotation occur in the midcarpal joint. Pronation and supination occur primarily at the proximal and distal radioulnar articulations.

Tendons

The long flexor tendons of the muscles of the forearm are enclosed in a common flexor tendon sheath that begins proximal to the wrist crease and extends to the middle of the palm (Fig. 1.6). Part of the common flexor tendon sheath lies in the carpal tunnel and is bounded anteriorly by the flexor retinaculum (a ligament that lies on the volar surface of the wrist). Thickening of the synovial membrane of the flexor tendons because of synovitis can cause carpal tunnel syndrome (see Ch. 3). The flexor tendons of the fingers are tethered close to the bones by slings of connective tissue termed 'pulleys' found at eight different locations that extend from the metacarpophalengeal (MCP) joints to the distal phalanx. Pulleys facilitate smooth gliding of the tendons, govern the flexor mechanism of the hand and wrist, and provide mechanical torque and pulling force when flexing. There are five pulleys in the fingers called annular pulleys (A1-5) and three *cruciate* pulleys (C1-3). Clinical syndromes attributed to problems with pulleys include 'trigger finger' and bow-stringing effect following traumatic rupture.

The extensor tendons of the forearm pass through fibro-osseous tunnels on the dorsum of the wrist. These tunnels, which are lined with a synovial sheath, are bounded superficially by the extensor retinaculum and on the deep surface by the carpal bones and ligaments. A depression over the dorsolateral aspect of the wrist when the thumb is extended and abducted is called the anatomical snuffbox.

It is formed by the tendons of abductor pollicis longus and extensor pollicis brevis muscles and is limited proximally by the radial styloid process. Tenderness in this region can be due to stenosing tenosynovitis of these tendons (a condition called de Quervain's tenosynovitis). In this condition, placing the thumb in the palm of the hand, flexing the fingers over the thumb and adducting the wrist will usually produce severe pain (Finkelstein's manoeuvre).

Essential immunology

The immune system has developed principally to help the host combat infections and provide internal immunosurveillance. The human body uses several ways to achieve this, some of which are inherent (innate) and non-specific, while others are exquisitely precise targeted processes that adapt to the inciting stimulus (adaptive).

Innate immune system

The innate response is the first line of host defence. Innate mechanisms are an evolutionary old, immediate, non-specific, first line of defence that avert a microbial infection. Various intrinsic mechanisms include the protective effects of intact skin and mucosa in combating microbe invasion. Normal skin acts as an impermeable barrier to most infectious agents. Mucus secreted by the membranes lining the inner surfaces of the body (e.g. nasal and bronchial mucosa) acts as a protective barrier that prevents bacteria from adhering to epithelial cells. Tears secreted by lacrimal glands protect the cornea of the eye from infection. Similarly, an acidic gastric pH eradicates any bacteria that may enter the upper gastro-intestinal tract. The passing of urine through the urinary track prevents urinary stasis and bacterial olonization.

A variety of white blood cells, including polymorpho-nuclear neutrophils (PMNs) and macrophages, can act as important first lines of defence against microbial attack. These cells, derived from bone marrow precursors, can eliminate microbes following their phagocytosis (uptake). The cells are rich in digestive enzymes that aid in the elim-

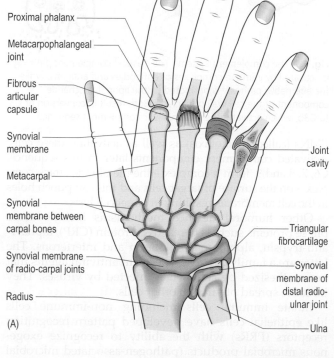

Proximal phalanx

Metacarpophalengeal joint

Fibrous articular capsule

Synovial membrane

Metacarpal

Synovial membrane between carpal bones

Synovial membrane of radio-carpal joints

Radius

(A)

Joint cavity

Triangular fibrocartilage

Synovial membrane of distal radio-ulnar joint

Ulna

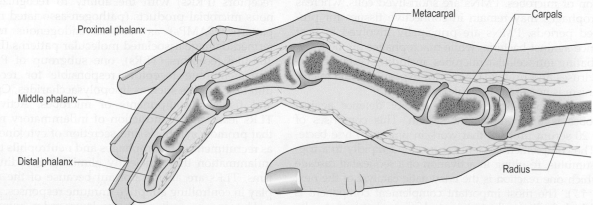

Proximal phalanx

Middle phalanx

Distal phalanx

(B)

Metacarpal

Carpals

Radius

Fig. 1.5 Relationship of the synovial membranes of the wrist and metacarpal joints with adjacent bones. (A) Dorsal view; (B) sagittal view showing proximal and distal interphalangeal joints.

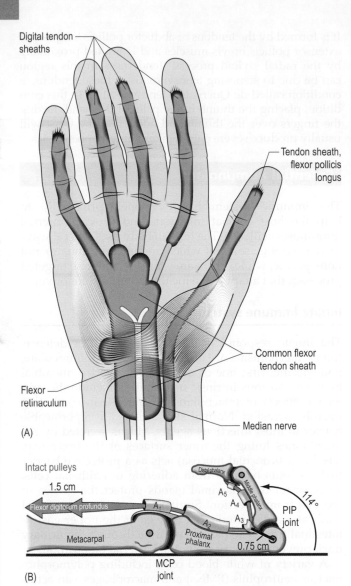

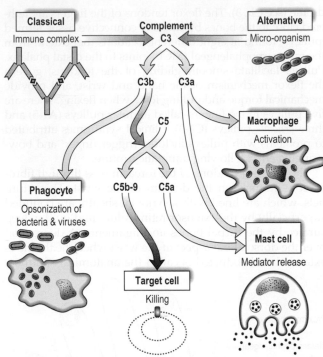

Fig. 1.7 The complement system. The classical complement pathway is activated by immune complexes of antibodies and antigens, while the alternative pathway is promoted by the lipopolysaccharide component of the cell wall of bacteria. Both result in conversion of C3 to C3b, which activates the terminal lytic complement sequence.

Fig. 1.6 (A) Palmar view of the hand showing distribution of the synovial sheaths and flexor tendons; (B) Location of A1–5 pulleys. *MCP*, Metacarpophalangeal; *PIP*, Proximal interphalangeal (From Neumann, D.A. (2017). Kinesiology of the Musculoskeletal System. St. Louis: Mosby).

ination of microbes. PMNs are short-lived cells, whereas macrophages may remain in connective tissues for prolonged periods. PMNs are principally involved in host defence against bacteria, while macrophages are better at combating intracellular microbes, including certain bacteria, viruses and protozoa. No prior exposure to the microorganism is necessary for leukocytes to act.

A more sophisticated innate line of defence against microbes is the complement system. This comprises of over 20 serum proteins that work in unison to lyse bacteria. The complement system can respond rapidly to a trigger stimulus, resulting in activation of a sequential cascade in which one reaction is the enzymatic catalyst of the next (Fig. 1.7). The most important complement component is C3, which facilitates the uptake and removal of microbes by enhancing their adherence to the surface of phagocytic cells. Biologically active fragments of C3–C3a and C5a can attract

PMNs (called chemotaxis) as well as activating these cells. Activated complement components later in this sequence, C6, 7, 8 and 9, form a complex – the membrane attack complex – on the surface of target cells and this can punch holes in the cell membrane, resulting in target cell lysis.

Other humoral defence mechanisms include acute phase proteins such as C-reactive protein (CRP), alpha-1-anti-trypsin, alpha2-macroglobulin and interferons. The latter are a family of broad-spectrum antiviral agents that are synthesized by cells when infected by viruses. They limit the spread of virus to other cells.

Innate immune cells including non-immune cells like epithelial cells have developed pattern recognition receptors (PRRs) with the ability to recognize exogenous microbial products (pathogen-associated microbial patterns (PAMPs) as well as endogenous molecules termed damage associated molecular patterns (DAMPS). Toll-like receptors (TLRs), one subgroup of PRRs, are transmembrane receptors responsible for recognizing different PAMPs such as lipopolysaccharides, CpG DNA and flagellin components of microbes. Activation of TLRs leads to the induction of inflammatory responses that promote synthesis and secretion of cytokines as well as recruitment of macrophages and neutrophils to sites of inflammation that efficiently eliminate invading organisms. TLRs are also important because of the role they play in controlling adaptive immune responses.

Humans as well as many lower-order animals have developed more selective mechanisms to adapt and combat infection, involving humoral (antibody) and cellular systems.

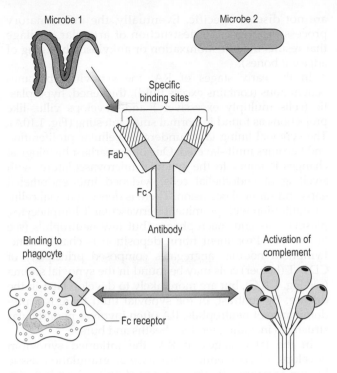

Fig. 1.8 The structure of an immunoglobulin. The antibody is an adaptable molecule able to bind specifically to microbial antigen 1, but not antigen 2, via its Fab end. The Fc end is able to activate complement and to bind to the Fc receptor on host phagocytic cells.

Adaptive immune system

Humoral immunity – antibodies

Antibodies are remarkable proteins produced by bone marrow-derived B lymphocytes, which differentiate into plasma cells and produce antibodies. Antibodies are adaptor molecules that are capable of binding to phagocytic cells, activating complement and binding to microbes. Each antibody has a unique recognition site for a particular microbe – the Fab end of the molecule, which binds non-covalently to matching amino acids on the surface of microbes (Fig. 1.8). Molecules in the microorganism that evoke and react with antibodies are called antigens. The Fc end of the antibody molecule contains domains capable of binding and activating the first component of complement as well as binding to phagocyte Fc receptors. There are five antibody subtypes, classified by variations in the structure of the Fab region: IgG, IgM, IgA, IgD and IgE.

There is an enormous variety of B lymphocytes, each programmed to synthesize a single antibody with sole specificity. These antibodies are expressed on the lymphocyte cell surface and act as a receptor for antigens. This process is highly selective; for example, antibodies that recognize tetanus toxoid antigen do not recognize influenza virus, and vice versa. On exposure to antigen, B lymphocytes with the corresponding cell surface antibody specificity, bind to the cell and deliver activation signals. This leads to their differentiation into plasma cells and synthesis and secretion of specific antibodies. The activated B lymphocytes also undergo proliferation, resulting in expansion of the number of clones capable of producing the same antibody. Antibody production in response to antigenic challenge is referred to as an acquired immune response.

Even after the elimination of a microbial antigen trigger, some B lymphocytes remain and have a 'memory' to this exposure. On subsequent challenge with the same antigen, the body responds by synthesizing antibody faster and in greater quantities than on the first exposure. This is the secondary immune response.

Antibodies can recognize a particular antigen that is foreign and discriminate between self-antigen and non-self (i.e. foreign) antigens. There is an active process by which self-antigen fails to induce an immune response, known as tolerance. In some circumstances, there is a breakdown in tolerance and the individual produces self-directed antibodies known as autoantibodies. These may give rise to autoimmune diseases. The prototype autoimmune disease, systemic lupus erythematosus, is discussed in Chapter 9.

Cell-mediated immunity

Many microbes live inside host cells and out of the reach of antibodies. Viruses can live inside host cells, such as macrophages, where they replicate. This form of immune evasion requires a different form of immune defence, known as cell-mediated immunity, to combat intracellular infection. This involves T or thymus-derived lymphocytes. T cells only recognize antigen when it is presented on the surface of a host cell. There are T cell receptors present on the T cell surface, distinct from antibody receptors, which recognize antigen. A further complexity is that antigen is recognized in association with another cell surface molecule known as the major histocompatibility complex (MHC) expressed on the target cell. The MHC plays an important role in organ transplant rejection.

A macrophage that has been infected with a virus is able to process small antigenic components of the virus and place these on its cell surface. A subpopulation of T lymphocytes, known as T helper (cluster of differentiation 4, CD4$^+$) cells, primed to that antigen, recognize and bind to the combination of antigen and MHC class II molecules. These T cells also secrete a range of soluble products known as lymphokines. The latter include interferon (IFN)-gamma, which stimulates microbiocidal mechanisms in the macrophage that help to kill the intracellular microbe. There are functional subtypes of T helper cells that under the influence of various transcription factors (T-bet, Gata3, RORgt, FoxP3,) shape the T cell repertoire to become Th1, Th2, T17 or Tregs, respectively. Th1 type cells produce pro-inflammatory cytokines such as IL-2, IFN-gamma and GMCSF, all of which are involved with host defence against intracellular viral and bacterial pathogens; Th2 cells produce IL-4, IL-5, IL-13 and are important in allergic responses and elimination of parasites; and T17 cells produce IL-17 and are involved in mucosal immunity and autoimmune disorders. Tregs comprise 5%–10% of total CD4$^+$ cells and are responsible for maintaining immune homeostasis via inhibition of differentiation and activity of pro-inflammatory T helper cells. FoxP3 expression is the most used marker for Treg cells.

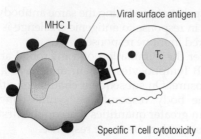

Fig. 1.9 Cytotoxic T cells are able to recognize viral surface antigen in association with MHC class 1 molecules and subsequently lyse the target cell.

There is another subpopulation of T lymphocytes, known as cytotoxic T cells (CD8⁺), which recognize antigen expressed on the surface of target cells in association with MHC class I molecules (Fig. 1.9). Cytotoxic T cells are responsible for the direct killing of damaged, infected and dysfunctional cells such a tumour cells. Just as is true for B cells, T cells selected and activated by binding antigen undergo clonal proliferation and mature to produce T helper and cytotoxic cells and produce memory cells. The latter can be reactivated upon further antigenic challenge.

For T cell activation and proliferation to occur second signals are required following antigen recognition. Without a secondary co-stimulatory signal, T cells remain in an anergic state. The second signal occurs with the binding of CD28 on T cells and B7 proteins on antigen-presenting cells. Along the path of activation and proliferation there are normal inhibitory checkpoint signals that play an important role in T-cell regulation, self-tolerance and immune surveillance. Certain tumours such as melanomas have recently been noted to influence checkpoint molecules and allow escape from immune-surveillance by preventing T cell activation. Examples of checkpoint protein markers found on T cells or cancer cells include PD-1/PD-L1 and CTLA-4/B7-1/B7-2. By releasing the blockade on T cell activation using monoclonal antibodies (e.g. Pembrolizumab, Nivolumab), the T cells are now able to recognize and attack tumours. This therapy is called immune checkpoint blockade.

In summary, a wide range of innate and adaptive immunological mechanisms has evolved to protect the host against microbial infection. In some circumstances, the host becomes a target for these responses, resulting in autoimmune disease.

Pathology

Synovitis

To gain a better appreciation of the processes occurring within an inflamed joint, it is necessary to understand synovial pathology. However, in clinical practice a synovial biopsy is not routinely performed as part of the diagnosis of inflammatory arthritis.

In RA, the classical example of an inflammatory arthropathy, the synovium undergoes histological changes that are not disease specific. Eventually, the inflammatory process progresses to destruction of articular cartilage that results in joint subluxation or ankylosis (bridging of adjacent bones).

In the early stages of RA, the synovium becomes oedematous (contains excess fluid), thickened, hyperplastic (cells multiply excessively) and develops villus-like projections as found in normal small intestine (Fig. 1.10A). The synovial lining layer undergoes cellular proliferation and becomes multi-layered. One of the earliest histological changes is injury to the synovial microvasculature, with swelling of endothelial cells, widened inter-endothelial gaps and luminal occlusion. There is dense synovial cellular infiltration with prominent perivascular T lymphocytes, plasma cells and macrophages, but few neutrophils (see Fig. 1.10B). Prominent fibrin deposition is characteristic. Lymphoid nodular aggregates composed principally of CD4⁺ T (helper) cells may be found in the synovial stroma (see Fig. 1.10C), but are more likely to develop later in the disease. By contrast, in the synovial fluid there is a predominance of neutrophils. RA often involves periarticular structures including tendon sheaths and bursae.

In the later stages of RA, the inflamed synovium develops a hyperaemic, fibrovascular granulation tissue known as pannus (Latin: 'piece of cloth'), which includes new blood vessel formation (angiogenesis). This spreads over and subsequently invades the articular cartilage. The pannus eventually destroys articular cartilage and invades bone, causing juxta-articular erosions and subchondral cysts. These can be seen on plain radiography and at an even earlier stage of disease using magnetic resonance imaging (MRI). It may lead to ankylosis and loss of joint mobility. Joint instability and subluxation (partial dislocation) may arise from damage to the joint capsule, ligaments,and tendons, as the inflammatory process extends. This may subsequently heal with fibrosis and lead to fixed deformities. The destruction of cartilage predisposes to secondary osteoarthritis.

Although RA predominantly involves synovial joints, it is a systemic disease and may affect many tissues and organs including skin, blood vessels, heart, lungs, muscles and eyes. The most characteristic extra-articular feature is the rheumatoid nodule, found in 25% of patients, typically in subcutaneous tissues over pressure areas. Rheumatoid nodules have a characteristic microscopic appearance, consisting of three distinct layers – a central zone of fibrinoid necrosis (pink-staining dead material) surrounded by palisading (fence-like) phagocytes arranged radially, and granulation tissue with inflammatory cells.

The synovium in the seronegative spondyloarthropathies may be difficult to distinguish microscopically from RA. Typically there is inflammation both in the synovium and bony entheses (the site of ligamentous and capsular insertion into bone) – enthesitis. The synovium does not usually develop extensive pannus formation and consequently, there is less invasion of bone and articular cartilage compared with RA. The enthesis becomes infiltrated by a non-specific granulation tissue. In severe forms of the disease, enthesopathy is followed by calcifi-

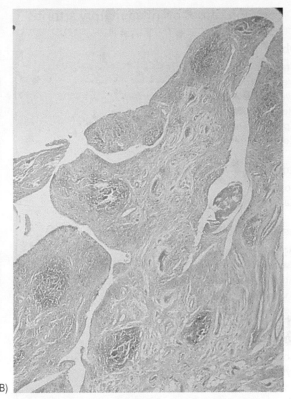

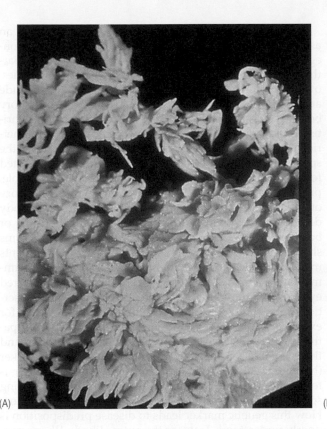

Fig. 1.10 Histopathology of a joint with rheumatoid arthritis. (A) Early disease: low-power micrograph of inflamed synovium; (B) Lymphoid nodular aggregates in synovial stroma; (C) Diagram of the histopathology of a rheumatoid joint.

cation and ossification, particularly in the spine and capsules of peripheral joints.

Differential diagnosis of inflammation of the synovium

Synovial joints are susceptible to inflammatory injury, probably because of their rich network of fenestrated capillaries. The synovium has only a limited number of ways in which it can respond to injury.

The synovium may be the target of a large number of insults that may arise from microbes, for example, *Staphylococcus aureus* leading to septic arthritis; crystals, for example, sodium urate leading to gouty arthritis; or autoimmune attack, for example, RA in which the trigger is unknown (Box 1.1).

Determining the aetiological basis for synovitis may be difficult. Tender soft tissue swelling and fluid (effusion) of synovial joints (as seen with Mrs Gale) indicates that the joint is inflamed, which is synovitis (see inset Case 1). Information on the following may enable a more precise diagnosis to be made: (a) the pattern and distribution of joint involvement (symmetrical vs asymmetrical); (b) the number of joints involved – one (monoarthritis), a few (<6 – oligoarthritis) or multiple (>6 – polyarthritis); (c) the duration of inflammation (days, weeks or months); (d) the type of trigger; and (e) the presence of extra-articular features, for example, fever, rashes. The sudden onset of painful swelling of one joint – monoarthritis – raises the possibility of infection. Microorganisms may lodge

Box 1.1 Common causes of inflammatory arthritis

Microbial

- *Staphylococcus aureus*
- *Neisseria gonorrhoeae*
- Lyme disease (*Borrelia burgdorferi*)
- Hepatitis B virus
- Epstein–Barr virus
- Ross River fever virus

Crystal

- Sodium urate
- Calcium pyrophosphate dihydrate

Seronegative spondyloarthropathies

- Ankylosing spondylitis
- Psoriatic arthritis
- Arthritis associated with chronic bowel inflammation – ulcerative colitis and Crohn's disease
- Reactive arthritis

Autoimmune

- Rheumatoid arthritis
- Systemic lupus erythematosus

Other

- Polymyalgia rheumatica

in the joint from a direct penetrating injury or, more commonly, by haematogenous (blood-borne) spread from a distant site during bacteraemia. Clinical pointers include fever and constitutional symptoms – sweating, rigors (shivers), malaise. However, these symptoms are not specific for infection and may occur in patients with gout or RA. A cutaneous source of infection may give a clue, for example, a boil or carbuncle. In the case of sexually active young adults, *Neisseria gonorrhoeae* infection needs to be considered. This subject is covered in more detail in Chapter 11.

Sudden onset of monoarthritis, particularly in the big toe, in an older male raises the suspicion of crystal-induced arthritis due to sodium urate deposition. Uric acid, the product of purine metabolism, may precipitate out of its usually soluble state, deposit in the synovium and produce acute inflammation. An acute attack is typically triggered by dehydration or agents that induce dehydration such as alcohol or thiazide diuretics that raise serum uric acid levels and precipitate sodium urate crystal deposition. Clinically, gout presents with the sudden onset of exquisite pain in a joint – frequently the first metatarsophalangeal joint. The patient exhibits the classic signs of inflammation – local heat, erythema (redness), tenderness, swelling and loss of function. Another type of crystal that commonly produces mono-arthritis is calcium pyrophosphate dihydrate. This usually affects middle-aged females and involves the knee joint. Crystal arthritis is covered in greater depth in Chapter 7.

Involvement of one or a limited number of joints in an asymmetric distribution raises the possibility of seronegative (i.e. rheumatoid factor (RF) negative) spondyloarthritis. The spondyloarthropathies, as the name implies, often have arthritis that involves the spine and include ankylosing spondylitis, psoriatic arthritis, inflammatory bowel disease associated arthritis and reactive arthritis. These conditions typically manifest as an asymmetric arthritis involving one or several joints, including the spine and/or sacroiliac joints. There are often associated features that give clues to the diagnosis, for example, presence of psoriasis (a red, scaly skin rash) or a history of inflammatory bowel disease (e.g. episodes of bloody diarrhoea). A recent episode of non-specific urethritis or bowel infection with *Salmonella* or *Shigella* microorganisms should raise the possibility of reactive arthritis. Patients may give a history of eye inflammation (e.g. iritis – inflammation of the iris) resulting in episodes of painful red eyes, or inflammation of ligamentous or tendinous insertions into bone (enthesitis) resulting in painful heels, for example. Patients with seronegative spondyloarthropathies frequently have a family history of the condition and there is an association with the white blood cell marker (histocompatibility locus antigen) HLA-B27. The latter is found in over 95% of Caucasian males with ankylosing spondylitis, but in only 6%–8% of the normal population. How this genetic marker leads to disease predisposition is poorly understood. Tests for the autoantibody RF are negative – hence the term seronegative.

The pattern of disease onset in RA is quite variable. Although it often presents insidiously with the development of a symmetrical inflammatory arthritis involving multiple joints over weeks to months, a monoarticular onset, especially involving the knee (as in Mrs Gale's case), may antedate the development of symmetrical arthritis. The joints most affected in polyarthritis with RA are the small joints of the hands (proximal interphalangeal and metacarpophalangeal joints), wrists, elbows, feet, knees and ankles. Later in the disease, large joints such as the hip and shoulder may be involved, but not usually at presentation. A family history of RA is often present. The patient usually complains of joint stiffness, especially in the morning, joint swelling and pain. The patient may also have systemic symptoms, such as weight loss and fatigue.

Polymyalgia rheumatica is a rheumatic condition that may precede RA. It is characterized by pain and stiffness, usually of sudden onset, predominantly affecting the limb girdle areas (shoulders and hips). It usually occurs in older subjects, is generally associated with a moderate to markedly elevated erythrocyte sedimentation rate (ESR) and CRP levels and is rapidly responsive to corticosteroids. It is also often associated with giant cell arteritis, especially in the temporal arteries but any artery can be affected. Headache is the most common symptom but visual symptoms suggesting arteritis include transient and permanent visual loss. Biopsies characteristically show infiltrations of macrophages, T cells and multinucleated giant cells, the hallmark of the disease.

Aetiopathogenesis of rheumatoid arthritis

There are a diverse range of causes for inflammatory arthritis – infection, crystal and autoimmune. The first two are discussed in the chapters on bone and joint infection (see Ch. 11) and crystal arthritis (see Ch. 7), respectively. Here, the aetiopathogenesis of RA is discussed (Fig. 1.11).

Although the cause of RA is unknown, genetic, microbial and immunological factors are thought to play a role in disease susceptibility. RA is one of a group of conditions in which immunogenetic responses are important. As such, it joins many autoimmune diseases in which genes known to exert influence on the immune response (immune response genes) are involved in disease pathogenesis. However, because the antigen(s) that trigger RA are unknown, the precise details remain elusive.

MHC genes, present on chromosome 6 in humans, are important in determining host immune responses to foreign antigens. They play a vital role in organ transplantation and determine whether rejection of a graft occurs. They are also involved in predisposition to other autoimmune diseases such as systemic lupus erythematosus, diabetes mellitus type 1 and multiple sclerosis. There is a linkage of certain genes in this complex, known as DR, with susceptibility to RA. The best-described association of RA is with HLA-DR4/DR1. Other genes identified include protein tyrosine phosphatase, non-receptor type 22 (PTPN22), Peptidyl Arginine Deaminase (PADI4), signal transducer and activator of transcription 4 (STAT4

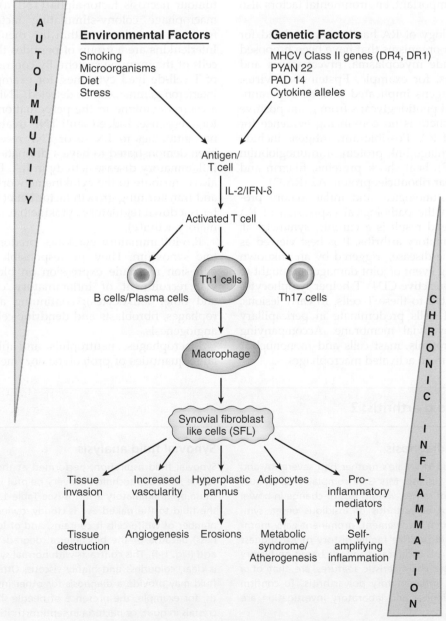

Fig. 1.11 Schematic diagram of the pathogenesis of RA.

T/C), cytotoxic T-lymphocyte-associated protein 4 (CTLA4), tumour necrosis factor-receptor associated factor 1 (TRAF1) and complement component 5 (C5), tumour necrosis factor (TNF) and others.

Family studies have found that HLA haplotype sharing (i.e. individuals sharing the same genetic markers) is increased in family members affected by RA. Molecular analysis of the DR alleles (variations at this gene locus) associated with RA suggests that the genetic contribution of MHC genes to RA is approximately 25%. Other genes thought to play a role in disease susceptibility to RA include immunoglobulin genes, genes controlling glycosylation patterns of immunoglobulin (i.e. the different type and amount of carbohydrate present) and T cell receptor genes. It must be remembered that RA has a complex multifactorial pathogenesis and, while immune response genes are important, environmental factors also play a role.

A microbial aetiology of RA has been postulated for many decades. Microorganisms that have been proposed to play a role include mycoplasma, mycobacteria and a number of viruses, for example, Epstein–Barr virus. Other microbial antigens implicated include superantigens, parvovirus and peptidoglycans from gram positive bacteria. However, there is no convincing evidence for a microbial cause of RA. Possible autoantigens include collagen type II, cartilage link protein, immunoglobulin binding protein (BiP), heat shock proteins, filagrin and heterogeneous nuclear ribonucleoprotein A2 (RA33).

The fact that immunological and inflammatory processes play a role in the pathological expression of RA is undisputed. The end result is a chronic, symmetrical, polyarticular, inflammatory arthritis. It is best viewed as being an autoimmune disease, triggered by an unknown antigen. The initiating event of joint damage is thought to be triggering of autoreactive CD4+ T helper lymphocytes by antigen(s) presented to these T cells. In early lesions, activated/memory T cells predominate in pericapillary sites beneath the synovial membrane. Accompanying the T cells are neutrophils, mast cells and mononuclear phagocytes that mature to activated macrophages.

In the earliest lesions, there is an increase in vascularity driven by angiogenesis-stimulating factors released from macrophages and fibroblasts. Both vessels and infiltrating cells have enhanced expression of intercellular adhesion molecules, especially intercellular adhesion molecule-1 (ICAM-1). As the lesion progresses, lymphoid cells organize into microenvironments like that seen in lymph nodes. Dendritic cells (specialized cells that present antigens to the immune system effectively) are found in these environments and are thought to provide the basis of local antibody production by B cells and ongoing T cell activation. Mature memory T cells promote antibody synthesis with little negative feedback.

Despite the importance of T cell involvement, the most active cells in synovial lesions are macrophages. The macrophage-derived cytokines IL-1, IL-6 and IL-8, tumour necrosis factor-alpha (TNF-α) and granulocyte-macrophage colony-stimulating factor (GM-CSF) are found in abundance within the rheumatoid synovium. Interleukins are a group of peptides that signal between cells of the immune system. By contrast, only low levels of T cell-derived cytokines, for example, IL-2, IL-4 and interferon-gamma, can be detected. TNF-α is thought to be a central cytokine in the perpetuation of the inflammatory response. Indeed, anti-TNF treatment by monoclonal antibodies to TNF-α or TNF receptor blockade has been demonstrated to have a dramatic effect in reducing inflammatory disease activity in RA. Fibroblast-like cells also contribute to the cytokine network, particularly IL-6 and transforming growth factor beta (TGF-beta). The later is a down regulatory cytokine (i.e. it decreases inflammatory activity).

Pro-inflammatory cytokines predominate in rheumatoid synovium. They are responsible for: activation of adhesion molecule expression on blood vessels; synovial recruitment of inflammatory cells (lymphocytes and other leukocytes); continuing activation of macrophages, fibroblasts and dendritic cells; and promoting angiogenesis.

Macrophages, neutrophils and fibroblasts produce large quantities of proteolytic enzymes including matrix

---

Case 1.1 Rheumatoid arthritis: 2

Establishing the diagnosis

It comes to light that Mrs Gale's mother had severe RA and was disabled by her disease. Mrs Gale complains of fatigue, but gives no history of rashes, weight loss or change in bowel habit. The history of polyarthritis of insidious onset, symmetrical pattern of joint involvement, prominent early morning joint stiffness and positive family history of RA suggest a diagnosis of RA. RA is a clinical diagnosis based on history and examination. The characteristic features are that of a chronic symmetrical, inflammatory polyarthritis. To confirm the diagnosis, radiological and laboratory investigation are undertaken.

Synovial fluid analysis

Synovial fluid aspiration, performed at the bedside, using a sterile no-touch technique is very helpful in determining the cause of inflammatory arthritis (see Table 1.1). Typically, in RA, the fluid to the naked eye is cloudy, owing to the increased number of white cells it contains, and of low viscosity (stickiness) because of the biochemical degradation of hyaluronic acid (Fig. 1.4). This contrasts with normal synovial fluid, which is clear, colourless and highly viscous. Other features of the fluid may provide a diagnosis for other inflammatory arthritis, for example, the presence of needle-shaped birefringent crystals in gout, or bacteria in septic arthritis.

Case 1.1   Rheumatoid arthritis: 2—cont'd

Table 1.1   Synovial fluid analysis in inflammatory arthritis

	Normal	*RA*	*Gout*	*Septic*
Colour	Colourless	Yellow	Yellow	Yellow
Clarity	Clear	Cloudy	Cloudy	Purulent
Viscosity	High	Low	Low	Low
White cell count (/mm³)	<1500	2–50 000	5–50 000	50–500 000
% neutrophils	<5	30–80	50–80	.95
Crystals	No	No	Yes	No
Bacteria	No	No	No	Yes

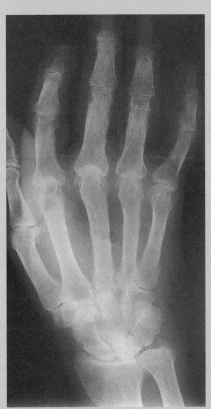

Fig. 1.12 X-ray showing bony erosion of metacarpophalangeal joint and proximal interphalangeal joint.

Joint X-rays

Plain X-rays of the hands and feet often provide useful diagnostic information in patients with inflammatory arthritis. The earliest changes in RA involving the hands are soft tissue swelling of proximal interphalangeal and metacarpophalangeal joints. This corresponds with synovitis of affected joints. There is periarticular osteoporosis (bone thinning) thought to be secondary to increased blood flow through inflamed joints and local release of cytokines (molecules that are released by activated cells and are involved in signalling to other cells). However, these changes are not specific for RA and simply reflect joint inflammation. The most characteristic feature is the development of bony erosions that start at the periphery of the joint where the synovium reflects off the joint capsule. Erosions correspond with the site of local invasion by inflammatory synovial tissue, known as pannus, which grows into the adjacent bone and cartilage (Fig. 1.12), discussed below.

metalloproteinases (MMPs) – enzymes that require cleavage by other proteases to become active. The MMPs – collagenase, gelatinase and stromelysin – mediate the degradation of joint tissues that accompanies the development of pannus.

Large quantities of antibody are present within the joint, including local production of RFs. The latter are autoantibodies of the IgM, IgG and IgA classes characterized by antigenic binding determinants on the constant region of human IgG. IgM RF are found in the serum of 70% of patients with RA and are associated with severe joint disease and extra-articular features, for example, vasculitis (inflammation of blood vessels). Patients who have IgM RF in their serum are said to be seropositive. RF may participate in some of the clinical phenomena that occur in RA,

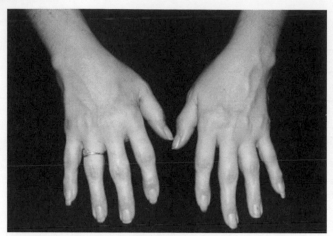

Fig. 1.13 The hands in rheumatoid arthritis.

for example, vasculitis leading to leg ulcers or nodules. However, they are not specific for RA and may occur in other autoimmune diseases such as Sjögren's syndrome, and/or occasionally in infectious diseases such as bacterial endocarditis. Another autoantibody has been described in the serum of patients with RA, namely anti-citrullinated protein antibodies (ACPAs). Citrullination is a biochemical process where the amino acid arginine is converted into the amino acid citrulline by the enzyme PAD. Citrullinated proteins are found in the synovium of patients with RA but are not unique to that site or to that disease. Detection of cyclic citrullinated protein antibodies have challenged RFs as the most valuable test in the diagnosis of RA and allow the diagnosis of RA to be made at a very early stage. It is postulated that the gram negative, anaerobic bacterium *Porphyromonas gingivalis* found in the oral cavity contain the enzyme PAD, which is involved in the citrullination of proteins such as vimentin, that leads to the production of ACPAs. These ACPAs then cross react with joint tissue and are believed to play a role in disease pathogenesis. The increased susceptibility of RA in smokers may be due to the upregulation of PAD enzyme induced by smoking.

Pathophysiological basis of symptoms and signs of rheumatoid arthritis

Although RA is an autoimmune multisystem disease, its primary clinical manifestation usually relates to the involvement of synovial joints. The clinical features vary in severity between patients, as well as fluctuate over time in individual patients. The initial presentation of the disease is most commonly as a symmetrical inflammatory polyarthritis involving the hands (Fig. 1.13). The patient experiences pain, stiffness and swelling in the joints that is characteristically worse in the morning. Joint swelling and pain are due to the presence of active inflammation in the synovium, that is, synovitis or effusion. Systemic symptoms may be due to the presence of circulating cytokines such as TNF-α.

Joint deformity is not a typical feature of early disease and usually occurs only after the disease has been present for some time. Deformity arises secondary to damage caused by the pannus invading cartilage and bone. Radiological bone erosions may not be present at the time of diagnosis, but usually develop over months, or longer, with ongoing active disease (Fig 1.12). They reflect invasion of bone by pannus. Typical deformities include ulnar deviation of the digits at the metacarpophalangeal joints and swan-neck deformities of the fingers. Ulnar deviation results from the fingers being pulled in the ulnar direction by the natural pull of the forearm muscles in the presence of subluxation (partial dislocation) at the metacarpophalangeal joints. In a swan-neck deformity, the proximal interphalangeal joint is hyperextended and the distal interphalangeal joint flexed.

The temporal pattern of these clinical manifestations varies between patients. About one-third experience prolonged periods of remission. Another third demonstrates fluctuating disease activity characterized by periods of active joint inflammation interspersed with periods of more quiescent disease. The remaining third manifest progressive deforming joint damage with declining functional status over time. Mortality rates are increased in those with the most severe forms of the disease.

Rheumatoid arthritis as a systemic disease

RA may be more accurately termed rheumatoid disease, as it is a multisystem disorder affecting multiple organs (Fig. 1.14), with the major clinical manifestation being polyarthritis. In addition to joint pain, stiffness and swelling, patients with RA often have systemic constitutional symptoms that can include fatigue, weight loss, low-grade fever and myalgia (muscle pain). Lymphadenopathy (enlarged lymph glands) is present in about 30% of patients with active disease, usually of axillary, epitrochlear (near the elbow) or inguinal regions, and biopsy shows reactive hyperplasia.

Patients often have a normochromic (normal colour), normocytic (normal-sized red blood cells) anaemia. This occurs commonly in patients with chronic inflammatory or infectious diseases and is due to ineffective bone marrow production of red blood cells. It is known as the anaemia of chronic disease. If the haemoglobin level drops below 10 g/L, other explanations besides RA, such as gastrointestinal blood loss from NSAIDs, should be considered and looked for. Thrombocytosis (elevation of platelet count), common in active disease, returns to normal when the arthritis is controlled. The ESR and serum CRP levels are often elevated and are used as markers of disease activity. The ESR is determined by counting the number of millimetres the red blood cells have settled from the top of the serum in a capillary tube after 60 minutes.

Rheumatoid nodules occur in 25% of patients, most commonly on the extensor surfaces of the hands (Fig. 1.15), but they can occur at any site where there is pressure (Fig. 1.16). Subcutaneous nodules are usually only

Case 1.1 Rheumatoid arthritis: 3

Case note: Management

Mrs Gale reports that she has noticed the development of small painless nodular lumps over the extensor surfaces of both elbows. Her general practitioner explains that she has RA and that the lumps are rheumatoid nodules. She will need to be treated with a comprehensive management programme. She is referred to the local branch of the Arthritis Foundation for information and is advised to attend their patient education programme. She is recommended to undertake a period of rest and commenced on an NSAID. She is referred to a rheumatologist for advice about the use of disease-modifying anti-rheumatic drugs.

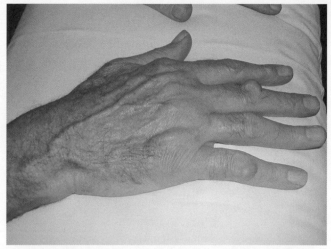

Fig. 1.15 Rheumatoid nodules in the hand over dorsum of fingers.

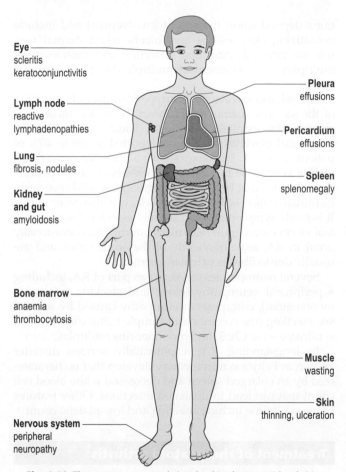

Eye
scleritis
keratoconjunctivitis

Lymph node
reactive
lymphadenopathies

Lung
fibrosis, nodules

**Kidney
and gut**
amyloidosis

Bone marrow
anaemia
thrombocytosis

Nervous system
peripheral
neuropathy

Pleura
effusions

Pericardium
effusions

Spleen
splenomegaly

Muscle
wasting

Skin
thinning, ulceration

Fig. 1.14 The organs commonly involved in rheumatoid arthritis.

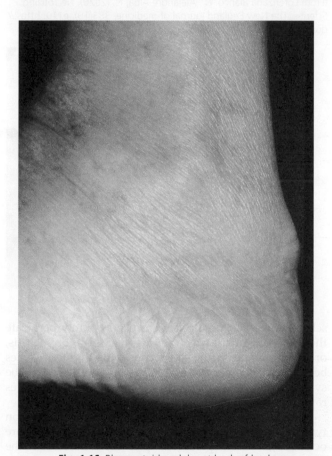

Fig. 1.16 Rheumatoid nodules at back of heel.

removed if they cause discomfort or become ulcerated. They may recur if the arthritis remains active. They may also occur in internal organs such as the lung and eyes. The most common respiratory manifestation of RA is pleural involvement, typically manifesting as an asymptomatic pleural effusion. Occasionally, it can produce frank pleurisy (pleuritis). Rheumatoid nodules may also be found in the lung and can be difficult to distinguish from other causes of pulmonary nodules. Pulmonary fibrosis may occur secondary to chronic lymphocytic and monocytic infiltrate in the pulmonary interstitium or rarely as an adverse reaction to treatment with agents such as gold or methotrexate. There are several types of eye involvement. Scleritis, or inflammation of the sclera, results in a painful, red eye. It can lead to thinning of the

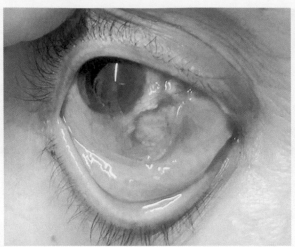

Fig. 1.17 Rheumatoid arthritis: scleritis with scleromalacia perforans. (From Lorenzana Blanco, N., Alejandre Alba, N. (2020). Necrotizing Scleritis. The New England Journal of medicine, 383(19), e110. https://doi.org/10.1056/NEJMicm2004836).

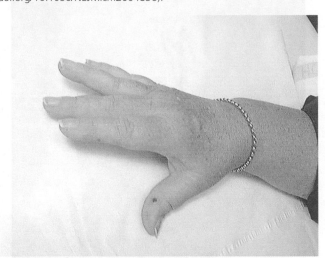

Fig. 1.18 Rheumatoid vasculitis in hand (small vessel).

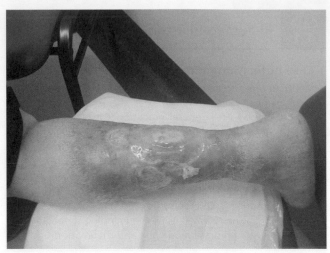

Fig. 1.19 Rheumatoid vasculitis in legs with ulcers.

sclera, called scleromalacia, which may rarely perforate the eye – scleromalacia perforans (Fig. 1.17). Episcleritis, or inflammation in the loose connective tissue that lies between the conjunctiva and the sclera, is less likely to be symptomatic or as serious as scleritis. It usually resolves rapidly with no residual abnormalities.

Vasculitis may occur in RA. The most common type is a mild obliterative endarteritis (the vessels are occluded), which produces painless infarcts in the fingernail beds and paronychia. These lesions frequently appear in crops, heal without tissue damage and, accordingly, do not require specific treatment (Fig. 1.18). Leukocytoclastic vasculitis (inflammation of small blood vessels with 'nuclear dust') in the skin may also occur and manifest as palpable purpura (small raised purple lesions). This type of vasculitis most commonly occurs in the legs and heals without scarring. The most serious type of vasculitis in RA is a necrotizing vasculitis of small to medium-sized arteries and requires aggressive treatment (Fig. 1.19). Vasculitic manifesta-

tions depend upon the site of involvement and include necrotizing skin lesions and ulcers when dermal vessels are affected, intestinal infarction and mononeuritis multiplex – involvement of multiple discrete peripheral nerves.

RA can also involve the heart, pericarditis (inflammation of the sac that surrounds the heart) being the most common cardiac manifestation. Small, usually asymptomatic, pericardial effusions have been reported in up to 40% of patients with RA. Histology shows a fibrinous pericarditis. Only a very small number of patients have larger pericardial effusions that become symptomatic. A mild myocarditis (inflammation of the heart muscle) can also occur in RA. It is rarely symptomatic and usually associated with a normal electrocardiogram. Valvular abnormalities occasionally occur in RA, most frequently of the aortic valve, and are usually due to fibrous valvular scarring.

Several neuropathies can occur as part of RA, including a peripheral neuropathy (glove and stocking pattern of involvement), entrapment neuropathy caused by soft tissue swelling (the commonest example being carpal tunnel syndrome – see Ch. 3) and mononeuritis multiplex.

In longstanding RA, a potentially serious disorder known as Felty's syndrome may develop that is characterized by an enlarged spleen and decreased white blood cell count that can lead to unabated infections. Other features of the syndrome include anaemia and low platelet count.

Treatment of rheumatoid arthritis

The management of patients with RA is complex. The paradigm is to treat early and aggressively aiming to stop the damage that results from prolonged inflammation. This section is restricted to a discussion on the principles guiding management rather than individual drugs and doses. For a more comprehensive coverage of this subject, the reader is directed to other textbooks of rheumatology.

Modern approaches involve recognition of the importance of the therapeutic team in the optimal management

Table 1.2	Principles of drug treatment in RA
Drug type	**Action**
Analgesics	Pain relief
Non-steroidal anti-inflammatory drugs	Reduce inflammation
Corticosteroids	Reduce inflammation
Disease-modifying anti-rheumatic drugs	Induce remission and prevent joint destruction
Biological therapy	Induce remission and prevent joint destruction

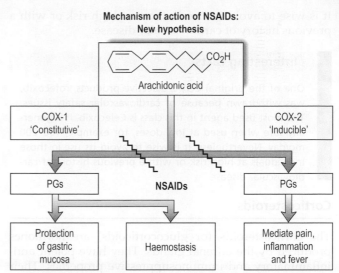

Fig. 1.20 The cyclooxygenase system. Arachidonic acid is converted to prostaglandins by the enzyme cyclooxygenase (COX). There are two forms of this enzyme: COX-1 and COX-2. *NSAIDs*, Non-steroidal anti-inflammatory drugs; *PGs*, Prostaglandins.

of patients with RA. The team comprises a rheumatologist (who usually acts as team leader), family physician, orthopaedic surgeon, allied health members including physiotherapist, occupational therapist, social worker, nurse and patient educator, the patient and his or her immediate family. While not all members of this team are required in the management of every patient, at times each may be called on to contribute his or her expertise.

Rest is therapeutic during periods of active disease. Controlled trials of rest therapy have demonstrated its therapeutic benefit. Therapy may simply involve rest periods taken during the day. Rest must be balanced with exercise, best supervised by an experienced physiotherapist. Exercises include passive joint movement during periods of active disease, which are used to preserve a full range of joint motion. Active exercises include isometrics to reverse muscle wasting. The latter often develops in muscles adjacent to inflamed joints because of disuse.

Patients often experience depressive symptoms, relationship disharmony and financial hardship because of having a chronic painful debilitating disease. The social worker can help with these aspects of the patient's care. In more advanced cases, the orthopaedic surgeon plays an important role, usually in performing synovectomy for a chronically inflamed joint that has failed to respond to medical therapy or in reconstructive surgery to replace irreversibly damaged joints.

Pharmacological treatment principles (Table 1.2) include providing analgesia, reducing joint inflammation, preventing joint damage and inducing remission with disease modifying drugs or biological therapies.

Analgesics

Analgesics, including paracetamol/acetaminophen, have no anti-inflammatory effects. They can be used every 4–6 hours for pain relief if necessary. They seldom produce side-effects and are well tolerated.

Non-steroidal anti-inflammatory drugs

Non-steroidal anti-inflammatory drugs (NSAIDs), of which aspirin is the historical prototype, act quickly (within hours

to a few days) and reduce joint inflammation by inhibiting the production of inflammatory cyclooxygenase products, particularly the prostaglandins – small lipid molecules with potent effects on many steps in the inflammatory process. Consequently, these potent anti-inflammatory agents provide temporary symptomatic relief, with a reduction in joint pain, stiffness and swelling. They do not prevent the development of joint erosions or damage. Commonly used drugs include diclofenac, naproxen, meloxicam, ketoprofen, piroxicam and ibuprofen. They vary in their plasma half-lives, potency and degree of gastrointestinal toxicity. NSAIDs are usually administered orally, in conjunction with food, sometimes as an enteric-coated formulation to reduce gastrointestinal toxicity. Several NSAIDs are available as gels that can be applied topically to inflamed joints.

As a class of drugs, their use has been limited by adverse effects, particularly upper gastrointestinal toxicity such as gastritis and peptic ulcer formation. In susceptible and elderly patients NSAIDs can also be nephrotoxic, by inhibiting prostaglandin-dependent compensatory renal blood flow. Two classes of cyclooxygenase enzymes have been described: COX-1 and COX-2. COX-1 enzymes are expressed constitutively in gastric mucosa, kidneys, brain and other organs and are not inducible. By contrast, COX-2 enzymes are not usually constitutively expressed in tissues but can be induced by certain molecules at sites of inflammation. Traditional NSAIDs, as described above, inhibit both COX-1 and COX-2 enzymes (Fig. 1.20). However, selective COX-2 inhibitors have been developed that have minimal effects on the COX-1 enzyme. These agents provide anti-inflammatory effects with less upper gastrointestinal toxicity. However, they may be associated with an increased risk of cardiovascular disease, particularly if used at high doses and in patients with a previous history of cardiovascular disease. The most commonly used agent in this class is Celecoxib used at low doses, for example, 200 mg/day.

It is wise to avoid its use in those at high risk or with a previous history of cardiovascular disease.

Interesting facts

One of the original COX-2 selective products, rofecoxib, was withdrawn because of cardiovascular safety issues. The most used agent in this class is Celecoxib. It is generally safe when used at low doses, for example, 100–200 mg/day. Nevertheless, it is wise to avoid its use in those individuals at high risk or with a previous history of cardiovascular disease.

Corticosteroids

The corticosteroids (or glucocorticoids) are hormones produced by the adrenal glands. They have potent anti-inflammatory and immunosuppressive properties. Their effect in RA, when used at high doses, is dramatic. Corticosteroid analogues have been produced synthetically by chemical modification of the natural hormone cortisol. This has resulted in a range of compounds with varying potencies and differential toxicities. The most used compound is prednisone, which is four times as potent as cortisol and has less mineralocorticoid activity, resulting in less fluid retention.

Prednisone is administered orally and acts rapidly to reduce inflammation, resulting in a lessening of joint swelling, pain and stiffness in RA. Corticosteroids bind to cytoplasmic cortisol receptors and are transported into the nucleus where they interfere with RNA processing of protein molecules. Corticosteroids act on a wide variety of target cells including leukocytes. They inhibit leukocyte chemotaxis (directed motion towards a stimulus), preventing circulating polymorphs, monocytes and lymphocytes from reaching sites of inflammation. They reduce vascular permeability and inhibit the production of cytokines and arachidonic acid metabolites, such as prostaglandins and leukotrienes.

Despite clinical efficacy, corticosteroids are harmful if used at high doses for prolonged periods. They affect bone metabolism resulting in osteoporosis and non-traumatic fractures (discussed in Ch. 5). They interfere with glucose metabolism and are diabetogenic. Corticosteroids cause salt and water retention and may precipitate or exacerbate hypertension. They interfere with ocular lens metabolism resulting in cataract formation. Their immunosuppressive action, while beneficial in reducing inflammation in RA, results in increased susceptibility to a wide range of bacterial and opportunistic infections, for example, herpes zoster virus and fungal infections.

In general, corticosteroid side-effects are dose- and time-related. To limit toxicity, corticosteroids should be used for as short a time and at as low a dose as possible to achieve an anti-inflammatory effect. In recent years, a few different regimens have been introduced to improve efficacy, while minimizing toxicity. These include the use of intermittent pulses of high-dose corticosteroids, for example, intravenous methylprednisolone. Continuous low-dose daily oral prednisone (<5 mg/day) retards the development of bony erosions with minimal toxicity.

Another route frequently used to administer corticosteroids is intra-articular injection of depot preparations. This approach aims to deliver a high dose of corticosteroid, which is retained within the joint and reduces local inflammation with limited systemic absorption. This approach is effective in controlling local disease activity.

In patients with life- or major organ-threatening rheumatoid vasculitis, high-dose systemic treatment with corticosteroids for prolonged periods is usually required. Drugs to protect against the development of osteoporosis, such as vitamin D and calcium, bisphosphonates or denosumab are all deserving of consideration (see Ch. 5).

Disease-modifying anti-rheumatic drugs

Conventional synthetic disease-modifying anti-rheumatic drugs

Conventional synthetic disease-modifying anti-rheumatic drugs (csDMARDs) are a group of disparate compounds that in general share an important feature – the potential to slow the progression of joint damage, reduce immune response, and retard the development of bony erosions in RA. Drugs in this category include the folic acid antagonist methotrexate (the most widely used), sulphasalazine, the anti-malarial drug hydroxychloroquine and the pyrimidine antagonist leflunomide. There is no single mechanism by which these agents work. In general, they have a delayed onset of clinical action, measured in weeks to months. They all have potential toxicity and require careful regular haematological and biochemical monitoring. Their initiation should be under the guidance of a rheumatologist. A detailed description of these drugs, their mechanism of action and toxicity profile is beyond the scope of this chapter.

The way in which anti-rheumatic drugs, especially the disease-modifying anti-rheumatic drugs (DMARDs), are used in RA has changed. It is now standard practice to introduce these drugs at the time of diagnosis. The radiological and clinical outcome of patients with RA treated with DMARDs early in disease has improved. DMARDs are now often used in combination rather than as single agents, much as oncologists use combina-

Case 1.1 Rheumatoid arthritis: 4

Case note: Corticosteroid treatment

Despite 2 weeks of complete rest and a course of naproxen Mrs Gale has only partly improved, remains in pain and cannot function effectively. After a telephone call by her general practitioner to a rheumatologist, she is advised to commence oral prednisone 20 mg/day as a morning dose, as a temporary measure to relieve the pain, until reviewed by the rheumatologist.

tion chemotherapy to treat haematological malignancy. Combinations of drugs with different mechanisms of action and different toxicity profiles are used. A combination shown to be superior to single-agent DMARD treatment is hydroxychloroquine, sulfasalazine plus methotrexate. This triple therapy has been achieved without greater toxicity than using methotrexate alone.

Biological treatments

A new era has arrived with the introduction of biological agents in the treatment of RA. These are now part of standard practice for RA patients with difficult to control disease. They are termed biologic agents because these compounds are derived from living sources such as cells in culture. They are most often monoclonal antibodies that can be directed against B cells (e.g. CD20; Rituximab), co-stimulatory molecules (e.g. Abatacept), pro-inflammatory cytokines (e.g. TNF-α, IL-17, IL-6) or cytokine receptors. These drugs are proving to be highly effective in both suppressing joint inflammation and in preventing the development of bony erosions.

Targeted synthetic DMARDs

The development of newer synthetic medications with specific mode of action have recently been developed, differentiating this group of molecules from the previous csDMARDs, which lack a specific mode of action. The targeted synthetic DMARDs (tsDMARDs) are orally bioavailable, synthetic compounds such as upadacitinib, baricitinib, tofacitinib, which inhibit the Janus kinase (JAK) pathway, and apremilast, which is a phosphodiesterase inhibitor. They are effective as biological therapies and are having a major impact on clinical practice.

In summary, the medical treatment of RA is complex and not for the occasional practitioner. It involves the use of specialized drugs with significant toxicity and requires considerable expertise in their appropriate use and monitoring. Detailed use of these drugs and side-effects are not discussed further in this chapter.

Case 1.1 | **Rheumatoid arthritis: 5**

Case note: Treatment with a disease-modifying anti-rheumatic drug

Mrs Gale has her first appointment with the rheumatologist. She has had a good symptomatic response to oral prednisone and has markedly reduced joint pain and stiffness. Nevertheless, the rheumatologist recommends that she be commenced on DMARDs. He discusses the various options available, and they decide on methotrexate 10 mg once a week, with folic acid supplementation, Sulphasalazine 1000 mg bd, and hydroxychloroquine 200 mg/day. She is told about possible adverse drug effects and the need for regular blood counts to monitor for toxicity, and a yearly opthalmological eye examination.

Case 1.1 | **Rheumatoid arthritis: 6**

Case note: Response to drug treatment

Six months later, Mrs Gale is managing moderately well on treatment and can help with the family business. However, there is persistent synovitis in her right knee and MCP joints in her hands. Her CRP level is elevated. It is decided to apply for a biological therapy, anti-TNF monoclonal antibody, to gain better control of her disease.

Interesting facts

Over the past two decades there has been a dramatic expansion in both the range of diseases in which biological and targeted DMARD therapies are being used. In the rheumatic field, this has broadened to include psoriatic arthritis, ankylosing spondylitis, microangiopathic polyarteritis and giant cell arteritis. These have expanded to include many other targets including B cells, IL-6 receptors and co-stimulatory molecules. The latest advance has been the development and clinical application of oral agents directed against JAK, which inhibit intracellular second messages and lead to reduced cytokine production.

Surgery for rheumatoid arthritis

A significant number of patients with RA require the skills of an orthopaedic surgeon at some stage of their disease. Two types of surgery are used – synovectomy and reconstructive or joint-replacement surgery.

Synovectomy is the surgical removal of synovium from an inflamed joint. It can be performed as an open procedure or by arthroscopy, depending on the joint involved and the skill of the surgeon. The main indication is persistent arthritis in a joint, which fails to settle despite medical therapy and repeated intra-articular depot corticosteroid injections. The site most treated is the knee. Less commonly treated are other joints or inflamed tendon sheaths – tenosynovitis sometimes requires synovectomy. Results are good with better symptomatic and radiographic outcome for an involved joint, compared with medical therapy, even after 3 years. Due to the good results from the use of biologic and targeted therapies, synovectomies are performed less frequently. Synovial tissue biopsies, however, are frequently performed to aid in diagnosis.

Reconstructive or joint-replacement surgery is reserved for patients with irreversibly damaged joints and severe articular cartilage loss, who are experiencing severe pain and limited mobility. The joints most commonly replaced are the knee, hip, shoulder and metacarpophalangeal joints of the hands. There are many types of artificial joints with different biomechanical properties. Some require the use of cement to hold the joint prosthesis in place, while uncemented prostheses have been developed. The results of surgery, particularly for knee and hip joint replacement, are excellent with markedly reduced pain and improved joint function. Half-lives for cemented knee and hip prostheses are approximately 8–10 years. Surgical revision is now a common procedure. The main local adverse outcomes of joint replacement surgery are cement loosening and, uncommonly, but seriously, secondary bacterial infection. It is hoped that the use of uncemented prostheses will eliminate loosening of prostheses and result in longer prosthetic half-life.

Other types of surgery performed less commonly on patients with RA, include bony fusion, particularly for unstable wrists, and carpal tunnel release for a median nerve entrapped in the carpal tunnel by persistently inflamed synovium (see Ch. 3).

Prognosis

The natural history of untreated RA is poor. It is associated with severe morbidity and shortening of life-expectancy by 7–10 years. In the past, patients died because of premature cardiovascular disease, infection or extra-articular complications involving lung and kidney. It has been claimed that the prognosis for untreated RA is like that of treated Hodgkin's disease. The introduction of methotrexate and other DMARDs slowed disease progression both clinically and radiologically. The change in treatment paradigm of using DMARDs early in the disease and the idea of inducing remission has substantially improved the long-term prognosis and reduced mortality. The introduction of biologic agents was revolutionary and changed the profile of the disease. Progress continues to be made in the introduction of targeted therapies.

Interesting facts

New treatments for rheumatoid arthritis

The last 10–15 years has seen a revolution in the treatment of rheumatoid arthritis. The application of monoclonal antibody technology and the use of targeted small molecules has transformed the way rheumatoid arthritis is treated. The application of these therapies has resulted not only in better control of the inflammatory process but helped prevent joint damage and deformities. These treatments have recently been shown to prolong life expectancy in patients with rheumatoid arthritis. Although these treatments do not represent a cure for rheumatoid arthritis, and are expensive, they represent a major advance in the way rheumatoid arthritis is treated.

Clinical skill 1 – assessing synovitis

One of the commonest clinical challenges in rheumatology is assessing whether the patient has active synovitis. A typical history includes the presence of prominent early morning joint stiffness (>60 minutes) and joint pain. It is important to distinguish whether this is due to osteoarthritis or an inflammatory arthritis. In either case, the joints may be tender. Distinguishing features include the distribution of joints involved. Osteoarthritis involves the distal interphalangeal and proximal interphalangeal joints. By contrast, in inflammatory arthritides such as rheumatoid arthritis typically, there is symmetrical involvement of metacarpophalangeal and proximal interphalangeal joints.

With a careful history and physical examination, it is usually possible to determine whether or not the patient has active synovitis. Palpating the joints can usually distinguish between osteoarthritis and inflammatory arthritis. In osteoarthritis, the swelling is bony hard while in inflammatory arthritis, the joint swelling is usually soft. In large joints (e.g. knees), swelling may be predominately due to excess joint fluid (effusion). This can be demonstrated with the bulge sign or patella tap. The former is usually helpful when there is a small effusion. The bulge sign is elicited by gentle pressure over the lateral aspect of the knee and observing a fluid wave move along the medial aspect of the knee. The technique requires practice. In patients with osteoarthritis, there are no extra-articular features. These may be present in patients with inflammatory arthritis, such as a scaly erythematous rash on extensor surfaces in psoriasis or painless nodules over the elbows (rheumatoid arthritis).

Clinical skill 2 – assessment for extra-articular disease

In patients with inflammatory arthritis, there are often clues from the clinical history as to the type of arthritis one is dealing with. Physical examination should include a general medical assessment looking for evidence of extra-articular features. This may provide clues as to whether the patient has rheumatoid arthritis, psoriatic arthritis or gout. The presence of extra-articular features such as nodules, tophi or psoriatic skin rash may be helpful in establishing the clinical diagnosis. Other manifestations on examination include erythematous rash over the cheeks and bridge of the nose (lupus), alopecia, mouth ulcers, scaly skin over hairline or inflamed red conjunctivae (reactive arthritis).

The number of abnormalities described in different rheumatic diseases is too numerous to elaborate here. The main message is that, in patients with an inflammatory arthritis, it is important to obtain a thorough history and perform a detailed and systematic physical examination.

Summary

This chapter provides a review of the basic sciences (anatomy and immunology) that underpin an understanding of the musculoskeletal system and the ways in which it is affected in inflammatory joint disease. The chapter outlines the clinical features of patients with inflammatory arthritis and the principles of treatment both pharmacological and surgical.

Further Reading

Bone and Spine. Flexor tendon pulley system of hand. Available from: https://boneandspine.com/flexor-tendon-pulley-system-of-hand/.

El-Zayat, S.R., Sibaii, H., Mannaa, FA 2019. Toll-like receptors activation, signaling, and targeting: an overview. Bull. Natl. Res. Cent., 43, 187. https://doi.org/10.1186/s42269-019-0227-2.

Hochberg, M.C., Silman, A.J., Smolen, J.S., Weinblatt, M.E., Weisman, M.H. (Eds.), 2008. Rheumatology, fourth ed. Mosby, Philadelphia.

Okada, Y., Eyre, S., Suzuki, A., et al. 2019. Genetics of rheumatoid arthritis: 2018 status. Ann. Rheum. Dis. 78, 446–453. https://doi.org/10.1136/annrheumdis-2018-213678.

Moore, K.L., Dalley, A.F. 1999. Clinically Oriented Anatomy, fourth ed. Williams & Wilkins, Baltimore.

Sun, C., Mezzadra, R., Schumacher, T.N. 2018. Regulation and function of the PD-L1 checkpoint. Immunity 48 (3), 434–452. https://doi.org/10.1016/j.immuni.2018.03.014.

T cell. Available from: https://en.wikipedia.org/wiki/T_cell.

SOFT TISSUE RHEUMATIC DISEASE INVOLVING THE SHOULDER AND ELBOW

2

Chapter objectives

After studying this chapter, you should be able to:

1. Describe normal shoulder and elbow anatomy and function.

2. Understand some of the common pathological processes involving the shoulder and elbow.

3. Appreciate rotator cuff pathology and treatment options.

4. Describe risk factors for rotator cuff disease and principles of treatment.

6. Understand common soft tissue conditions affecting the elbow.

Terence Rae Moopanar

Introduction

Rheumatic diseases are diseases that affect joints, ligaments, tendons, bones and muscles. Sometimes, this group of diseases is referred to as musculoskeletal disease and is used to describe over 100 diseases and conditions. We can divide rheumatological diseases into diseases that affect bone and cartilage (hard tissue) and diseases that affect the soft tissue (muscles, tendons, ligaments, bursae and capsule, etc.). 'Fibromyalgia' is also sometimes included under this heading, as diagnosis involves pain in the neck, shoulder and upper arm but will be considered separately in Chapter 8. Upper limb pain in general, and shoulder pain in particular, is commonly due to disease of these soft tissues. When considering making a diagnosis, careful history-taking and specific examinations often provides a provisional diagnosis. Physical examination should be both general and specifically directed towards the most likely site/s of pathology. This involves general inspection (assessing asymmetry, muscle loss and deformity); palpation (assessing anatomical points of tenderness); and observation of movement to assess global range and weakness. Special provocative tests are also performed by the clinician to reproduce pain and/or weakness, which identify the specific sites of pathology in the shoulder and elbow. Investigations include plain X-rays, ultrasound, computed tomography (CT) scans and magnetic resonance imaging (MRI) and are used judiciously to help confirm the diagnosis. Multiple modalities of treatment should be considered and may be employed simultaneously. These include rest, activity modification to avoid aggravating symptoms, physical modalities (such as ice and heat), physiotherapy, specific exercise programmes (including stretching and strengthening) and both non-steroidal anti-inflammatory medication and corticosteroids by injection. Surgery is sometimes the definitive treatment, and in appropriate cases should not be delayed unduly.

Case 2.1   Rotator cuff injury: 1

Case history

Mr Jones, a 50-year-old self-employed carpenter, presented with a 10-week history of gradually increasing right shoulder pain. The pain began when he suddenly took the full weight of a cupboard which he was carrying with his workmate. Initially the pain was of nuisance value only, but more recently it had interfered with sleep and various activities of daily living (washing, dressing, hair care and driving a car). Over the last few weeks, Mr Jones had been unable to continue to work as a carpenter, because of both activity-related pain and, more recently, increasing shoulder weakness when working overhead. Pain was maximal at the front of the shoulder, but occasionally radiated to the deltoid insertion and beyond. The hand was uninvolved.

This chapter uses rotator cuff pathology (tendonitis, impingement and tear) as a model for discussing soft tissue disorders, and reviews normal shoulder anatomy and function. Common soft tissue conditions of the elbow are also considered.

Anatomy of the shoulder

The shoulder joint is a ball-and-socket joint formed from the articulation of the head of the humerus and the glenoid cavity of the scapula, and is functionally considered a diarthrodial, multiaxial joint (Fig. 2.1A). The articular surfaces of the glenoid and the humeral head are lined by articular cartilage. The glenoid socket is deepened by a fibrocartilaginous labrum or rim which surrounds its edge. The joint is lined by synovium and enclosed by a fibrous capsule.

The scapula also contains the acromion, which articulates with the clavicle and the axial skeleton through the sternoclavicular joint.

The attachment of the arm to the trunk is almost totally dependent on musculature. The scapula is held on and moves on the chest wall. This connection is called the 'scapulothoracic articulation'. Shoulder movement occurs simultaneously at both the glenohumeral and the scapulothoracic joints, in a ratio of approximately two to one.

While the glenohumeral joint may be seen as a 'ball and socket joint', the socket is very shallow and flat. The static (ligaments, labrum, capsule) and dynamic (periarticular musculature) stabilizing structures allow for extreme degrees of motion in multiple planes of the body that predisposes the joint to instability events.

There are multiple synovial bursae present around the shoulder as well. These bursae act as a cushion between joint structures, such as tendons and include the subacromial, subcoracoid and subscapular bursae. The most clinically significant is the subacromial bursa which lies between the deltoid muscle and joint capsule in the superolateral aspect of the shoulder joint.

Interesting facts

Although many animals have supra- and infraspinatus tendons, true rotator cuffs (the fusion of supra- and infraspinatus tendons to form a single 'tendon sheet') are unique to animals which are able to reach overhead – mainly the advanced primates.

The rotator cuff muscles

The rotator cuff refers to four muscles that stabilize the shoulder and allow for its extensive range of movement (Fig. 2.1C). These are the supraspinatus, infraspinatus, teres minor and subscapularis muscles. Although supra- and infraspinatus and teres minor are separate muscles, their flat sheet-like tendons of insertion blend with each other as they approach the humeral head to form a cuff that holds the humeral head in place and assists with active elevation and external rotation of the shoulder. More specifically, they act as a dynamic stabilizer of the humerus during abduction and external rotation. The supraspinatus muscle comes from the dorsal (superficial) surface of the scapula above its spine (hence, *supra*spinatus). Its tendon passes over the *top* of the glenohumeral joint to the front of the greater tuberosity of the humeral head. Infraspinatus and teres minor arise from the dorsal surface of the scapula *below* its spine, and cross over the back of the glenohumeral joint to the back of the (greater tuberosity of the) humeral head.

The fourth cuff muscle (subscapularis), which inserts onto the lesser tubercle of the humerus, is a powerful internal rotator of the shoulder and together, the cuff muscles act synergistically to prevent sheer forces within the joint and assist the other muscles such as the deltoid, pectoralis major and latissimus dorsi muscles in the complex wide range of movements of the shoulder.

Other muscles of the shoulder

The scapular motors are large muscles which stabilize and move the scapula on the chest wall. They include the serratus anterior, which protracts the scapula and the trapezius, levator scapulae and rhomboids, which elevate and rotate it (Fig. 2.1B). Paralysis of the serratus produces 'winging' of the scapula. Paralysis of the trapezius allows the shoulder to 'drop', and this may stretch the brachial plexus.

Two large muscles, latissimus dorsi and pectoralis major, cross from the trunk to the humerus, bypassing

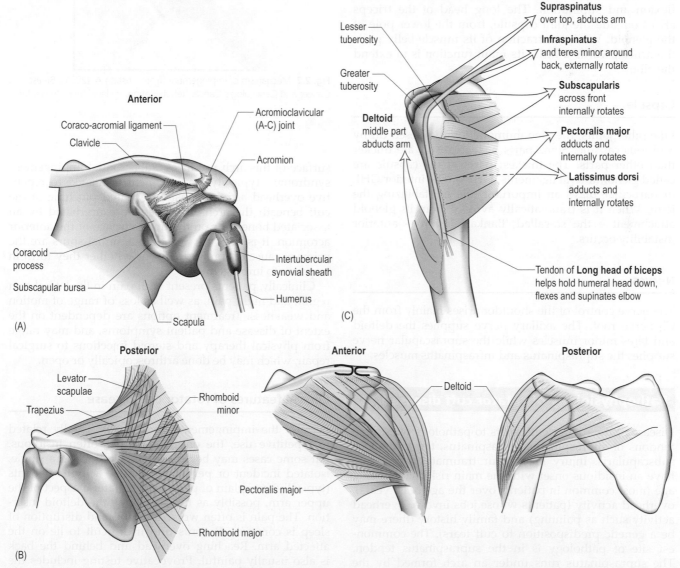

Fig. 2.1 Anatomy of the shoulder. (A) Anterior view of shoulder showing bones, synovial membrane, bursae and ligaments; (B) view showing serratus anterior, trapezius, levator scapulae, rhomboids, latissimus dorsi and pectoralis major; (C) diagram of rotator cuff.

the scapula. Both adduct the arm to the trunk and can rotate it internally. The scapulothoracic motors, together with latissimus and pectoralis major, provide the gross control of the shoulder.

A number of other muscles connect the humerus to the scapula and provide fine control. The largest of these is the deltoid. The deltoid can be regarded in three parts: anterior, middle and posterior. Anterior deltoid (between clavicle and acromion superiorly and humerus inferiorly) can forward-flex the humerus. The lateral deltoid (arising from the side of the acromion), helps abduct the arm. The posterior deltoid extends the arm. All three parts act together to pull the arm up and abduct it.

Various other muscles also affect shoulder function. The tendon of the long head of biceps arises inside the glenohumeral joint, at the top of the glenoid, and crosses over the humeral head before leaving the joint and passing into the biceps groove. It helps hold the humeral head down, but its main function is in elbow flexion and supination. The long head of the triceps arises outside the joint capsule, from the lower pole of the glenoid. While contraction of its muscle belly pulls the arm upwards a little, its main function is to extend the elbow.

Capsule

Like other joints, the glenohumeral joint is closed off by a fibrous capsule. Some parts of the capsule are thicker than other parts. The thickest parts of the capsule are called glenohumeral ligaments (GHLs). The inferior GHL in particular plays an important role in stabilizing the joint. When it is traumatically avulsed from its glenoid attachment – the so-called 'Bankart lesion' – anterior instability occurs.

Nerves

The nerve control of the shoulder arises mainly from the C5 nerve root. The axillary nerve supplies the deltoid and teres minor muscles while the suprascapular nerve supplies the supraspinatus and infraspinatus muscles.

Pathophysiology of rotator cuff disease

Disease of the rotator cuff refers to pathology within the tendons of supraspinatus, infraspinatus, teres minor or subscapularis. Injury may occur traumatically or may have an insidious onset with the main risk factors being age (most common in patients over the age of 60 years), overhead activity (patients whose jobs involve overhead activity such as painting) and family history (there may be a genetic predisposition to cuff tears). The commonest site of pathology is in the supraspinatus tendon. The supraspinatus runs under an arch formed by the coracoid, the coracoacromial ligament and the anterior acromion (Fig. 2.2). Rubbing of the tendon on the under-

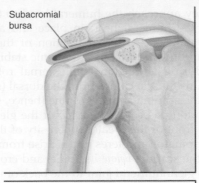

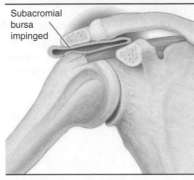

Fig. 2.2 Mechanism of impingement (from Cristian A. (2021). Breast Cancer and Gynecologic Cancer Rehabilitation. Philadelphia: Elsevier Inc.).

surface of this arch produces 'subacromial impingement syndrome'. Typically, impingement is related to repetitive overhead activity causing repeated pinching of the cuff beneath the arch. This may be exacerbated by an associated bone spur on the undersurface of the anterior acromion. It is not clear whether acromial spurs are the primary cause of impingement or whether they form in response to impingement.

Clinically, patients present with pain in the lateral arm region and night pain, as well as loss of range of motion and weakness. Treatment options are dependent on the extent of disease and patient symptoms, and may range from physical therapy and steroid injections to surgical repair, which may be done arthroscopically or open.

Clinical features of rotator cuff disease

Because the impingement syndrome is usually related to repetitive use, the onset of pain is often insidious, but some cases may begin suddenly following a single, isolated incident or period of overuse activity. Patients (typically) complain of pain over the lateral aspect of the upper arm, possibly as far distally as the deltoid insertion. The pain is often worse at night, and disruption of sleep is common. Patients find it difficult to lie on the affected arm. Reaching overhead and behind the back is also usually painful. Provocative testing includes the 'empty can test' in the plane of the scapula and this classically reproduces symptoms. The investigation of choice is an MRI, which shows the extent of the tear and helps guide surgical treatment (anatomy of the tear for surgical planning vs the tear not being surgically reparable in some instances).

Clinical aspects of shoulder pain

Due to the broad range of movement of the shoulder and number of structures responsible for achieving this (bones, muscles, tendons, etc.), multiple structures may be attributed to causing pain in the clinical setting. In considering a patient's history, the patient's age, the mechanism of pain onset, the progression of the symptoms, the site of pain and the nature of any resultant disability all provide an insight into the responsible pathology. The mechanism of onset provides some clues. Sudden onset, associated with a single traumatic event (such as trying to catch a falling cupboard), suggests a mechanical event, such as a tendon tearing. A more insidious onset suggests degenerative disease, or possibly repeated micro-trauma.

Perhaps the most useful information about the source of pathology is surprisingly the age of the patient! Younger patients are more likely to have instability and inflammation of structures (such as bursitis and tendonitis), while older patients are more likely to have degenerative joint disease such as osteoarthritis. Rotator cuff pathology usually begins as 40 years of age and starts with cuff tendinitis and mild abrasions due to potential impingement. This may be activity related such as for those who perform repetitive overhead activities (such as throwing in sport or painting). This insult to the rotator cuff progresses in time and by the age of 60, partial or full thickness tears are more common.

In cases of sudden onset (usually related to a traumatic event), the position of the arm and the nature of the initial injury may provide some clue. If the arm was forced into abduction and external rotation, anterior subluxation or dislocation is of concern. If the arm was at or near the side at the time of onset, or if the mechanism involved contraction of the shoulder muscles against resistance, an injury to the rotator cuff mechanism is more likely.

The progression of symptoms helps diagnosis. Increasing pain implies progressive pathology. Increasing weakness may be due to painful inhibition of shoulder activity. If the loss of strength is profound, this suggests progressive disruption of a muscle–tendon unit, possibly the rotator cuff. Increasing stiffness (loss of range) suggests an inflammatory process, possibly adhesive capsulitis (frozen shoulder).

The site of pain is important. Subacromial pain is usually felt at the front of the shoulder. Radiation of pain to the deltoid insertion is common but non-specific, as it also occurs with glenohumeral pathology and cervical pathology, especially a C5 radiculopathy (nerve root lesion). Involvement of the trapezius, the parascapular muscles and the side of the neck are also common

but relatively non-specific. Pain over the posterior joint line is frequently glenohumeral in origin. Involvement of the hand may suggest neurological or neurovascular pathology, including neck pathology, thoracic outlet syndrome or even carpal tunnel syndrome (see Ch. 3). Regional pain syndromes may also involve both shoulder and hand.

It is important to assess the patient's degree of disability when taking a history of shoulder pain. It is also important to address the patient's ability to perform routine daily activities (such as brushing their hair, dressing themselves and feeding themselves and being able to perform their tasks at work. An inability to attend to activities of daily living, and particularly an inability to sleep at night, warrants serious attention, as does any condition which affects the patient's occupation. For a keen sportsperson, an inability to throw or to serve at tennis may be equally distressing. The use of patient questionnaires and visual analogue scales aids assessment. A typical patient-questionnaire directed at the assessment of shoulder pain is shown below (Fig. 2.3) and may be repeated at a later stage to guide progress.

Inspection and palpation are best carried out with the examiner standing behind the seated patient. When present, significant wasting of the rotator cuff muscles will be obvious in all but the most obese patients. The best-known tests for subacromial impingement are the Neer and Hawkins tests (Fig. 2.4). In both, the greater tuberosity, the attached supraspinatus tendon, the overlying bursa and the adjacent biceps tendon are compressed beneath the coracoacromial arch. If either manoeuvre recreates typical symptoms, this suggests cuff impingement but may also reflect biceps pathology. Yergason's test for biceps tendinitis is less sensitive but moderately specific (Fig. 2.5).

Differential diagnosis

Common pathologies to consider in a patient with shoulder pain are shown in Box 2.1. Each of these will briefly discussed to help differentiate between clinical presentations.

Calcific tendonitis is a condition that results in the calcification and degeneration of usually the supraspinatus tendon at its site of insertion. It usually occurs between the ages of 30 and 60 and is more common on women. X-rays usually demonstrate calcium deposits. Laboratory tests usually do not reveal any abnormality of calcium or phosphate metabolism. Treatment is usually nonoperative involving non-steroidal anti-inflammatory drugs (NSAIDs), physiotherapy, physical therapy, steroid injection and needle barbotage. Surgery is indicated when there is a progression of symptoms or the condition is refractory to nonoperative measures.

Subacromial bursitis is a common cause of shoulder pain resulting from inflammation of the bursa due to abutment between the humerus and the rotator cuff and the acromion. In the shoulder, an extensive bursa lies

SHOULDER QUESTIONNAIRE

Date: / /

Name: .... Date of Birth: / /

Are you right-handed ☐ / left-handed ☐ / ambidextrous ☐ ?

Which shoulder is currently troubling you? Right ☐ / Left ☐ / Both ☐

Usual Occupation.. Sports..

Is your shoulder comfortable when your arm is by your side when using a knife and fork?	Yes ☐ / No ☐
Can you lie on affected shoulder at night without waking?	Yes ☐ / No ☐
Can you reach your back pocket and/or tuck your clothes in?	Yes ☐ / No ☐
Can you comb your hair/reach your head with affected arm?	Yes ☐ / No ☐

Can you use your arm (e.g. put a coin in a slot) with your arm straight (elbow not bent) at shoulder height

(A) In front of you?	Yes ☐ / No ☐
(B) To your side?	Yes ☐ / No ☐
Can you lift a full 600mL milk container (or equivalent) to shoulder height without bending your elbow?	Yes ☐ / No ☐
Can you carry a suitcase or a heavy shopping bag with your arm by your side (without help from the other hand)?	Yes ☐ / No ☐
Can you throw a tennis ball overarm or use a hair dryer?	Yes ☐ / No ☐
Can you wash the opposite shoulder and armpit?	Yes ☐ / No ☐

Please circle the number on the scale at the point which best depicts your situation.

Shoulder comfort with arm at rest

No pain   1   2   3   4   5   6   7   8   9   10   Very painful

Shoulder comfort during sleep

No pain   1   2   3   4   5   6   7   8   9   10   Painful/wakes me

Ability to use arm at work or play

Little or no problem to use it   1   2   3   4   5   6   7   8   9   10   Painful/cannot

Effect of shoulder on overall quality of life

Little or no problem   1   2   3   4   5   6   7   8   9   10   Very bad

Fig. 2.3 Shoulder questionnaire.

between the acromion, the coracoacromial arch and the deltoid muscle 'above' and the underlying humeral head and attached rotator cuff tendons 'below'. Chronic irritation (rubbing) of a bursa produces inflammation (called bursitis) in the bursa which becomes swollen with synovial fluid. In the shoulder, this bursa (known variously as the subacromial or subdeltoid bursa) may be irritated by subacromial impingement or other pathologies affecting synovial tissues.

Adhesive capsulitis (frozen shoulder) is characterized by chronic pain and marked global restriction of shoulder movement. While most cases are idiopathic, some are secondary to conditions that cause immobility such as a stroke or occur as a late complication of rotator cuff lesions. Three phases are usually recognized: 'freezing' (capsulitis causing pain, especially at the extremes of range when the capsule is stretched and progressive restriction of movement); 'frozen' (capsulitis causing mainly immobility with lessening of pain); and 'thawing' (involving gradual recovery of the range of movement). Treatment involves steroids, physical therapy and physiotherapy and medical management of underlying disease if present (diabetes, thyroid disorder). Surgery is reserved for cases that are recalcitrant to non-operative measures and involves arthroscopic capsular release and shoulder manipulation under anaesthesia.

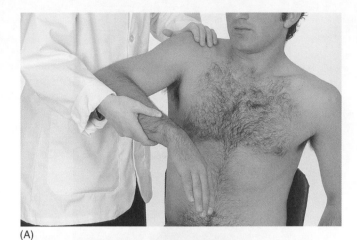

(A)

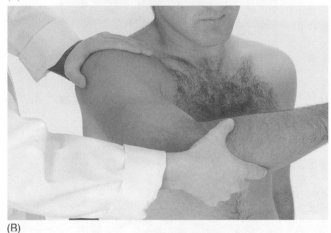

(B)

Fig. 2.4 Neer and Hawkins tests. (A) The Neer test is performed by the examiner lifting the patient's arm in front of the patient with the elbow bent. At the same time, the examiner presses up on the elbow with one hand and places counterpressure on the top of the shoulder. (B) In the Hawkins test, the arm is brought by the examiner into the Neer position and then internally rotated (the hand of the patient is brought downward) as the elbow is pushed up. Both should 'pinch' the rotator cuff tendons if impingement is present.

The distinction between **cervical disease** and shoulder pathology is not always easy. Pain involving the upper arm, especially the region of the deltoid muscle insertion, can be due to shoulder pathology or cervical radiculopathy involving the fifth cervical nerve root. Similarly, spondylotic (osteoarthritic) changes involving the cervical spine can also produce pain in the trapezius muscle, the supraclavicular region and the shoulder. Cervical disc degeneration is usually associated with restricted neck movement and also possibly neurological signs, if there is nerve compression.

Polymyalgia rheumatica (PMR), an inflammatory condition predominantly affecting the proximal limb girdles (shoulders and hips), usually occurs in older patients. It is usually associated with bilateral shoulder symptoms, prominent early morning stiffness and often fever and weight loss. PMR is thought to be idiopathic and may be brought on by a viral or bacterial illness and is treated with oral steroids.

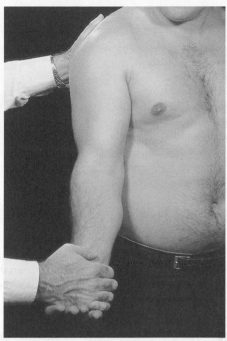

Fig. 2.5 Yergason's sign. With the patient's elbow held at his side and flexed to 90 degrees, the forearm is supinated against resistance while shaking hands.

Case 2.1 Rotator cuff injury: 2

Case history

On examination, Mr Jones appeared a healthy man, slightly overweight, who held his right arm carefully by his side. Shaking hands was painful. With Mr Jones seated, inspection from above and behind revealed obvious wasting of the right supraspinatus muscle belly. Gentle palpation suggested that infraspinatus was also significantly smaller on the right than on the left, despite Mr Jones' right-handedness. Examination of range of movement produced pain in the mid-arc of forward flexion. The pain settled in part, but not completely, as flexion progressed to its limit of 160 degrees (180 degrees on the left). Abduction was similarly painful, but full. The range of external rotation in both adduction and abduction was almost normal, but internal rotation was markedly limited. Active range of movement was more limited, with Mr Jones unable to actively flex more than 80 degrees against gravity, even with the elbow bent to reduce the lever-arm. Strength of external rotation in adduction was markedly weaker on the right than on the left. Pain precluded testing internal rotation. Palpation of the shoulder revealed exquisite tenderness over the greater tuberosity and some tenderness over the biceps groove at the front of the humeral head. A number of specific tests were carried out, including the impingement test (which was severely painful), and various biceps provocation tests which were also somewhat uncomfortable. There was however no evidence of biceps disruption, and the subscapularis appeared intact.

A tentative diagnosis of subacromial pathology, possibly subacromial impingement or a full thickness cuff tear, was made.

Box 2.1 Common causes of shoulder pain

- Rotator cuff impingement (with or without cuff tear)
- Subacromial bursitis
- Bicipital tendonitis
- Calcific tendonitis
- Polymyalgia rheumatica
- Adhesive capsulitis
- Acute myocardial ischaemia
- Cervical disc disease

Interesting facts

The incidence of 'idiopathic' frozen shoulder (adhesive capsulitis) is much higher in diabetics than in non-diabetics. Any patient presenting with a frozen shoulder should have a fasting blood sugar test to check for underlying diabetes.

Investigations

Plain X-rays of the shoulder are often normal in patients presenting with shoulder pain but are useful to exclude certain pathologies. In general, one should seek at least three standard views: anteroposterior, supraspinatus outlet (lateral) and axillary, taken at right angles to each other. With an incomplete series of radiographic views, one might well miss significant pathology such as an acromial spur. If posterior dislocation is ever a consideration, the multiple views are mandatory, as it is possible to miss a posterior dislocation on a single anteroposterior view.

When expertly performed, shoulder ultrasound is a valuable modality for assessing the rotator cuff for impingement or tears (Fig. 2.6). It is, however, very operator-dependent. Ultrasound can also give some indication as to the extent of any fatty degeneration of the supraspinatus and infraspinatus muscles, and the extent of retraction of any torn tendons. This is important information if a rotator cuff repair is contemplated, as an excessively retracted cuff may be irreparable. Double contrast arthrography, the injection of air and dye into the shoulder, followed by radiography, looks for leakage through a cuff tear and has been useful in the diagnosis of full thickness rotator cuff tears.

MRI scanning is now more widely used and is regarded as the gold standard of investigation. It allows more accuracy in the assessment of tear size, and particularly the extent of any tendon retraction, and is also useful in assessing atrophy and fatty degeneration of the muscles. Combined with intra-articular gadolinium, it is also useful in assessing pathology involving the labrum of the glenoid and the biceps tendon origin. It is, however, an expensive investigation. Before the advent of

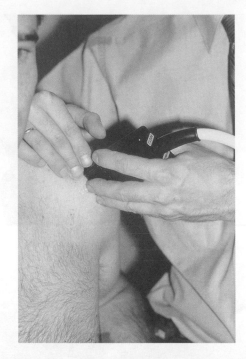

(A)

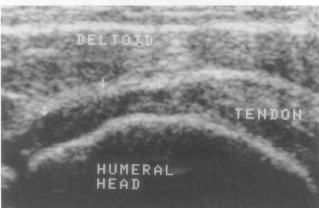

(B)

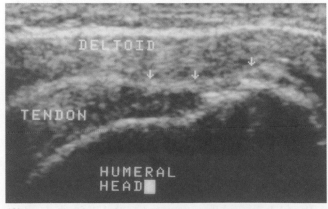

(C)

Fig. 2.6 Ultrasound of rotator cuff tear. (A) Ultrasound technique; (B) normal transverse view of supraspinatus; (C) normal longitudinal view of supraspinatus.

<table>
<tr><td>

Case 2.1

</td><td>

Rotator cuff injury: 3

</td></tr>
</table>

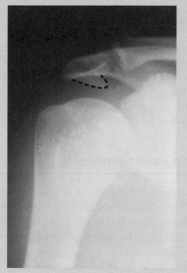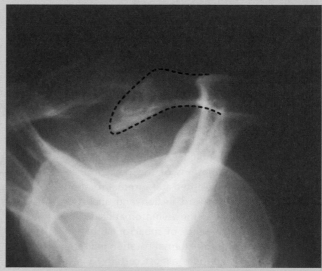

(A)   (B)

Fig. 2.7 Plain radiographs of the shoulder. (A) Anterior view of acromial spur; (B) outlet view of acromial spur.

Case history

In Mr Jones' case, there was a full and pain-free range of cervical spine movement, and no neurological abnormality (motor, sensory or reflex) in the upper limb.

Plain radiographs of the shoulder were obtained (Fig. 2.7). The anteroposterior view showed chronic changes at the site of cuff insertion to the greater tuberosity, and some minor degenerative arthritis of the acromioclavicular joint. Specifically, there was no evidence of supraspinatus or subscapularis calcification, and acromiohumeral height (the distance between the acromion and the humeral head) was not reduced, as might have occurred in the presence of a major cuff disruption. Nor was there any obvious osteophyte formation or reduction in glenohumeral joint space, to suggest glenohumeral arthritis.

The lateral view did show a spur on the undersurface of the anterior acromion, consistent with possible subacromial impingement. The axillary view (not shown here) showed no evidence of os acromiale, a relatively common congenital variant often associated with subacromial impingement and cuff pathology.

Since the local radiologist had no particular expertise in dynamic ultrasound of the shoulder, an MRI was obtained.

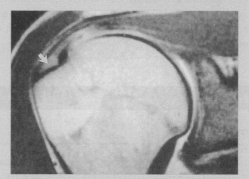

Fig. 2.8 Magnetic resonance imaging (MRI) showing a partial-thickness tear of supraspinatus.

This showed a partial thickness deep surface tear of the cuff, without any full thickness extension (Fig. 2.8).

Because of a family history of rheumatoid arthritis, Mr Jones was referred for a full blood count, erythrocyte sedimentation rate (ESR) and rheumatoid factor (see Ch. 1), but these were all normal. A high ESR would also be expected in polymyalgia rheumatica (PMR).

A definitive diagnosis of partial thickness deep surface cuff tear was made.

MRI, CT arthrography (the combination of a CT scan with intra-articular contrast) was often used to assess labral integrity, but CT scan of the shoulder is now mainly used for detailed assessment of bone pathology, or in the planning of surgical intervention. In general terms, soft tissues are better assessed by MRI scan and bone by CT scan.

Radionucleotide bone scan, usually using [99m]Technetium, is useful in the assessment of bone vascularity (or avascularity) and areas of increased or decreased osteoblastic activity. It is also useful in localizing metastatic disease. In soft tissue pathology it may show increased activity (vascularity) at sites of enthesopathy (abnormality of bone–tendon junctions).

Case 2.1 Rotator cuff injury: 4

Case history

With a provisional diagnosis of subacromial pathology, including but not necessarily limited to a partial thickness deep surface rotator cuff tear, Mr Jones was given an injection of local anaesthetic and corticosteroid to his subacromial space. The corticosteroid was included to help relieve, at least temporarily, the subacromial impingement component of Mr Jones' symptoms. Within minutes, the local anaesthetic produced almost complete pain relief, and, with the pain gone, Mr Jones was able to demonstrate a virtually full active range of shoulder movement. Some secondary inflammation and tightness of the posterior capsule of the shoulder joint prevented full internal rotation. However, the strength of forward flexion and abduction was noticeably less than that on the asymptomatic side. The pain relief confirmed the presence of subacromial pathology and the normal strength of external rotation indicated that the infraspinatus tendon was almost certainly intact. The significance of this is that the infraspinatus and teres minor tendons form the posterior half of the rotator cuff. If they are intact, any cuff tear is limited to the anterior half of the cuff, and thus not massive, and if necessary, is surgically reparable.

Treatment

Corticosteroids

Corticosteroid injections are commonly used in the treatment of musculoskeletal conditions. They act by reducing local inflammation, thus directly reducing pain and local swelling. In subacromial bursitis, in addition to the corticosteroids' direct effect on inflammation and pain, the reduced swelling of the supraspinatus tendon may be important. The impingement process involves a vicious cycle of 'rub, inflammation, swelling, increased rub, increased inflammation, increased swelling, etc.' By breaking the cycle at the inflammation/swelling stage, corticosteroids can sometimes be virtually curative. There are, however, potential problems associated with injectable steroids. First, any steroid injection into a joint or bursal space carries a small risk of infection, and needs to be performed with appropriate attention to sterility. Second, the effects of corticosteroids on connective tissue are well documented. The repeated use of corticosteroids may produce atrophy and weakening of connective tissues, an obviously undesirable effect in an already damaged structure such as the supraspinatus tendon. There is no consensus regarding how much is safe, but most authorities agree that two injections of steroids to any one site in any 6-month period are not deleterious. As there is a suggestion that steroids produce particular weakening of the soft tissues in the first 24–48 hours after injection, it may be wise to avoid strenuously exercising the injected area for a day or possibly two after a steroid injection.

Interesting facts

Small and medium-sized cuff tears are often compatible with pain-free function. Many older citizens have such tears in one or both shoulders without being aware of 'anything wrong'. Large cuff tears predispose to 'cuff arthropathy', a form of severe secondary shoulder osteoarthritis.

Physiotherapy and exercises

A strong rotator cuff helps hold the humeral head down and away from the coracoacromial arch, reducing the risk of further impingement and improving overall shoulder function. The lines of pull of both infraspinatus and subscapularis are downwards and medial. Increasing the tone of these muscles may produce an increased downward force vector on the humeral head, further reducing subacromial impingement between the acromion and the humeral head ('inner range internal and external rotator strengthening'), at least while the muscles are 'firing'. Exercises designed to strengthen external rotators (especially infraspinatus) and internal rotators (especially subscapularis) can be performed by keeping the elbow flexed at 90 degrees by the side and rotating the shoulder outwards or inwards, respectively, while holding onto the end of an elasticized band of suitable thickness for resistance. Anatomical studies have shown that the posterior capsule of the glenohumeral joint holds the humeral head up, and that a tight posterior capsule exacerbates subacromial impingement of the rotator cuff. Posterior capsule stretching exercises help lower the humeral head and reduce subacromial impingement.

Increasing the strength of those muscles which move the scapula is of particular help. Shoulder movement occurs at both the glenohumeral and scapulothoracic articulations in an approximate ratio of two to one. By increasing the strength of the scapular muscles ('scapular stabilizing'), better shoulder flexion and abduction can be achieved with scapulothoracic movement, placing less demand on the glenohumeral component of shoulder function and resulting in less subacromial impingement and pain. The stretching of injured joint capsules, ligaments and tendons is an integral part of systematic rehabilitation.

Applied physiology

Connective tissues, which include joint capsules, tendons, ligaments and the fascia covering muscles, contain collagen and elastin fibres. Collagen provides tensile strength and elastin provides elasticity. The higher the

Case 2.1 Rotator cuff injury: 5

Case history

Two days after the steroid injection, Mr Jones was started on a programme of shoulder exercises. A physiotherapist instructed him in a home programme of posterior capsule stretching, inner range internal and external rotator strengthening and scapular stabilizing exercises. He was also instructed in supraspinatus-tendon-stretching techniques.

Mr Jones' shoulder was surprisingly comfortable for 4 days after the steroid injection. Two days after commencing his home exercise programme (5 min, three times a day), Mr Jones again developed shoulder discomfort and nocturnal pain. These increased for a week or so, but just as Mr Jones was about to give up his exercise programme, the pain started to settle. Mr Jones was still not able to return to work, but 8 weeks after starting his exercise programme, his symptoms were at least 75% less severe than they had been. He was given another subacromial corticosteroid injection, and increased the strengthening component of his exercise programme. At 10 weeks after the first corticosteroid injection, Mr Jones returned to work on restricted duties, working mainly at a bench top, and avoiding strenuous and repetitive forward reaching and overhead activity, especially lifting.

He managed well for about 2 months, but then developed sudden severe pain while lifting his toolbox from the boot of the car one evening. The next day, Mr Jones noticed quite marked weakness of forward flexion and especially of external rotation. He had developed a full thickness cuff tear. The surgeon discussed the various treatment options with Mr Jones. Potential advantages of cuff repair included definitive pain relief and return of strength. Disadvantages included the lengthy convalescent period required and a further 2–3 months of physiotherapy and exercise before Mr Jones could return to even light duties as a carpenter. Mr Jones initially opted for ongoing non-operative treatment. Non-steroidal anti-inflammatory medication was added to his regime, and after several days of rest, Mr Jones returned to his exercise programme. Because of a past history of peptic ulcer, Mr Jones was prescribed a specific COX-2 inhibitor anti-inflammatory drug (see Ch. 1). This produced some reduction in pain, but Mr Jones remained frustrated by shoulder weakness and, after a further month, opted for rotator cuff repair.

At surgery, the acromial spur seen on preoperative radiographs was resected as part of an anterior acromioplasty (removal of the under-surface of the anterior acromion to enlarge the space between the bone and the underlying rotator cuff, reducing the risk of tendon-on-bone impingement). There was a large amount of synovial fluid present in the subacromial space, subdeltoid bursa and the shoulder joint, reflecting an ongoing inflammatory process. The full thickness rotator cuff tear was only 2 cm in diameter, but it was in continuity with an interlaminar defect which extended a further centimetre into the rotator cuff tendon posteriorly. The biceps tendon, seen at the front of the rotator cuff defect, was very inflamed. So too was part of the adjacent subdeltoid bursa. Part of the inflamed bursal tissue was resected, together with the inflamed edges of the cuff defect. The interlaminar defect was repaired and the cuff was reattached to the bone of the greater tuberosity.

ratio of elastin to collagen in the capsule of a joint, the greater that joint's range of movement. The basic unit of contraction in muscle is the sarcomere (see Ch. 8). Once a muscle is maximally stretched, with the sarcomere fully stretched, connective tissues take up the slack. In this process, fibres are aligned in the direction of tension. Proprioceptors relay information from the tendon and the muscle–tendon junction to the central nervous system. One important proprioceptor is the Golgi tendon organ, which is sensitive to changes in tension (see Ch. 8). The mechanical behaviour of non-contractile tissue depends on the proportion of collagen and elastin present. In general terms, increased age is associated with decreased maximal tensile strength and increased risk of injury and tear in soft tissues, including tendons and ligaments. Active muscle contraction and passive stretching of muscles is associated with elongation of the connective tissue elements at the ends of the muscle (i.e. tendon and muscle–tendon junction). Regular stretching of connective tissue such as a joint capsule helps alter static (resting) forces on a joint and may actually alter the resting position of the joint and enhance proprioception and joint control.

Surgery

Rotator cuff tears may be repaired arthroscopically or by open surgery. Impingement beneath an acromial spur is often part of the pathology and it may be worthwhile removing the subacromial spur early, by arthroscopic acromioplasty. This is a relatively benign procedure, performed as day surgery and requiring a short convalescence, which may allow return to work within 2 weeks of surgery. However, this procedure does not correct any partial thickness cuff tears, which will continue to predispose to further cuff pathology.

The inflammation of the biceps tendon alerts the clinician to the likely cause of anterior shoulder pain. The biceps tendon runs immediately in front of the anterior margin of the supraspinatus, between it and the subscapularis, until it exits the shoulder joint. It too can impinge on the undersurface of the acromion and the coracoacromial ligament, and the clinical picture of subacromial impingement is often that of combined supraspinatus and bicipital tendinitis. Supraspinatus changes usually predominate, but occasionally isolated biceps tendinitis occurs, sometimes even progressing to rupture of

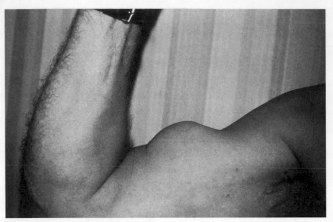

Fig. 2.9 Popeye sign.

the tendon of the long-headed biceps, with the result-ant well-recognized 'popeye sign' (Fig. 2.9). Biceps rup-ture is a good example of a tendon rupture which does not always require repair. A progressively painful biceps tendinitis suddenly becomes pain-free when the tendon finally ruptures. The resultant weakness affects mainly supination, and elbow flexion is often surprisingly little affected.

Rehabilitation and outcome

Socioeconomic factors are important in the management of 'soft-tissue rheumatism'. An uninsured self-employed contractor may be more willing or likely than some to return to work early, or before complete resolution of symptoms. The use of specialized rehabilitation services is now widespread in industry, and in some places man-datory, to help plan return-to-work programmes, with hour modifications, task modification and retraining each being relevant in certain situations.

The benefits of exercise programmes are never instan-taneous. The first week or two of an exercise programme is often associated with increased discomfort, and patients need to be forewarned of this and encouraged to persist with their programme for several weeks before assessing its efficacy.

Patients should also be warned of danger signs. In this case, the sudden loss of strength indicated a major exten-sion of the initially incomplete cuff tear. This suggested possible urgency to surgical repair, before cuff retraction and muscle atrophy precluded a good surgical result. Not all rotator cuff tears need surgery. In fact, many rota-tor cuff tears are asymptomatic. Post-mortem studies suggest that 50% or more of 70-year-olds have partial or full thickness tears involving one or both rotator cuffs. That is, like cervical spondylosis, rotator cuff pathology is often asymptomatic and may not require treatment, conservative or surgical. The presence of a damaged rotator cuff however does increase the risk of further ten-don injury.

Case 2.1	Rotator cuff injury: 6

Case history

Mr Jones' first postoperative week was difficult. To mini-mize postoperative stiffness, especially due to adhesions between the cuff repair and the overlying acromion and deltoid, *passive* mobilization of the shoulder was nec-essary. At the same time, *active* flexion and abduction were avoided to minimize the risk of disrupting the ten-don repair. Six weeks postoperatively, Mr Jones' sling was removed and a programme of *active-assisted* exercises was commenced. In this, Mr Jones employed a pulley, initially raising his right hand with considerable help from the left, but gradually doing more and more of the raising using the muscles of the right shoulder. He also added rotation exercises to his regime. Twelve weeks postoperatively, a more strenuous *'active-resisted'* programme was started, aimed at strengthening the rotator cuff and deltoid muscu-lature in particular. He returned to work 16 weeks postop-eratively, initially avoiding the heaviest of forward-reaching and overhead activities, and minimizing any impact-loading (jarring) on the shoulder. Six months postoperatively, he was coping with unrestricted work activities and sleeping well at night, but was vaguely aware of some mild discom-fort with overhead activity.

Anatomy of the elbow

The elbow is a hinge joint composed of three articula-tions, ulnohumeral (the principal articulation), radio-humeral and proximal radioulnar. All these articulations are enclosed by the capsule in a common synovial joint cavity. The synovial membrane is usually only palpa-ble posteriorly. One large bursa (olecranon) and several small bursae lie about the elbow (Fig. 2.10). The tendi-nous attachments of muscles to the medial and lateral epicondyles of the humerus are common sites of local-ized tenderness. These joints allow for the functional range of the elbow which is between 30 degrees and 130 degrees of flexion and 50 degrees of supination and pro-nation. In loading the elbow, 60% of weight goes through the radiohumeral joint and the rest through the ulno-humeral joint. Finally, ligamentous and bony stabilizers of this complex joint allow for this wide range of stable movement. Primary stabilizers include the coronoid process of the ulna and the medial and lateral collateral ligament complexes. Secondary stabilizers include the radiocapitellar joint, the joint capsule and the common flexor and extensor origins.

Lateral epicondylitis (tennis elbow)

Lateral epicondylitis or 'tennis elbow' is generally an overuse phenomenon reflecting inflammation of the

<table>
<tr><td>Case
2.1</td><td>Rotator cuff injury: 7</td></tr>
</table>

Case history

Mr Jones' physiotherapy regime, was tailored to the expected course of tendon-healing. Initial passive mobilization should not strain the healing bone–tendon junction. By 12 weeks postoperatively, it was hoped that the collagen fibres crossing the healing bone–tendon junction, initially haphazardly, would be at least partly 'realigned' perpendicularly to the bone surface, in the 'line of pull' of the tendon. This should provide sufficient strength to allow active and active-resisted exercise.

The success rate of surgery depends on how it is measured. If measured in degrees of motion, or absolute units of strength, recovery is rarely complete. The best measure of success is patient satisfaction. Recent trends in musculoskeletal outcome studies have been directed towards parameters determined by the patient (relief of pain, return to normal work and sport activities, ability to perform activities of daily living, etc.) rather than more quantifiable parameters, measured by the examiner, such as range-of-motion or kilopascals of strength. Measured in terms of patient satisfaction, rotator cuff repair is successful in over 90% of non-compensable patients. The reported success rate in compensable patients is significantly lower. In addition to the obvious explanations concerning motivation and secondary gain, this may be in part due to the younger age group and the more strenuous activities required.

<table>
<tr><td>Case
2.2</td><td>Tennis elbow: 1</td></tr>
</table>

Case history

Mrs Smith, 50 years old, gives a history of pain in the lateral aspect of her left elbow, especially when reaching for objects with her left hand, such as when doing the ironing or lifting a kettle of water. She consults her local doctor who elicits tenderness over the lateral epicondyle of the elbow and pain on resisted extension of the wrist. He diagnoses 'tennis elbow'. Mrs Smith asks how could that be, stating that she does not play tennis.

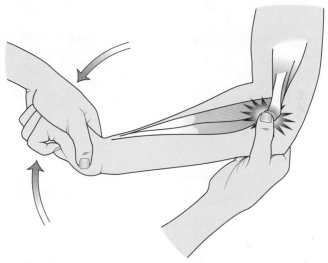

Fig. 2.11 Provocation test for lateral epicondylitis.

common extensor tendon, which inserts at the lateral epicondyle of the humerus (Fig. 2.11). The main muscle affected in tennis elbow is extensor carpi radialis brevis (ECRB). Extensor digitorum communis, extensor carpi radialis longus and extensor carpi ulnaris are also often involved. Clinical signs include marked localized tenderness over the epicondyle and pain on resisted extension of the wrist or middle finger. Investigations often used include X-ray, ultrasound and MRI studies. These are not necessary for the diagnosis, however MRI may show thickening, degeneration and tissue oedema while ultrasound may be used to confirm a hyperechoic tendon. Treatment is most often nonoperative with activity modification, physical therapy, NSAIDs, steroid injections (up to three) and bracing (counter-force brace). Rarely, for cases recalcitrant to nonoperative measures, surgical intervention is required with excision of the degraded portion of the tendon.

Medial epicondylitis (Golfer's elbow)

Similar to its lateral counterpart, medial epicondylitis is an overuse syndrome caused by an eccentric overload

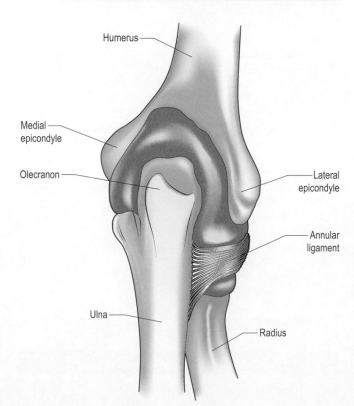

Fig. 2.10 Anatomy of the elbow (posterior view).

Humerus

Medial epicondyle

Olecranon

Lateral epicondyle

Annular ligament

Ulna

Radius

of the flexor-pronator mass at the medial epicondyle. It is much less common than tennis elbow (5–10 times less common) and predominantly affects the dominant arm (75% of cases). Again, the diagnosis is made clinically with aggravation of systems on resisted wrist flexion and is treated largely nonoperatively. Treatment involves rest, ice, activity modification, anti-inflammatory medication and physical therapy. Surgery is reserved for cases that have failed substantial nonoperative measures for at least six months.

Further reading

Moore, K.L., Dalley, A.F., 2006. Clinically Oriented Anatomy, fifth ed. Williams & Wilkins, Baltimore.

Post, M., Bigliani, L.U., Flatow, E.L., et al., 1998. The Shoulder: Operative Technique. Williams & Wilkins, Baltimore.

NERVE COMPRESSION SYNDROMES

David Stewart

3

Chapter objectives

After studying this chapter, you should be able to:

1. Understand normal peripheral nerve anatomy and function, including electrophysiological testing.

2. Appreciate the aetiopathogenesis of the most common entrapment syndromes.

3. Assess the risk factors commonly associated with carpal tunnel syndrome.

4. Understand the general principles of medical and surgical treatment of entrapment neuropathies and their complications.

Introduction

Nerve compression (entrapment) syndromes are a common cause of limb pain. The most common of these is carpal tunnel syndrome in which the median nerve is compressed at the wrist. Other examples include cubital tunnel syndrome due to compression of the ulnar nerve at the elbow, tarsal tunnel syndrome due to entrapment of the posterior tibial nerve at the ankle and meralgia paraesthetica due to entrapment of the lateral cutaneous nerve of the thigh in the inguinal region. Understanding these syndromes requires knowledge of nerve anatomy, the classification and pathophysiology of nerve injury and the causes of nerve injury. Electrophysiological examination is the main investigation used to support or clarify clinical diagnoses based upon history taking and careful examination. Treatment of individual patients may vary according to the duration and severity of symptoms and signs, age and general medical condition. When present, reversible causes must be addressed.

This chapter will focus on nerve compression syndromes in the diagnosis of hand and upper limb pain and will review normal peripheral nerve anatomy and physiology.

Peripheral nerve anatomy

Peripheral nerves emerge from the spinal intervertebral foramina and travel to their endpoint structures, sensory receptors and neuromuscular junctions. The axon is a peripheral process from the nerve cell body in the anterior horn of the spinal cord (motor neuron) or the dorsal root ganglion (sensory neuron). Neurons and muscle fibres communicate with each other at synapses. The first cell communicates with the second by releasing neurotransmitters. The synapse between a motor neuron and a skeletal muscle fibre is called the neuromuscular junction, and the neurotransmitter is acetylcholine (see Ch. 8 for further discussion).

The axon is surrounded by Schwann cells and, together, axon and Schwann cells make up a nerve fibre. Myelinated fibres are those in which each axon is surrounded by single Schwann cells arranged longitudinally to form a continuous chain. Non-myelinated fibres contain multiple axons within the cytoplasm of a surrounding Schwann cell.

Peripheral nerve fibres are usually classified into three types in relation to their conduction velocity, which is generally proportionate to size (Table 3.1).

Nerve fibres are gathered into groups called fascicles and are surrounded by a mechanically strong membrane, the perineurium. Within the fascicles, nerve fibres lie within connective tissue called endoneurium. The fascicles themselves are embedded in an internal epineurium surrounded by an external loose epineurial connective tissue layer (Fig. 3.1). Nerves, such as the sciatic nerve, contain a greater percentage of connective tissue in relation to axonal substance. However, most people experience the sensation of leg and foot numbness following prolonged periods of sitting, especially on unyielding objects, when the protective benefit of the connective tissue cushion is overcome.

The nerve trunk receives a segmental vascular supply. Extrinsic vessels run parallel to the nerve providing branches that lie within the epineurium, perineurium and endoneurium in a longitudinal pattern in each layer, with interconnecting branches between layers. Those vessels passing through the perineurium into the endoneurium often lie obliquely, creating a valve mechanism, which is vulnerable to pressure (Fig. 3.2).

Case 3.1 **Carpal tunnel syndrome: 1**

Case history

Mrs Fotini, aged 55 years, is a production line worker in a factory with a packaging company. She works an 8-hour day in four shifts divided by half-hour rest periods between shifts.

She presented complaining of pins and needles in both hands, which wake her at night and occur intermittently during the day. She also describes neck stiffness and discomfort with pain radiating from her left shoulder to her hand and swelling in both hands, more so in the early mornings.

She was diagnosed as having late-onset diabetes 2 years earlier, which has been reasonably controlled by diet and oral hypoglycaemic medication. She also takes non-steroidal anti-inflammatory medications for osteoarthritis affecting the small joints in her hands, neck and back.

Examination of her hands reveals no swelling of her joints and a normal range of movement. However, sustained wrist flexion for 1 min reproduced her symptoms of numbness affecting both hands.

The history and examination findings suggest a diagnosis of bilateral carpal tunnel syndrome, and her GP recommended she wear a wrist splint at night to keep her wrist in the neutral position.

Table 3.1 Classification of nerve fibres

Group	Function
Group A: up to 20 µm diameter, myelinated, subdivided into:	
α: 12–20 µm	Touch and proprioception (Ia and Ib)
β: 5–12 µm	Touch, pressure and proprioception (II)
γ: 5–12 µm	Fusimotor to muscle spindles (II)
δ: 1–15 µm	Touch, pain and temperature (III)
Group B: up to 3 µm diameter, myelinated	Preganglionic autonomic
Group C: up to 12 µm diameter, unmyelinated	Postganglionic autonomic, and touch and pain (IV)

3

Nerves span joints with varying ranges of motion. On the outside of the nerve trunk, a conjunctival adventitia allows movement of the nerve trunk within its soft tissue surroundings. In deeper layers, fascicles can slide against each other. This allows movement of approximately 50 mm within the brachial plexus during abduction and adduction of the shoulder, 10 mm of the ulnar nerve at the elbow during flexion and extension, and 9 mm of the median nerve at the carpal tunnel with wrist flexion and extension.

Pathophysiology and classification of nerve injury

The endoneurial environment of the nerve is preserved by a combination of a blood–nerve barrier, in which the endoneurial vessels do not allow extravasation of proteins, and by the diffusion barrier of the perineurial sheath. The tissue pressure inside fascicles is slightly positive, providing a normal and healthy mechanical stiffness of fascicles.

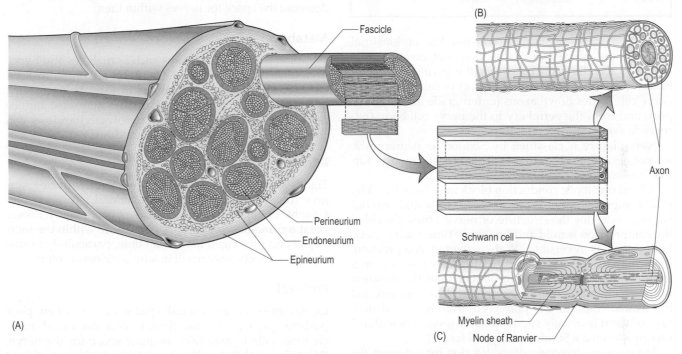

Fig. 3.1 Microanatomy of a peripheral nerve and its components. (A) Fascicles surrounded by perineurium are embedded in a loose connective tissue, the epineurium. The outer layers of the epineurium are condensed into a sheath. The expanded views show the appearance of (B) unmyelinated and (C) myelinated fibres.

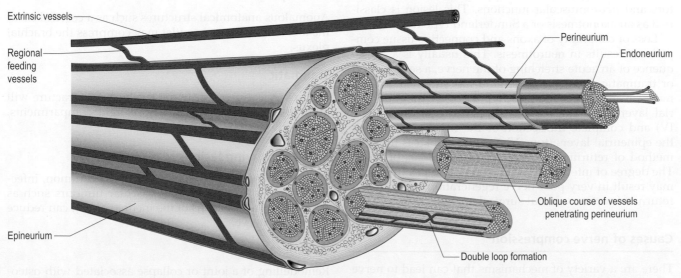

Fig. 3.2 Vascular supply of a peripheral nerve. Vessels are abundant in all layers of the nerve; extrinsic vessels support, via regional feeding vessels, the epineurium, perineurium and endoneurium.

Table 3.2 Classification of nerve injury

Sunderland	Seddon	Spontaneous recovery
Grade 1	Neurapraxia	Yes
Grade 2	Axonotmesis	Sometimes
Grade 3	Axonotmesis	Unlikely
Grade 4	Axonotmesis	Very unlikely
Grade 5	Axonotmesis	Very unlikely
Grade 6	Neurotmesis	Never

When oedema is introduced into the endoneurial space of the nerve trunk, this may not escape easily owing to the diffusion barrier of the perineurial membrane. Consequently, axonal transport of substances from nerve cell bodies down axons (anterograde axonal transport) and from the periphery to the nerve cell body (retrograde axonal transport) is impaired.

Nerve injury is classified by Seddon as neurapraxia, axonotmesis and neurotmesis. This classification is further broken down by Sunderland (Table 3.2).

A local metabolic conduction block may be induced by mild compression but is physiological only and without consequences for the structure of nerve fibres. Provided the compression is mild and limited in time, such a metabolic block is reversible. With extended compression, there may be oedema within the fascicles resulting in a local conduction block lasting longer than the duration of the precipitating cause. The myelin sheath is damaged but axonal continuity is preserved. This is termed neurapraxia and is usually spontaneously reversible within 3 months (termed a Sunderland type I lesion).

More severe compression or traction may disrupt the continuity of axons. Provided the endoneurium is intact, regenerating axons are maintained within the correct tubes and are guided to the appropriate sensory receptors and neuromuscular junctions. This lesion is classified as an axonotmesis or a Sunderland type II lesion.

Loss of continuity of axons and connective tissue components results in neurotmesis. This usually is a consequence of an acute stretching of the nerve, a severe crush or traumatic division. Sunderland has subdivided these more severe lesions into three types: loss of the endoneurial layer (type III), loss of the perineurial layer (type IV) and complete transection of the nerve with loss of the epineurial layers (type V). Surgical repair is the only method of returning some function in the last of these. The degree of internal disorganization in types III and IV may result in very poor nerve regeneration and minimal return of function without surgical repair.

Causes of nerve compression

There are a variety of mechanisms that can lead to nerve compression and several factors may be present at the same time, especially at the carpal tunnel.

Anatomical

Unyielding anatomical structures, such as within the carpal tunnel, allow little increase in pressure before the median nerve is compressed.

Inflammatory

Synovial compartments will be affected most commonly by inflammatory diseases such as rheumatoid arthritis. However, any cause of tenosynovitis will increase the size of contents of anatomical compartments and decrease the space for nerves within them.

Metabolic

Common metabolic problems such as diabetes and hypothyroidism can be associated with an alteration in fluid balance. Physiological alterations in fluid balance, such as in pregnancy and premenstrually, may also induce carpal tunnel compression. Mucopolysaccharidosis can cause carpal tunnel syndrome in children.

Iatrogenic

Tight plasters and dressings or compression during surgery from retraction or other mechanical injury are preventable but all too common causes of nerve injury. Poorly fitted tourniquets, inappropriate pressure within the tourniquet and prolonged tourniquet time, particularly in susceptible subjects, may result in iatrogenic nerve injury.

Postural

Compromise of anatomical spaces occurs when poor posture, perhaps in association with decreased muscle tone, fails to maintain adequate space for the nerve. Repetitive activities placing joints in extreme positions may also compromise the environment of the nerve.

Developmental

Anomalous anatomical structures such as a cervical rib at the level of the thoracic outlet may compress the brachial plexus.

Traumatic

Any injury causing soft tissue swelling or a fracture will affect the pressure, particularly in tight compartments, such as the carpal tunnel.

Space occupying lesions

Tumours, of which ganglia are the most common, infections such as an abscess, and vascular tumours such as aneurysm or thrombosis of the median artery, can reduce space for a nerve.

Degenerative

Remodelling of a joint or collapse associated with osteoarthritis, osteophyte formation and instability of joints may result in nerve compression.

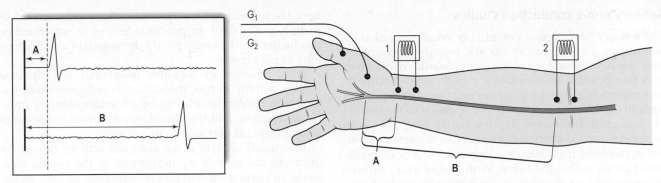

Fig. 3.3 An electrical stimulus is given over the wrist (1) or elbow (2) and measured by recording electrodes at G overlying the abductor pollicis brevis muscle. The time taken to travel from 1 to G1 is the distal motor latency A and that from 2 to G2 is the proximal motor latency B. (Based on Hilburn, J.W. 1996. General principles and use of electrodiagnostic studies in carpal and cubital tunnel syndrome: with special attention to pitfalls and interpretation. Hand Clinics 12 (2), 212, Fig. 4.)

Neuropathic

A nerve already damaged, either by a disease such as diabetic neuropathy or by a proximal compressive lesion, renders the nerve more irritable and more likely to be susceptible to compression at other sites. The latter lesion is sometimes called a double crush syndrome, as there are both proximal and distal lesions. For example, a patient with C5/C6 radiculopathy is more at risk of carpal tunnel syndrome.

Electrophysiology

Nerve conduction studies and electromyography often provide the only objective evidence of a neuropathic condition. It is necessary to understand the concepts and terminology of nerve physiology, pathology and methods of electrodiagnostic studies in order to evaluate the results of these studies.

Electrodiagnostic studies can help confirm the clinical compression of a compression neuropathy with a high degree of sensitivity and specificity, but there are some pitfalls.

Both nerve and muscle cells have a relative negative electrical charge inside them compared with the extracellular environment by virtue of a much higher concentration of potassium within the cells and a lower concentration of sodium and chloride. Electrical stimulation of the cells causes depolarization and generates an action potential. During depolarization, there is an opening of sodium channels in the cell membrane leading to an increase in sodium permeability and creation of an electric current by this rush of positively charged ions into the cell. Current then flows along the path of least electrical resistance, the length of the axon. Myelinated nerve fibres provide a mechanism for regenerating the charge of current (saltatory conduction). The myelin acts as an insulator to prevent current leakage. The myelin sheath indents at intervals, creating tight gaps that expose the axon, called nodes of Ranvier (Fig. 3.1). The action potential is propagated down the axon and exits

at the node completing the electrical circuit through the extracellular fluid. This repeats the process of depolarization and perpetuates regeneration of the longitudinal current. However, there is a delay in the process at each node. Conduction velocity is faster with fewer nodal delays, the large-diameter nerves having the greatest internodal distances and therefore the fastest conduction speeds. These fibres include the alpha motor neurons and the sensory fibres transmitting light touch and proprioceptive (joint position) sensations. Pain and temperature and autonomic functions are conducted by slower, smaller myelinated or unmyelinated fibres.

When the action potential from the motor neuron arrives at the neuromuscular junction, it is transmitted chemically to the muscle. The electrical current is measurable and allows objective measurements of nerve function.

Nerve conduction studies

Motor nerve conduction studies

Motor nerve conduction studies assess the lower motor neurons from the level of the anterior horn to the muscle. The principle will be illustrated by reference to the median nerve (Fig. 3.3). A supramaximal electrical stimulus depolarizes all axons of the nerve and results in an action potential that travels in the normal physiological direction (orthodromically) down the nerve and is measured by recording electrodes overlying the thenar muscle belly. The distal motor latency is the time in milliseconds (ms) that it takes the impulse to travel from the stimulation point at the wrist to the recording electrode, say 3 ms. If the nerve is then stimulated at the elbow and the response follows after 7 ms, the motor conduction velocity is estimated by subtracting the distal motor latency from the proximal motor latency (i.e. 7 - 3 = 4 ms) and dividing the result by the distance between the two stimulating points (240 mm), i.e. a motor conduction velocity of 60 m/s. The shape of the wave is also important. A drop in amplitude indicates a conduction block, whereas an increase in duration indicates a lack of uniform conduction along the axons.

Sensory nerve conduction studies

The sensory nerve action potential is usually recorded by stimulating a distal sensory site and recording proximally over a mixed or sensory nerve (orthodromic conduction). It is also possible to stimulate a mixed nerve proximally and record at a distal site where only sensory axons are present (antidromic conduction, or opposite to the normal physiological direction of impulse transmission). As with motor conduction studies, the sensory nerve action potential is recorded from only the largest 15%–20% of myelinated axons within the nerve. With loss of axons (axonal degeneration), or blocking of conduction owing to demyelination, the amplitude of the action potential decreases.

Estimation of the F wave and H reflex provides additional information. The F wave is a late muscle response from the anterior horn cells in response to the same stimulus that evoked the early direct muscle response. It results in a discharge that sends an impulse back down the same motor axon. Thus the stimulus to the median nerve at the wrist resulted in a direct thenar muscle response after 3 ms and a later response, the F wave, giving the conduction time from the wrist to the spinal cord and back again. The F wave latency gives an indication of the state of the nerve proximally and, if prolonged significantly, one may suspect proximal compression.

The F wave should not be confused with the H reflex, another late response. This is obtained by a submaximal stimulation of the nerve (i.e. a stimulus too low to excite the nerve directly) and results in proximal propagation of a sensory nerve action potential to the spinal cord and a measurable monosynaptic return to the muscle. This is helpful, particularly, in assessing radiculopathies (spinal nerve root lesions).

There are pitfalls of nerve conduction studies. Both motor and sensory studies measure velocity in the largest-diameter and fastest-conducting nerve fibres only. Measurements will be normal if these nerve fibres remain intact. In addition, there is a wide range of normal values for motor conduction velocity of nerves. Operator error may be a factor. Some nerves are located within deep tissues and are less accessible for surface electrode stimulation. The stimulus intensity necessary to depolarize these nerves causes such a spread of current through the intervening tissues that the exact point of stimulation cannot be determined and the measurements are thus less reliable. Radiculopathies (compression at the nerve root origin) and plexopathies (compression of junctions or networks of several nerve roots, e.g. the brachial plexus) are poorly demonstrated on nerve conduction studies. Nerve conduction velocity diminishes with lower temperatures, with increased height of the individual and increased finger circumference. Age is also a factor in determining nerve conduction speed, which is slower in newborns–3 years of age and in older age groups.

Electromyography (EMG)

Motor unit potentials can only be recorded accurately by means of a needle electrode inserted within the muscle tested. Even with fine needles, the associated discomfort may compromise the ability to achieve reliable informa-tion. The technique does, however, offer significant information, particularly in proximal lesions in which nerve conduction studies may poorly demonstrate a radiculopathy or plexopathy.

It is possible to measure insertional activity (see below), activity at rest, the size and configuration of the motor unit potentials elicited by minimal voluntary muscle contraction, and the abundance of active motor units (recruitment) at maximal contraction.

Insertional activity is the electrical activity caused by injury to the muscle by movement of the needle electrode. In normal muscle this persists only as long as the needle is being advanced. With denervation, insertional activity is increased and prolonged.

Activity at rest is normally that of relative electrical silence or of endplate noise. Fibrillation potentials are action potentials of single muscle fibres that occur spontaneously and with needle insertion. They appear several weeks after a nerve injury and are also seen in myopathic disorders. Fasciculation potentials have the dimensions of motor unit potentials and can be benign spontaneous discharges or a sign of anterior horn cell disease. Polyphasic motor units, if numerous and of increased duration and amplitude, are indicative of chronic denervation with reinnervation by adjacent sprouting nerve

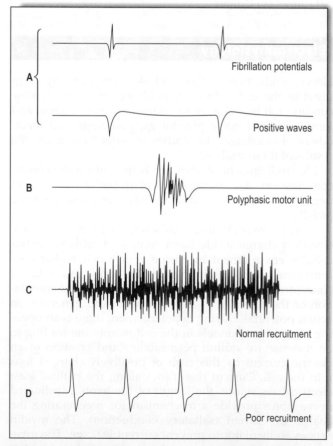

Fig. 3.4 Abnormal findings with electromyography. (Based on Hilburn, J.W. 1996. General principles and use of electrodiagstudies in carpal and cubital tunnel syndrome: with speattention to pitfalls and interpretation. Hand Clinics 12 (2), 211, Fig. 3.)

terminals. The nerve injury is relatively chronic but there is some reinnervation. Recruitment of motor units is a measure of the number of motor units activated (recruited) by maximum muscle contraction. Reduction is present with denervation (Fig. 3.4).

Electromyographic investigation is dependent upon the experience of the electrophysiologist and there is significant interobserver variability in interpretation. Anatomical placement of the needle needs to be precise and it may be necessary to sample multiple areas of each muscle to describe a muscle abnormality. It is important to realize that the EMG will be normal in neurapraxic lesions because of the absence of denervation and that the changes measured by EMG are delayed for 3 weeks following axonotmesis or neurotmesis when anterograde (Wallerian) degeneration of the axons detached from their cell bodies has occurred. The use of EMG for diagnosis of muscle disorders is discussed again in Chapter 8.

Carpal tunnel syndrome

Carpal tunnel compression is the most common of the nerve compression syndromes, with an incidence of approximately 99 in 100,000. It is more common in females (65%–75%), more common in middle age and bilateral in up to 50% of cases.

Anatomy of the carpal tunnel

The floor of the carpal tunnel is formed by the concave arch of the carpal bones covered by the extrinsic palmar wrist ligaments. The roof is the transverse carpal ligament (flexor retinaculum), which is attached to the scaphoid and trapezium bones radially and on the ulnar side to the pisiform and the hamate (Fig. 3.5).

The tunnel contains nine flexor tendons and their vascular synovium, and the median nerve, which may be accompanied by a persistent median artery. Within the carpal tunnel, the nerve lies superficial to the flexor ten-

dons beneath the flexor retinaculum in the radial aspect of the tunnel. The ulnar nerve and artery do not lie within the carpal tunnel but are covered by the palmar carpal ligament extending from the superficial aspect of the flexor retinaculum to the pisiform.

The palmar cutaneous branch of the median nerve takes origin from the radial side of the nerve approximately 5 cm above the wrist, pierces the antebrachial fascia at the distal wrist crease and lies superficial to the flexor retinaculum, supplying sensory fibres to the skin overlying the thenar eminence (Fig. 3.6). The median nerve proper usually divides at the distal end of the carpal tunnel into radial and ulnar portions and then lies deep to the palmar aponeurosis and the superficial palmar arch. The radial division of the nerve gives rise to the thenar motor branch, which innervates the abductor pollicis brevis muscle, opponens pollicis muscle and usually a large part of the flexor pollicis brevis muscle.

Pathophysiology and causes

Any one of the causes of nerve compression outlined previously may be responsible for carpal tunnel syndrome. On occasions, the aetiology is multifactorial. However, in most, the cause is unknown and is termed idiopathic. The increased incidence in perimenopausal

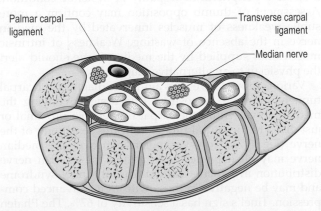

Fig. 3.5 Cross-sectional anatomy of the carpal tunnel. The tunnel contains the median nerve and nine flexor tendons. The transverse carpal ligament forms the palmar surface of the carpal tunnel and the dorsal boundary of the distal ulnar tunnel. The palmar carpal ligament forms the volar boundary of the distal ulnar tunnel.

Palmar carpal ligament
Transverse carpal ligament
Median nerve

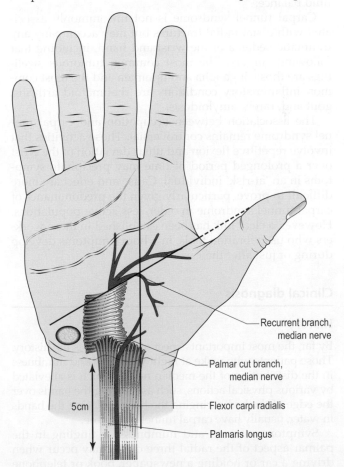

Recurrent branch, median nerve
Palmar cut branch, median nerve
Flexor carpi radialis
Palmaris longus
5cm

Fig. 3.6 Anatomy of the palmar cutaneous branch and thenar branch of the median nerve.

Carpal tunnel syndrome: 2

Case note: Surgical referral

Mrs Fotini had only partial relief of her symptoms from the wearing of night splints and she was referred to a hand surgeon. On further history taking, she stated that she woke nightly, on at least one occasion with numbness in both hands. She was unable to define which parts of the hands were affected but indicated that she often rose to make herself a cup of tea, during which time the symptoms disappeared.

Her hands were puffy in the mornings, as if 'full of fluid'. Stiffness in the hands improved during the day but was replaced by an aching pain, which was diffusely related to the left wrist and increased towards the end of her working day. Pins and needles occurred in both hands when driving home from work. She also described an aching pain in the neck with radiation to the left shoulder and arm during packaging, particularly towards the end of her working day.

women suggests an alteration in hormonal balance as a causative factor, perhaps in association with alteration in fluid balance.

Carpal tunnel syndrome is not uncommonly associated with distal radial fractures but may accompany any traumatic oedema of the wrist and hand, including that following surgery. The most common tumorous swellings are those of ganglia and lipomata and the most common inflammatory conditions are rheumatoid arthritis, gout and, rarely, amyloidosis.

The association between occupation and carpal tunnel syndrome remains controversial. Those activities that involve repetitive flexion and ulnar deviation of the wrist over a prolonged period of time may precipitate symptoms in an 'at-risk' individual. Cause and effect are more difficult to prove, particularly given the predominance of carpal tunnel syndrome in older, less active populations. However, a clear link has been established in those workers who use vibration tools, in whom symptoms develop during or just after their use.

Clinical diagnosis

History

By far, the most important aspect of diagnosis is the history. Those patients who wake at night with pain and numbness in the distribution of the median nerve, which is alleviated by various physical actions, such as hanging the hands over the edge of the bed, wringing the hands, placing the hands in water, usually have carpal tunnel syndrome.

Symptoms of pain and numbness or tingling in the palmar aspect of the radial three digits may occur when driving a car or holding a newspaper, book or telephone

for prolonged periods of time. Patients may not be able to describe a precise distribution of discomfort and may include the little finger in their description and the palm of the hand overlying the thenar eminence as being symptomatic. The former is supplied by the ulnar nerve and the latter by the palmar cutaneous branch of the median nerve, which does not pass through the carpal tunnel.

Patients with carpal tunnel syndrome may describe discomfort radiating proximally as far as the shoulder. Clumsiness and the complaint of dropping objects are more often associated with sensory disturbance than motor weakness, but may be a consequence of both. Those who do not present with the above symptoms are much less likely to have carpal tunnel syndrome. Clinical examination and electrophysiological testing are used to confirm the diagnosis. Although carpal tunnel syndrome is usually idiopathic, the examining physician should consider the multiple but less common causes that are described above.

Examination

In severe cases, the patient may be able to precisely map an area of numbness – the radial three digits and radial half of the ring finger on the palmar aspect to perhaps the distal palmar crease proximally and the level of the proximal interphalangeal joint dorsally. The examiner should attempt to differentiate normal and abnormal sensation within the distribution of the median nerve proper and that of the ulnar nerve, the palmar cutaneous branch of the median nerve, the superficial radial nerve and the lateral cutaneous nerve of the forearm.

Both hands should be examined for wasting, particularly within the thenar musculature. Wasting, if present, should be differentiated from combined thenar and finger intrinsic wasting, indicating a first thoracic (T1) nerve root lesion or a combined median and ulnar nerve lesion. Degenerative osteoarthritis of the basal thumb joints may cause thenar wasting, despite normal median nerve function. Generalized wasting may indicate a peripheral neuropathy or systemic condition. Assessment of thumb opposition may confirm a more subtle weakness of muscles innervated by the median nerve in the absence of wasting. Weakness of intrinsic muscles not supplied by the median nerve should alert the physician to an alternative diagnosis.

Various provocative tests aid in the diagnosis of carpal tunnel syndrome. A positive Tinel's sign overlying the median nerve within the carpal tunnel, just proximal or just distal to the carpal tunnel indicates sensitivity of the nerve (Fig. 3.7). However, percussion over the median nerve may elicit paraesthesia within the median nerve distribution in patients without carpal tunnel syndrome and may be negative in those with more advanced compression. Tinel's sign has a sensitivity of 67%. The Phalen test places the wrist in acute flexion and should be performed bilaterally (Fig. 3.8). This is the test performed by Mrs Fotini's general practitioner (GP) (Case 3.1: 1).

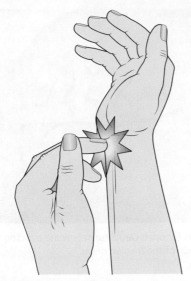

Fig. 3.7 Percussion over the median nerve to elicit Tinel's sign. Tinel's sign is positive when percussion over the nerve elicits a tingling sensation distally.

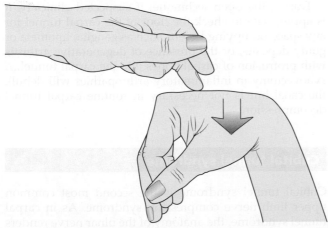

Fig. 3.8 The patient is asked to flex both wrists maximally and keep them flexed for at least 60 s – Phalen's test.

The timing of the development of symptoms is of value, particularly in comparison. Onset of numbness in less than 1 minute is suggestive. Durkan's test involves the examiner pressing over the carpal tunnel and applying pressure for 30 seconds to elicit median nerve paraesthesia.

Investigations

Radiographs of the wrist are usually unhelpful but may demonstrate degenerative arthritis or calcified tumours. The carpal tunnel radiological view is of value in demonstrating the presence of abnormal radiopaque structures within the carpal tunnel. Ultrasound, computed tomography (CT) and magnetic resonance imaging (MRI) examination may be appropriate when space-occupying lesions are suspected. Measurements of the carpal tunnel volume and pressure are rarely indicated.

Case 3.1 **Carpal tunnel syndrome: 3**

Case note: Examination
On examination, diffuse swelling was present around the dorsal aspect of Mrs Fotini's left wrist. Bony swelling (Heberden's nodes) was present in the distal interphalangeal joints. The bases of both thumbs were swollen and the thenar eminence was wasted bilaterally. Sensory testing indicated a constant alteration in touch sensibility in the thumb, index and middle fingers of the left hand, but not elsewhere. The Tinel and Phalen tests were positive bilaterally. Muscle power of the thenar eminence muscles was considered normal in spite of the thenar eminence wasting.

There was no evidence of a generalized lymphoedema in the feet or hands; however, Mrs Fotini was significantly overweight.

It is uncommon for electrophysiological investigations to make a diagnosis of carpal tunnel syndrome in a patient whose history taking and physical examination have not done so. However, it is interesting that as many as 38% of patients presenting with unilateral carpal tunnel syndrome may be asymptomatic on the opposite side but have abnormal nerve conduction tests.

Baseline electrophysiology is still appropriate to distinguish a compressive lesion from a peripheral neuropathy secondary to diseases such as diabetes; to provide objective evidence of a nerve disorder and its site of compression; and to provide comparative figures against which to measure improvement or lack of improvement. In general, distal motor latencies of more than 4.5 ms and distal sensory latencies of more than 3.5 ms are considered abnormal.

Treatment of carpal tunnel syndrome

Conservative therapy

If a reversible cause of carpal tunnel syndrome can be identified, attention must be directed to this. The use of diuretics when fluid retention is present is considered to be an aetiological factor.

Splinting of the wrist is effective, particularly in milder cases with nocturnal symptoms. Placement of the wrist in a neutral position avoids extreme positioning during sleep, preventing the increase in carpal tunnel pressure. It is most effective if applied within 3 months of onset of symptoms. Most pregnant women who develop carpal tunnel syndrome gain relief after giving birth. A corticosteroid injection in combination with local anaesthetic is a reasonable method of treatment in many patients. Its method of action is unclear but it will be effective in any inflammatory conditions through its anti-inflammatory effect, and possibly also from causing atrophy of synovium within the carpal tunnel.

Carpal tunnel syndrome: 4

Case note: Investigations

The symptoms and signs indicated that Mrs Fotini was suffering from bilateral carpal tunnel syndrome and that this was the primary cause of her presenting complaints. However, the presence of possible contributory factors such as diabetes and the association of pins and needles in the hands with neck, wrist and thumb pain and generalized osteoarthritis required further investigation.

The following investigations were therefore requested. X-rays of the cervical spine and hands revealed a generalized degenerative arthritis affecting the cervical spine, particularly the C5/6, C6/7 and C7/T1 intervertebral disc spaces and foraminal spaces. However, there was no significant encroachment of osteophytes or narrowing of the intervertebral foramina. X-rays of the hands revealed osteoarthritis.

Nerve conduction tests revealed a delay in sensory and motor conduction velocities bilaterally, moderate on the left side and mild on the right. There were prolonged motor and sensory latencies bilaterally. Electromyography did not reveal motor axonal degeneration. Normal studies of radial and ulnar nerves and of the common peroneal nerve of the right lower limb ruled out the possibility of a diabetic neuropathy.

Tests of serum iron and ferritin levels, performed to rule out haemochromatosis, were normal. This condition is characterized by excessive deposits of iron in the body and is associated with liver insufficiency and degenerative arthritis affecting the metacarpophalangeal joints of index and middle fingers, in combination with skin pigmentation and diabetes.

Following the above investigations, the hand surgeon was able to inform Mrs Fotini that there was clinical and electrophysiological evidence of bilateral carpal tunnel syndrome. The neck stiffness and shoulder discomfort were probably consequent upon the cervical spondylosis (degenerative arthritis). It is interesting that bilateral thenar eminence wasting was present. However, motor power was retained, and therefore this wasting was apparent rather than real and consequent upon the carpometacarpal joint degenerative arthritis.

Surgery

In patients unresponsive to the above measures, the mainstay of treatment is surgery. The indications for this are symptoms that interfere with sleep and activities, clumsiness associated with numbness and weakness and the prevention of progressive axonal degeneration.

Carpal tunnel surgery can be open or endoscopic. Endoscopic surgery through one or two small incisions rather than a longitudinal incision over the carpal tunnel (Fig. 3.9) is associated with less postoperative discomfort and a more rapid return to manual work, but the long

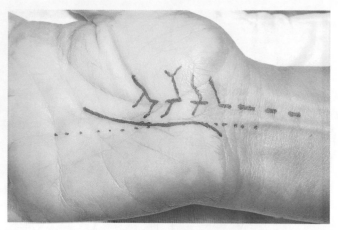

Fig. 3.9 Incision for open carpal tunnel release avoiding the palmar cutaneous branch of the median nerve.

term results are the same. One disadvantage of endoscopic carpal tunnel release is the inability to assess the anatomy of the carpal tunnel and to visualize effectively the nerve itself.

During the open technique, if suspected clinically, it is appropriate to check the floor of the carpal tunnel for any space-occupying lesions such as ganglia, lipomata or gouty deposits, or the presence of degenerative arthritis with protrusion of carpal bones into the carpal tunnel. A synovectomy in inflammatory arthropathies will debulk the canal but is not necessary in routine carpal tunnel decompression.

Cubital tunnel syndrome

Cubital tunnel syndrome is the second most common upper limb nerve compression syndrome. As in carpal tunnel syndrome, the anatomy of the ulnar nerve renders it susceptible to pressure and injury. Pain and dysfunction can be significant.

Anatomy of the cubital tunnel

The ulnar nerve is the main branch of the medial cord of the brachial plexus, arising from the C8 and T1 nerve roots. The nerve reaches the elbow lying behind the medial epicondyle and enters the forearm through the cubital tunnel (Fig. 3.10). The cubital tunnel is formed by the tendinous arch joining the humeral and ulnar heads of attachment of flexor carpi ulnaris. The ulnar nerve branches in Guyon's canal at the wrist into superficial and deep branches, the former predominantly providing sensory fibres to the ulnar one and one-half digits and the latter providing motor fibres to the intrinsic muscles of the fingers, adductor pollicis, and often part of flexor pollicis brevis. In the forearm, the nerve supplies motor fibres to flexor carpi ulnaris and flexor digitorum profundus of the ring and little finger.

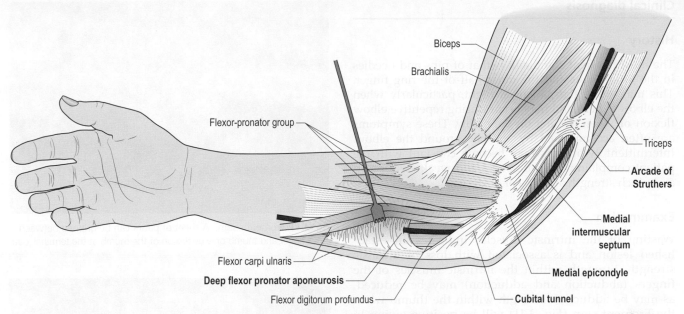

Fig. 3.10 Five sites of compression of the ulnar nerve about the elbow (seen in bold).

Pathophysiology and causes

There are five common sites of ulnar nerve compression (Fig. 3.10), but there may be no obvious reason for compression at any of these five sites (idiopathic). However, direct injury, external compression, space-occupying lesions, degenerative or inflammatory arthritis, a valgus-flexion deformity of the elbow or systemic diseases such as diabetes, chronic alcoholism or renal failure may render the nerve at risk.

Normally, the ulnar nerve is subject to compression, traction and friction. Pathology about the elbow may affect the nerve by limiting its excursion, increasing its required excursion and destabilizing or constricting it.

Dynamic irritation of the nerve occurs during repetitive elbow flexion and extension as the nerve is compressed by the medial epicondyle. During flexion of the elbow, the cross-sectional geometry of the cubital tunnel alters from a circular configuration to a flattened and triangular configuration, decreasing the volume of the tunnel by 55% and increasing intraneural pressure. Contracture of the flexor carpi ulnaris may further increase the pressure and if extraneural fibrosis is present, usually secondary to external trauma, excursion of the nerve will be limited, leading to compression associated with stretching of the tendon. Anterior subluxation (partial dislocation) over the medial epicondyle during flexion may injure the nerve. This is a normal finding in a small percentage of the population (16.2%) without symptoms; however, chronic changes can occur within the nerve secondary to trauma from repetitive subluxation. Alterations in pressure, resultant ischaemia, oedema and fibrosis lead to ulnar nerve symptoms and signs.

> ### Case 3.1 — Carpal tunnel syndrome: 5
>
> #### Case note: Management
>
> The surgeon advised Mrs Fotini to consider surgical decompression of her left carpal tunnel. In view of the moderately severe pressure in the left wrist, it was thought unwise to consider non-surgical management for fear of possible axonal degeneration if the pressure were not removed from the median nerve. However, the surgeon considered that surgery to decompress the right median nerve was not necessary as the symptoms and electrophysiological change were mild.
>
> The surgeon advised Mrs Fotini that her night symptoms should be relieved by surgery, but that the neck pain and stiffness would not respond and that the discomfort she had at the base of both thumbs and within the small joints of the hand would continue, because they were associated with her degenerative arthritis.
>
> The surgeon requested Mrs Fotini to stop taking aspirin 12 days prior to surgery and to discontinue her non-steroidal anti-inflammatory medication 2 days prior to surgery to prevent the possibility of postoperative bleeding.

A valgus deformity of the elbow may be a normal variant or secondary to previous injury around the elbow, particularly in childhood with growth deformation. Osteoarthritis may result in a flexion deformity. Furthermore, osteophytes may intrude into the cubital tunnel.

Failure to protect the elbow during surgery, in a comatose patient or in those confined to bed, may result in irritation of the ulnar nerve because of either a persistent flexion position or external pressure.

Clinical diagnosis

History

The most frequent complaint is that of pins and needles in the little finger and the ulnar half of the ring finger. This may wake the patient at night, particularly when the elbow is bent and may occur during repetitive elbow flexion or when leaning on the elbow. These symptoms are often accompanied by an ache around the elbow. Intermittent symptoms may become constant with the patient complaining of numbness and weakness of grip and pinch strength and loss of dexterity.

Examination

Wasting of the intrinsic muscles indicates an established lesion and is associated with loss of intrinsic strength. Strength within the intrinsic muscles of the fingers (abduction and adduction) may be reduced, as may be adduction strength within the thumb when the Froment sign (Fig. 3.11) will be positive owing to diminished strength in adductor pollicis and the first dorsal interosseous. During an attempt to maintain adduction of the thumb against the index finger, flexor pollicis longus flexes the interphalangeal joint to compensate for loss of power in these two muscles. Intrinsic weakness may be accompanied by diminished power in flexor digitorum profundus to the little finger and perhaps the ring finger. Loss of intrinsic finger function causes clawing of the ring and little fingers because the primary metacarpophalangeal joint flexors are absent (Fig. 3.12).

In those with constant sensory symptoms, it will be possible to demonstrate altered sensibility in the ulnar one and one-half digits supplied by the digital nerves proper, and the dorsal branch of the ulnar nerve will be affected, with alteration in sensation over the dorsal ulnar aspect of the hand and fingers. Persistent dorsal sensation and loss of little and ring finger sensation suggests a more distal compression at the wrist.

The nerve is often tender at the elbow and there may be evidence of flicking (subluxation) of the nerve over the medial epicondyle during flexion. The Tinel sign is positive when the ulnar nerve is percussed at the site of compression. Maintaining both elbows in the flexed position for up to 3 minutes is equivalent to the Phalen test for carpal tunnel syndrome and may reproduce symptoms.

The symptoms and signs of cubital tunnel syndrome must be differentiated from those accompanying cervical disc disease, thoracic outlet syndrome and compression of the ulnar nerve at the wrist. Cervical disc disease affecting the C8 and/or T1 nerve roots will usually present with a sensory deficit in a dermatomal distribution, weakness in the intrinsic muscles innervated by the median nerve, as well as in muscles innervated by the ulnar nerve, neck discomfort and restriction of motion.

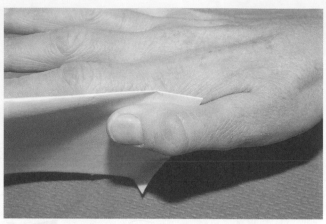

Fig. 3.11 Froment's sign. A sheet of paper can be gripped between index finger and thumb only by flexion of the thumb at the terminal joint.

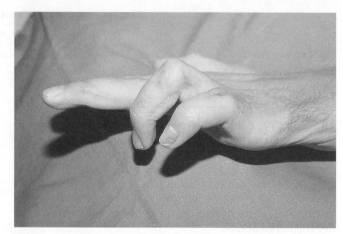

Fig. 3.12 Ulnar claw.

Interesting facts

The commonly used term 'Tinel's sign' is a misnomer. Jules Tinel, a French neurologist, and Paul Hoffmann, a German physiologist, served as physicians for opposing sides during the First World War. Tinel, in 1915, checked the level of nerve damage and progress of nerve healing after gunshot wounds by pressing over the nerve. Hoffmann, in the same year 1915, did so by tapping. So, what is generally described as the Tinel sign should better be described as the Hoffmann–Tinel sign. Phalen's sign was described in the mid-twentieth century by George Phalen, an American orthopaedic surgeon at the Cleveland Clinic.

Investigations

Electrodiagnostic studies should be performed in an attempt to provide objective evidence of nerve compression at the elbow and to rule out more proximal or distal lesions. However, normal electrodiagnostic studies do not exclude a diagnosis of cubital tunnel syndrome, nor prevent consideration of surgery, as neurophysiologically normal patients with a clinical diagnosis of nerve compression have still been shown to improve after surgery.

Radiological examination will indicate the presence of degenerative changes. A cubital tunnel projection provides good imaging of the cross-section of the tunnel. Ultrasonography is helpful in delineating nerve swelling and significant areas of constriction, as also is nuclear magnetic resonance imaging.

Treatment

Splinting appears to be effective in patients with mild to moderate symptoms and signs. The splint aims at preventing repetitive flexion of the elbow and resting the nerve in an optimal position, preventing friction, tension or compression, maintaining the elbow at 30 degrees of flexion from the fully extended position. The splint should be worn at night and as often as possible during the day for a period of 4 weeks. The patient should avoid leaning on the elbow. Aggravating factors such as repetitive elbow flexion are avoided. Modification of the work environment may be necessary.

Most would consider that those with severe signs and symptoms, those with electrodiagnostic evidence of nerve damage and those who fail to respond to non-surgical methods should undergo operative treatment to prevent long-term nerve damage and dysfunction. Many surgical procedures have been described. The least invasive is a simple decompression of the ulnar nerve within the cubital tunnel.

Tarsal tunnel syndrome

The tibial nerve can become compressed behind the medial malleolus at the ankle. A flexor retinaculum also known as the laciniate ligament passes from the malleolus to the medial and upper calcaneus and distally to the navicular. This structure holds in place the tendons of tibialis posterior, flexor hallucis longus and flexor digitorum longus. The space deep to the retinaculum is the tarsal tunnel, which also contains the tibial nerve and posterior tibial artery.

As with other compression neuropathies, the nerve can be compressed in this location by a space-occupying lesion, a nearby fracture (e.g. of the calcaneus) or the compression can be idiopathic.

Clinically, the patient will complain of pain on the plantar aspect of the foot. There may be paraesthesia in the distribution of the branches of the tibial nerve but not always and the syndrome must be distinguished from plantar fasciitis as a cause of pain. Tarsal tunnel syndrome can have a positive Tinel sign and tenderness along the path of the nerve. Nerve conduction study and EMG studies can be helpful but are often negative. There is some evidence to support calf stretching and tibialis posterior strengthening as a conservative therapy for tarsal tunnel syndrome. For persistent cases surgery is indicated to release the retinaculum and decompress the nerve.

Meralgia paraesthetica

Compression of the lateral femoral cutaneous nerve (LFCN) will result in pain and dysaesthesia in the anteromedial thigh. The name is derived from the Greek *meros* (thigh) and *algos* (pain). The LFCN arises from the L1, L2 and L3 nerve roots and emerges laterally from the psoas muscle. It then passes retroperitoneally to the anterior superior iliac spine (ASIS). It then enters the thigh by passing variably below, through, or above the inguinal ligament and it is here that the nerve most commonly becomes compressed.

Meralgia Paraesthetica can be classified as either spontaneous or iatrogenic. Spontaneous cases can be related to pregnancy, ill-fitting clothing or pelvic masses. Metabolic conditions including diabetes mellitus and alcoholism are also related. Iatrogenic causes are any surgery in the area of the lateral inguinal ligament or procedures requiring lengthy positioning that compresses the nerve, especially external rotation of the hip.

Patients will typically have a characteristic distribution of sensory symptoms and a positive Tinel sign 1 cm medial to the ASIS. Electrodiagnostic testing can help in the diagnosis as can a local anaesthetic block that relieves the symptoms.

Nonoperative management consists of addressing underlying causes. Weight gain should be addressed, tight clothing avoided, non-steroidal anti-inflammatories can alleviate an inflammatory cause of compression. In persistent cases, surgical decompression of the nerve, including release of the compressing part of the inguinal ligament has a high rate of success in relieving symptoms.

Further reading

Hilburn, J.W., 1996. General principles and use of electrodiagnostic studies in carpal and cubital tunnel syndrome: with special attention to pitfalls and interpretation. Hand Clinics 12 (2), 205–221.

Louis, D.S., Calkins, E.R., & Harris, P.G., 1996. Carpal tunnel syndrome in the work place. Hand Clinics 12 (2), 305–308.

Lundborg, G., 1988. Nerve Injury and Repair. Edinburgh: Churchill Livingstone.

Phalen, G.S., 1966. The carpal-tunnel syndrome: seventeen years' experience in diagnosis and treatment of six hundred and fifty-four hands. Journal of Bone and Joint Surgery 48A (2), 211–228.

Seddon, H., 1943. Three types of nerve injury. Brain 66, 237–288.

Stevens, J.C., Sun, S., Beard, C.M., et al., 1988. Carpal tunnel syndrome in Rochester, Minnesota, 1961 to 1980. Neurology 38 (1), 134–138.

Sunderland, S., 1951. A classification of peripheral nerve injuries producing loss of function. Brain 74, 491–516.

Tetro, A.M., Pichora, D.R., 1996. Cubital tunnel syndrome and the painful upper extremity. Hand Clinics 12 (4), 665–677.

von Schroeder, H.P., Botte, M.J. (1996). Carpal tunnel syndrome. Hand Clinics 12 (4), 643–655.

LOWER BACK PAIN

4

Christopher Needs and Manuela Ferreira

Chapter objectives

After studying this chapter, you should be able to:

1. Understand the normal anatomy and biomechanical function of the lumbar spine.

2. Impart an assessment method for patients presenting with acute low back pain that includes an evaluation for possible serious spinal disorders ('red flags').

3. Recall the natural history of low back pain syndromes.

4. Understand which low back pain syndromes relate to specific spinal morphological changes, such as radicular pain and which pain syndromes are not associated with specific spinal pathology.

5. Appreciate and assess the relevance of psychosocial factors ('yellow flags') to the prognosis of acute low back pain.

6. Describe the general principles of management of acute and chronic low back pain.

Introduction

Back pain is a universal human experience and represents a significant burden of illness in the community because of its frequency, poor recovery rates and its propensity among people aged 20–50 years, thus exacting economic and physical consequences.

Low back pain (LBP) is a syndrome not a disease. LBP cannot always be attributed to specific anatomical structures and locations, as such there is poor correlation between LBP symptoms and changes demonstrated on spinal imaging. There are a series of influences that contribute to LBP and its associated disability that include genetic, biophysical and psychosocial factors in addition to co-morbidities from other diseases. As well, there is variability in the prevalence of LBP-related disability between countries due to differences in health care systems, expected social behaviours and the various legal contexts within which LBP occurs.

The overwhelming majority of LBP is due to unspecified musculoskeletal causes, referred to as non-specific LBP or sometimes called mechanical LBP. Importantly, LBP may be the presenting symptom of a number of serious medical conditions. It is vital to have a consistent evidenced-based approach to the assessment of LBP such that serious conditions are excluded and psychosocial factors in the patient's environment that may be impediments to recovery are identified.

Normal lumbar spine anatomy

Vertebrae and sacrum

There are five lumbar vertebrae, numbered from proximal to distal. The vertebrae have a triple joint complex comprised of two zygapophyseal (ZA) joints, and the fibrocartilaginous intervertebral disc. They are articulated above and below such that each lumbar segment contributes to the summation of lumbar spinal movement. Traditionally, each vertebra is divided into its anterior and posterior elements, which are joined by the vertebral pedicles. The anterior element, or vertebral body, is a kidney-shaped prism of bone, with superior concavity directed posteriorly and flat superior and inferior surfaces called endplates (Fig. 4.1). A small rim of bone makes up the outer margin of these surfaces which is where the outer part of the intervertebral disc attaches.

The pedicles are thick projections that originate nearer the superior part of the vertebral body at the posterolateral corners. The posterior elements are those structures that lie behind the pedicles. Viewed from above, posterior elements, pedicles and the posterior sweep of the vertebral body form a protective ring that encloses the central vertebral canal contents. The vertebral canal is occupied by the spinal cord above L1/2 level and the spinal nerve roots (cauda equina) below this. The posterior components of the vertebral canal are comprised of the vertebral lamina with the pedicles connecting the lamina to the vertebral body. A bony plate oriented in the sagittal plane develops from the fusion of the laminae and is known as the spinous process.

Arising superiorly from the junction of each pedicle and its lamina, are the two superior articular processes. These present a relatively smooth curved surface posteriorly. From the lower corner of each lamina, there are matching inferior articular processes, whose smooth curved surface is presented anteriorly. Together, these processes make up the posterior intervertebral joint between adjacent vertebrae (Fig. 4.2). Arising from the side of the lateral aspects of the pedicles are the transverse processes (see Fig. 4.1).

The nerve roots exit the vertebral canal through the intervertebral foramen bounded by the vertebral body and disc anteriorly and the ZA joint posteriorly and the pedicle below. Prior to leaving the vertebral canal the nerve root marginalizes laterally at the level above its exit canal.

The sacrum is a triangular bone at the base of the spine, providing both the base of the spine and uniting the pelvic ring. Its superior components are a flat kidney-shaped surface to match the L5 vertebral body and a superior articular process on each side to form the L5/S1 ZA joints. The vertebral canal continues into the sacrum, allowing passage of the sacral nerve roots through the bone before they exit through the sacral foramina (Fig. 4.3).

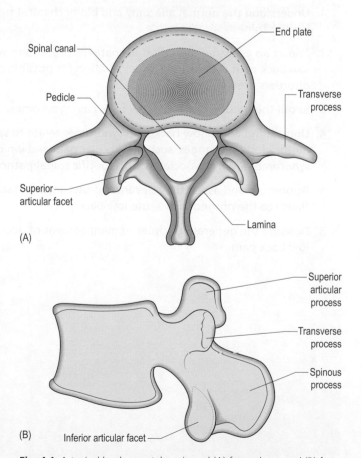

Fig. 4.1 A typical lumbar vertebra viewed (A) from above and (B) from the side.

Intervertebral discs

Between each pair of lumbar vertebrae, and between L5 and S1, lie the lumbar intervertebral discs. They have three components, an outer ring or annulus fibrosus and a central core, the nucleus pulposus and the cartilaginous disco-vertebral endplates (Fig. 4.4). Like peripheral joint articular cartilage the nucleus pulposus is composed of hydrophilic macromolecules known as aggrecan. This hydrophilic jelly contains up to 80% water due to the hydrostatic forces generated by hyaluronic acid chains of aggrecan units being constrained within a collagen and elastin matrix, thereby endowing the intervertebral disc with its unique biomechanical properties. Aggrecan, in turn, is composed of proteoglycans that are concentrated in the centre of the nucleus where the collagen is more scant. There is no blood supply to the nucleus pulposus in the adult, as well the intact nucleus is not innervated.

The annulus fibrosus comprises alternating layers of obliquely oriented collagen fibres (Fig. 4.5), with the outer layers anchoring to the vertebral bodies above and below. The central concentric layers constrain the nucleus pulposus. The outer one-third of the annulus fibrosus has nerve fibres and endings, so that this part of the disc may be a source of pain production.

The cartilaginous vertebral endplates are less than 1 mm thick separating the nucleus and annulus from the vertebral body. Disruption or calcification of the endplate cartilage is associated with impaired nutrition to the nucleus.

Lumbar zygapophyseal joints (facet joints)

Anatomically, the zygapophysis refers to any of the articular processes of the neural arch of a vertebra and their connection with the vertebrae above and below being the zygapophyseal joints. Recently it has become customary to refer to these joints as facet joints (less commonly apophyseal, or Z-joints). We have elected to refer to them as zygapophyseal (ZA) joints. These synovial joints are formed by the superior articular process of the lower vertebra and the inferior articular process of the upper vertebra (see Fig. 4.2).

Due to its morphology, the lumbar ZA joint allows for a restricted range of movement. The curved, opposing surfaces limit rotation and anteroposterior translation of adjacent vertebrae. However, gliding of the

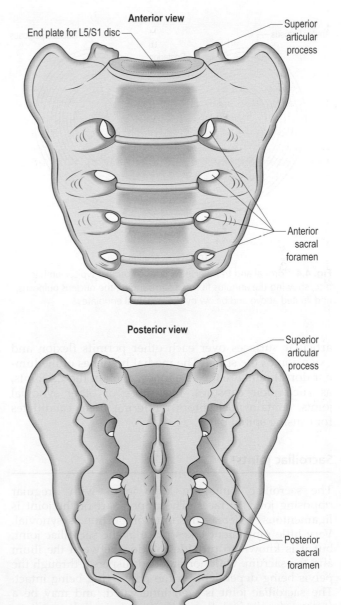

Fig. 4.3 Anterior and posterior views of the sacrum.

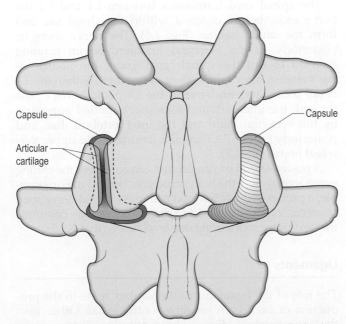

Fig. 4.2 Posterior view of two adjacent vertebrae showing the lumbar zygapophyseal joints. On the left, the capsule is drawn intact. On the right, the posterior capsule has been removed to demonstrate the articular cartilage covering the joint surfaces.

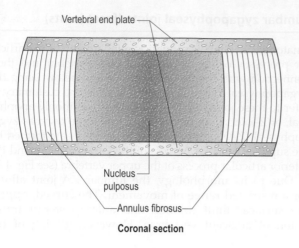

Coronal section

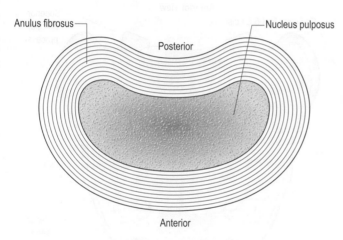

Transverse section

Fig. 4.4 Coronal and transverse sections through a typical lumbar disc, showing the annulus fibrosus surrounding the nucleus pulposus, and limited above and below by the vertebral endplates.

articular surfaces over each other permits flexion and extension of the spine. The medial branches of the lumbar dorsal rami are the sole innervation of the ZA joints, as such their capsules, like those of other synovial joints, contain nociceptors rendering them candidates for causing spinal pain.

Sacroiliac joints

The sacroiliac joints are large joints with irregular opposing joint surfaces. The upper part of the joint is ligamentous, whereas the inferior portion is synovial. Very little movement takes place at the sacroiliac joint, but it is known to provide rotation between the ilium and the sacrum. with normal load dispersal through the pelvis being dependent on the pelvic ring being intact. The sacroiliac joint is well innervated, and may be a source of pain in inflammatory and non-inflammatory conditions.

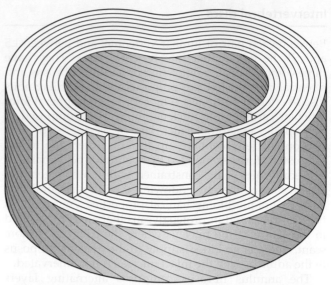

Fig. 4.5 Structure of the annulus fibrosus. The individual collagen fibres are organized into a series of concentric rings. In each ring the fibres are arranged obliquely, at about 25 degrees to the horizontal, with the direction alternating from one ring to the next.

Lumbar nerve roots and spinal cord

Typically, irritation of the lumbar nerve roots causes pain and neurological symptoms and signs in the leg. Pain associated with nerve root compression pain may be manifest as either radicular pain (pain in a lumbar dermatomal distribution) or radiculopathy (dermatomal pain accompanied by loss of neurological function of the involved lumbar nerve root)

The spinal cord terminates between L1 and L2 the nerve roots below descend within the dural sac and form the cauda equina (Fig. 4.6). The nerve roots lie posteriorly in the vertebral foramen, before running forward to exit the spinal canal under the pedicle of the vertebra after which they are named, either the L4 nerve root enters underneath the L4 pedicle. They pass through the intervertebral foramen, bounded anteriorly by the vertebral body and the intervertebral disc, and posteriorly by the ZA joint and lamina of the upper vertebral body (Fig. 4.7).

A posterolateral prolapsed disc can compress the exiting nerve root against the bony structures behind it. For example, a prolapse at L4/5 would compress the L4 nerve root, however, a more central L4/5 disc prolapse may compress the next nerve root exiting one level below, that is L5.

Ligaments

The role of the ligaments of the lumbar spine in the production of back pain remains controversial. Other than the intervertebral discs, whose annulus fibrosus may be considered a ligament, there are four main ligaments that link adjacent vertebrae (Fig. 4.8). The anterior longitudinal ligament covers the anterior and intervertebral

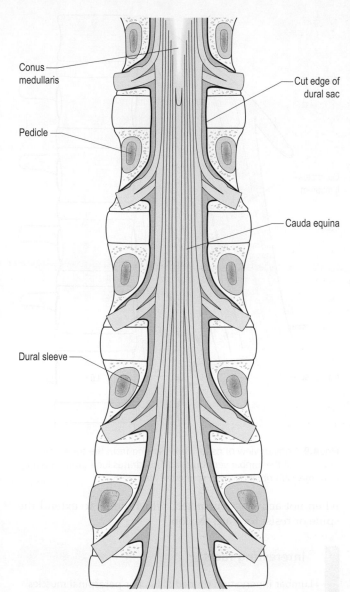

Fig. 4.6 The lumbar nerve roots within the dural sac. The nerve roots arise from the cord and descend within the dural sac, which is drawn out with each root to form the nerve root sheath before the root exits under the pedicles.

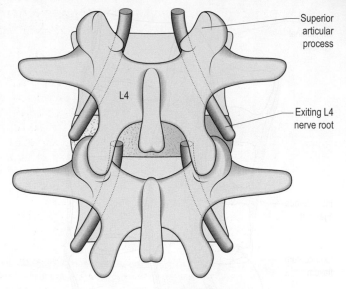

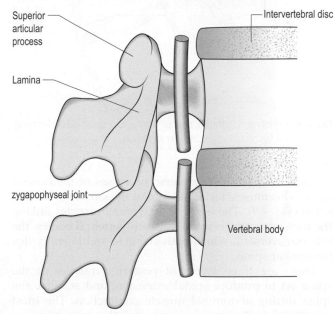

Fig. 4.7 The intervertebral foramen, through which the nerve roots exit the spinal canal. Above, the intact vertebra is viewed from the rear, showing the exiting nerve root crossing the posterolateral corner of the intervertebral disc. Below, the nerve roots are viewed from within the vertebral canal demonstrating the structures surrounding and making up the intervertebral foramen.

discs. The vertical fibres orientation functions to resist separation from adjacent vertebral bodies. The posterior longitudinal ligament runs inside the vertebral foramen functioning to resists separation during spinal flexion. The ligamentum flavum is a series of small ligaments joining the laminae of adjacent vertebrae. Its role is to preserve the shape and smoothness of the vertebral foramen during spinal movements, and prevent compression of the neural structures. The spinal ligaments may be subjected to degenerative change that may result in thickening, loss of elasticity and ossification. Thickening of the ligamentum flavum can contribute to a narrowing of the vertebral foramen in symptomatic lumbar canal stenosis.

Muscles

Flexion and rotation is achieved through contraction of the abdominal muscles, psoas major and quadratus lumborum. The psoas major muscle arises from the transverse processes of the lumbar vertebrae and the lateral margins of the vertebral bodies before inserting into the lesser trochanter of the hip. The psoas may be both a hip and lumbar spinal flexor, depending upon the position of the hip joint. Quadratus lumborum is a broad, flat muscle that attaches to the iliac crest, the inferior margins of

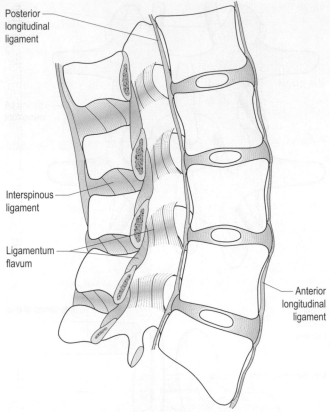

Posterior longitudinal ligament

Interspinous ligament

Ligamentum flavum

Anterior longitudinal ligament

Fig. 4.8 A midline, sagittal section of the lumbar spine demonstrating the principal ligaments. (See text for details.)

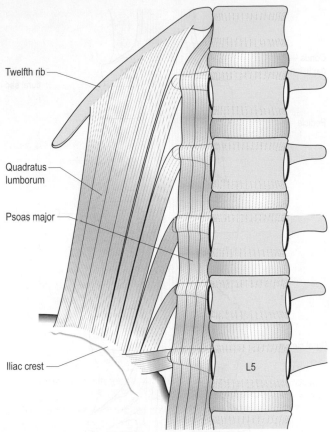

Twelfth rib

Quadratus lumborum

Psoas major

Iliac crest

L5

Fig. 4.9 Anterior view of psoas major, arising from the transverse processes of the lumbar vertebrae, and quadratus lumborum, arising from the 12th rib and inserting into the iliac crest.

the 12th rib and the transverse processes of the lumbar spine. This muscle facilitates lateral flexion of the lumbar spine (Fig. 4.9). There are several small muscles linking the transverse processes of adjacent vertebral bodies, the intertransversarii, which both stabilize and laterally flex the lumbar spine.

There are three layers of posterior muscles of the spine act to produce spinal extension, and stabilize the spine during abdominal muscle contraction. The most superficial of the spinal extensors is the erector spinae. This muscle is complex and made up of several parts. Part of this muscle group acts between the lumbar transverse processes and the iliac crest, part between the thoracic spine and the sacrum, and part from the ribs to the sacrum and iliac crest. Deep to that are the interspinales, connecting the spinous processes of adjacent vertebrae, the intertransversarii mediales, connecting the accessory/mammillary processes of adjacent vertebrae and the multifidus which consists of many distinct fibres with different origins and insertions. The largest parts of the multifidus muscle originate from the spinous processes and course downwards and obliquely to insert into the iliac crest and sacrum. These muscle groups are separated by sheets of fascia. Recent research has suggested that the posterior muscles have very little capacity to rotate the lumbar spine. In combination with the fascial layers, these muscles have passive elastic recoil even

when not actively contracted, which helps to extend the spine or resist forward flexion.

Interesting facts

Lumbar innervation of medial lumbar paraspinal muscles extends across multiple vertebral levels. For example, for a L5/S1 disc herniation causing a single nerve root lesion of the L5 or S1 nerve root, a needle electromyography (EMG) of the medial paraspinal muscles reveals pathological spontaneous activity at one to three vertebral levels cranial to the disc herniation. This is in contrast to single nerve root innervation in the lower limb muscles.

Biomechanics of the lumbar spine

The lumbar spine's primary function is weight bearing while allowing bending and rotations and at the same time distributing compressive loads. This is evidenced by the broad, flat surfaces of the vertebral bodies. Compression forces will raise the pressure in the nucleus pulposus, which will distend and tension the annulus fibrosus. Over 70% of the lumbar load is carried through the intervertebral disc, the remainder via the ZA joint, which increases as the disc height is reduced by degenerative changes.

Approximately 33% of the dynamic compressive load and 35% of the static load are sustained by the ZA joints

Flexion movements between the vertebrae are tolerated through the posterior annulus tightening and the anterior annulus buckling, while the weight continues to be transferred through the nucleus pulposus. The arrangement of the fibres within the annulus fibrosus of alternating obliquely oriented layers means that only half of them can resist rotation in one direction. The other half of the fibres are actually being relaxed during rotation (Fig. 4.10). Therefore, a combination of movements that involve flexion, lifting and rotation places increased load on the annulus rendering it vulnerable to tear and breaching the disc's integrity. The posterior annulus is subjected to greater forces and this is the area of the annulus that will commonly tear and then may lead to nuclear material being extruded from the disc (Fig 4.11).

Epidemiology of low back pain

Incidence and prevalence

LBP is an increasing worldwide problem impacting all nations. It affects all age groups and is associated with sedentary occupations, smoking, obesity and low socioeconomic status. Years lived with disability caused by LBP have increased by more than 50% since 1990. LBP is currently ranked the number one cause of disability in the world, measured as years lived with disability. Although this is a condition that affects all ages, recent studies show both the prevalence and severity of LBP symptoms increase with age. The peak rate of LBP prevalence globally in 2019 was observed at 80–89 years of age. Older people are also more likely to experience poorer outcomes in terms of both pain and disability compared to younger counterparts. LBP is extremely

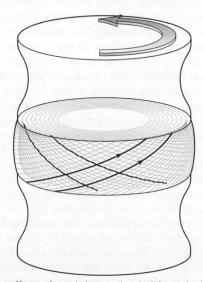

Fig. 4.10 The effects of a twisting motion (axial rotation) on the intervertebral disc. Half of the fibres are being stretched, while the other half are being relaxed.

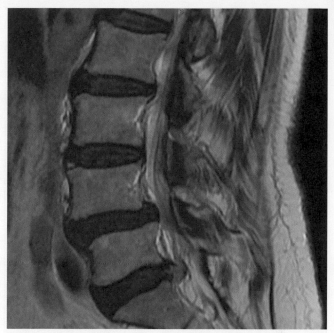

Fig. 4.11 L5 annulus tear with nuclear extrusion.

common. Population data indicate an incidence in the order of 1%–4%. The prevalence of back pain is 5%–10%, with a lifetime prevalence of 80%. In any 1 year, there is a 15%–20% chance that an adult will experience an episode of LBP.

Natural history

The natural history of LBP is best viewed as a condition with varying exacerbations and remissions, with some recovering completely while others have fluctuating pain of low to moderate pain. For those people with an episode of acute low back pain (ALBP), 40% of people will have recovered within a few weeks but 48% may still have pain and disability at 3 months. Patients who are destined to recover tend to do so relatively early. In the case of Mr CK (Case 4.1: 1), these natural history data can be offered as reassurance that his pain is likely to ease, and that movement will not cause harm.

It is well-recognized, however, that although over one-third of patients with an acute episode will recover in the first 9 months, for many, LBP will reoccur. In fact, one in five people who recover from an acute episode of LBP will seek care for a new episode within 12 months.

LBP is frequently associated with depression with rates 2.5 times higher in people with LBP than in those without. One of the most significant recent contributions to the conservative management of ALBP has been the understanding of the impact that psychosocial factors (termed yellow flags) has on prognosis. Yellow flags (Box 4.1) are potential barriers to recovery from ALBP so their early recognition and treatment may avoid ALBP transitioning to chronic back pain when the levels of

Low back pain: 1

Case history

Mr CK is a 54-year-old self-employed green grocer. He has been quite well in the past and rarely sees his local doctor. Three days ago, while lifting a 10-kg box of eggplants, he experienced the sudden onset of pain in his lower back and right gluteal region. He dropped the box and had to lie down. The severe pain settled a little over the next 24 hours but it was still present 3 days later, albeit improving a little each day. He described the pain as a deep-seated dull ache that was worse when he bends forward. When severe, the pain spread into his right buttock and down the back of the right thigh, to his knee, where it has the characteristics of a dull ache. He had been able to sleep with the pain and had kept working a few hours each day, despite the pain. He has not had any lower limb weakness, numbness or tingling in his legs, and has had no change to his bladder or bowel function. He has not had any weight loss, nor any fevers or night sweats.

On examination, he sat uncomfortably in the surgery, wanting to get up and move around. He has minor restriction of forward lumbar flexion but extension of the lumbar spine is restricted by localized back pain. There are no power or reflex losses in his legs, and sensory examination of his lower limbs was normal. The straight leg raise was 80 degrees on each side. The rest of his general physical examination was normal.

This history is important for the relevant negatives as much as for any positive feature. This patient has acute (lasting less than 3 months) low back pain. The history has excluded any 'red flags' and there were no neurological symptoms or signs. The history suggested a mechanical cause, a lifting injury, and there was no historical or examination evidence of any serious disorder or radiculopathy. Therefore, he was classified as having non-specific low back pain..

In practical terms, Mr CK should be asked about any fears, concerns or anxieties that he has about his pain, and be encouraged to resume normal activities as soon as possible.

recovery and the effectiveness of most treatments for acute pain are small. A biopsychosocial model of health, when applied to the assessment and management of LBP, brings together the links between the biological, behavioural, psychological and social factors and how these impact the risk of persistence of pain and disability.

Pain sources from the lumbar spine

Nociceptive neurons from the various lumbar spinal structures demonstrate a high degree of convergence within the nervous system. As a result, pain from lumbar origin tends to be experienced diffusely across the spinal and often into the gluteal region. That is somatically referred away from the pain's origin. Pain may be generated from a degenerative intervertebral disc, ZA

Box 4.1 Yellow flags

1. Belief that pain and activity are harmful
2. 'Sickness behaviours' (e.g. rest is best)
3. Low or negative moods, social withdrawal
4. Treatment that does not fit best practice
5. Problems with workers' compensation or insurance claims
6. History of back pain, time-off work
7. Poor job satisfaction
8. Heavy work, unsociable hours
9. Overprotective family or lack of social support

joint, the dural structures, nerve root or vertebral body but there are no pathognomonic clinical features that allow one to attribute the pain to a specific structure. Likewise, the presence of abnormal radiographic features alone does not implicate such changes to the cause of pain.

Intervertebral disc

Degenerative changes in the intervertebral disc, called lumbar spondylosis, occur with ageing and have genetic, mechanical, traumatic and nutritional factors that may contribute to such changes. Spinal radiographic features of disc degeneration include a reduction in disc height often accompanied by adjacent osteophytosis. The degenerative process involves structural change involving the annulus along with changes in the composition and functionally of nucleus pulposus. Within the annulus, early degenerative changes involve radial fissuring. Later, circumferential fissures develop in the outer annulus which, being innervated, may result in pain. The disruption of the annular layers allows nuclear material to track between and sometimes rupture through the layers of the annulus. Eventually, the movement of nuclear material through the confines of the annulus will cause the disc to fail in its biomechanical mission. The resulting extrusion or protrusion of nuclear material may then cause nerve root compression. Other consequences follow disc failure, including reduction in disc height and osteophyte formation also vertebral body bone marrow oedema may be seen on magnetic resonance imaging (MRI) and referred to as Modic changes. Modic changes refer to subchondral bone marrow oedema on MRI at the disco-vertebral junction and are classified into type 1, type 2 and type 3 based on differing signal on T1 and T2 images. (Box 4.2) A systematic review concluded that Modic type 1 changes may be associated with LBP, however, the true clinical relevance of Modic changes to patient's symptoms and prognosis is currently unclear.

Postmortem studies have also suggested that vascular ingrowth into damaged discs is accompanied by nerve fibre ingrowth, providing a nociceptive path beyond the outer one-third of the disc for a degenerative disc to

Box 4.2 Modic changes on MRI of lumbar spine

Modic type 1 changes
(Low signal in T1-weighted sequences, but high signal in T2-weighted sequences)
Are associated with fissuring of the cartilaginous endplate and increased vascularity within the subchondral bone on histological examination, and corresponding to endplate oedema.

Modic type 2 changes
(High signal in T1-weighted sequences and either high or intermediate signal in T2-weighted sequences)
Reflect fatty replacement of the adjacent marrow.

Modic type 3 changes
(Low signal in T1-weighted sequences and either low signal in T2-weighted sequences)
Are observed in vertebral bodies with sclerotic changes.

cause pain. Consensus opinion regarding the symptoms that may be attributed to disc disease is lacking despite the general acceptance that it may be a source of pain. As well, no characteristic image changes can be anchored down to specific symptom clusters.

Zygapophyseal joints

The lumbar zygapophyseal joints are susceptible to the conditions that might affect other synovial joints, such as inflammatory arthritis and osteoarthritis. Tropism of the ZA joints (difference between the angle of orientation between the right and left ZA joints, that is asymmetry in orientation of the ZA joints) may be factor in their development of osteoarthritis and lumbar canal stenosis.

Due to the increased incidence of ZA, osteoarthritis changes with age, as with the disc, it is not possible to clinically attribute pain to radiographic features. The judicious use of local anaesthetic blocks does, in some cases, allow the clinician to prove pain causation arising from a specific ZA joint.

Interesting facts

Despite ZA joints being synovial joints, it is rare that they are involved in rheumatoid arthritis. Other inflammatory arthropathies such as ankylosing spondylitis and less commonly crystal arthropathies may involve the ZA joints.

Sacroiliac joint

The sacroiliac joint has been shown to be a source of pain in inflammatory spondyloarthropathies or less commonly as a result of a haematogenous borne infection. If the pelvic ring becomes unstable, for example as may occur during pregnancy or in the post-partum period due to symphysis pubis disruption, then the sacroiliac joint may become painful. The pain is usually experienced in the buttocks and posterior thigh.

Other structures

In addition to pain referred to the lumbar region from intra-abdominal and pelvic structures, the lumbar musculature may be a source of traumatic lumbar pain, especially myotendinous junctions. Pathological processes causing pain involving the dura and fascia have been proposed but are difficult to prove or disprove.

Lumbar pain syndromes

Leg pain and disorders of the lumbar spine

There are two mechanisms by which lumbar structures may cause patients to experience leg pain. The first is through somatic referred pain from the spine into the leg, and the second by irritation and/or compression of a lumbar nerve root, that is radicular pain.

Somatic referred pain

Somatic referred pain occurs when pain is perceived in a region topographically displaced from the source of the pain. It is due to convergence of nociceptive stimuli from the spinal structures with neural input from cutaneous dermatomes that are then centrally processed resulting in the spinal pain being experienced from those dermatomal sites. The gluteal region is a common cutaneous site for somatic referral. Somatic referred pain has the characteristics of being dull, deep, aching and is rare that it would cause pain to be felt below the knee. This is the type of pain described by Mr CK.

Radicular pain

Radicular pain occurs because of irritation and/or compression of a nerve root. Such compression may be the result of a disc herniation, bony encroachment within narrow spinal canals (neural foramen, central spinal canal or lateral recess) or from a synovial cyst. This pain is typically lancinating in quality, shooting down the leg like an electric shock. It affects a narrow band and has both deep and cutaneous components. It is often made worse by coughing or sneezing or any activity that raises intradiscal pressure. The pain may be associated with neurological signs, then referred to as a radiculopathy. While back pain is also present, the dominant pain component in lumbar radicular pain is the leg pain.

Radicular pain: 1

Case history

Mr SH is a 40-year-old financial controller who presented with lancinating left leg pain after starting his poorly serviced lawn mower. He was pulling the starter cord when he felt something 'give' in his back. The following day he became aware of a severe, shooting pain down the back of his left leg and into his foot. The outside of his left foot felt tingly and the symptoms were much worse when he strained or sneezed. Lumbar flexion was severely restricted and painful while lumbar extension was less painful as was laterally flexing the lumbar spine to the right. Neurological examination revealed mild weakness of left foot dorsiflexion and loss of sensation over the lateral aspect of his left foot. Straight leg raising on the left side was limited to 30 degrees before the pain was aggravated.

After 4 weeks of treatment with anti-inflammatory medication and supervised exercise, his symptoms had not improved and he was frustrated he was unable to resume work. An MRI scan was performed that revealed a large focal posterolateral disc herniation at the left L4/5 level compressing the left L5 nerve root as it descended to exit below (Fig. 4.12). The L4 nerve root was able to exit the canal just above the prolapsed disc. A CT-guided left L5 perineural injection of soluble corticosteroid was undertaken. This resulted in a significant diminution of his left leg symptoms and normalization of the left foot dorsiflexion weakness. Four days later he had residual left sided lower back pain but was able to resume his work.

This case is a typical story for acute disc prolapse. The lag between the inciting event with the onset of back pain to the development of radicular pain is not uncommon. The natural history is generally favourable. The use of selective CT-guided nerve root sleeve injections have been demonstrated to decrease the need for surgery and hasten recovery.

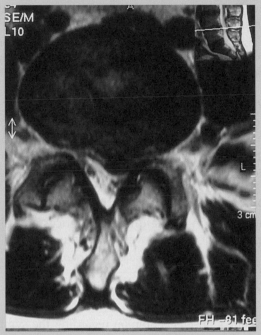

Fig. 4.12 A T2-weighted MRI scan (water appears white) demonstrating a large, left posterolateral disc herniation of the L4/L5 intervertebral disc compressing the descending intervertebral left L5 nerve root and deforming the dural sac. The MRI is reported as being viewed from below. Therefore, the left side of the image represents the right side of the patient. Note the descending sacral nerve roots, which appear as black dots in the white cerebrospinal fluid within the dural sac. The right L5 nerve root is seen as a black dot in the upper right part of the dural sac (left side of the image).

Lumbar radicular pain may also occur without a compressive cause such as in diabetic neuropathy, autoimmune demyelination, viral infections and vaccine-associated neuritis. EMG combined with NCS may be useful in such settings.

Acute versus chronic low back pain

Traditionally, LBP is divided into acute, subacute (6 weeks to 3 months) and chronic LBP. Acute back pain is defined as lasting less than 3 months and will respond to graduated activities and analgesics whereas chronic persists past 3 months with less predictable responses to analgesics and physical therapy. This rather arbitrary division fails to take into account the role psychosocial factors (yellow flags) may play in the overall prognosis. Attention has now focused on the identification and treatment of such factors with the intent of preventing the transition of acute to chronic back symptoms, also bearing in mind that chronic pain is often accompanied by the development of adverse psychological health.

In chronic low back pain (CLP), there is debate regarding the relative continuing contributions from peripheral nociception, which dominate acute pain, in addition to the changes in the central pain processing that occurs from the limbic and cortico-striatal pathways. As such the development of self-sustaining pain may arise following the initial normal activation of nociceptor pathways that later become autonomous and independent from the originating nociceptive event.

As such, a more pragmatic approach to chronic back pain is to identify what are the persisting nociceptive drivers and what are the psychosocial factors that are contributing to the pain. So treatment should be guided by the relative pain contributions from nociceptive drivers and psychosocial factors in each individual, rather than the duration of pain determining the therapy.

Assessment of acute low back pain

After a history and examination, including a lower limb neurological examination, the aim of assessing people

Box 4.3 Red flags

Cauda equina syndrome
History of malignancy
Significant trauma
Systemic symptoms of fever, weight loss
Risk factors for infection, e.g. intravenous drug use
Osteoporosis or history of long-term corticosteroid therapy
Symptoms of an inflammatory spinal arthropathy
Repeat presentations to the emergency department

with ALBP is to be able to triage them into one of three groups. The first priority of the assessment is to consider the possibility that serious disease may be causing the pain, that is to exclude red flags (Box 4.3). The second grouping are those with back and leg pain with or without neurological signs. The third group comprises those people with back pain alone and are referred to as having non-specific back pain. The assessment also will give consideration to back pain originating from non-spinal sources (*see section on back pain from extra-spinal sources*).

In the primary care setting non-specific LBP accounts for 90% of presentations. Non-specific LBP has a good prognosis and spinal imaging does not improve outcomes.

Indeed, unnecessary imaging may trigger a cascade of additional medical care causing avoidable anxiety to the patients involved. In this group, changes seen on spinal imaging can be rarely correlated with the person's symptoms, thus raising the possibility that reading a radiology report could provoke unnecessary fear. Also, patients with stable radicular neurological signs may not require imaging at the initial consultation. Only if improvement is slow or if there is progressive neurological loss would imaging be considered.

A recent emergency department study showed 6.7% of people presenting with ALBP had serious pathology. This fact should not produce complacency but rather a diligent approach to history and examination along with follow up to ensure serious pathology is considered and clinically evaluated. As such, exclusion of serious pathologies is the prime focus of the initial consultation

Positive responses to any of the red flag questions will prompt further assessment and investigations. The presence of possible cauda equina compression is signalled by saddle anaesthesia along with urinary retention and bowel dysfunction (reduced anal sphincter tone is not always present) and must be considered early in the assessment and, if present, requires urgent imaging and a surgical opinion. A previous history of malignancy is the strongest predictor of vertebral malignancy. Infection or osteomyelitis is a less common cause of back pain.

A recent history of intravenous drug use, immunosuppression, recent surgical procedures, intravenous cannula insertion or interventions including spinal injections should raise the suspicion of infection as the cause of pain. The presence of fever or raised inflammatory mark-

ers will lend weight to this consideration. Previous bone infection elsewhere in the body is another risk factor for spinal infection. Vertebral osteomyelitis follows haematogenous spread from an extraosseous source in 40% of patients. Infections of the musculoskeletal system are discussed in more detail in Chapter 11.

Inflammatory arthropathies of the spine include ankylosing spondylitis, psoriatic arthritis, colitis associated spondylarthritis and reactive arthritis. These processes selectively affect the sacroiliac joints. The characteristic history is of insidious onset of LBP associated with marked early morning stiffness lasting for 1 hour. The pain and stiffness is relieved by exercise, but recurs after resting. These conditions are often associated with the presence of the histocompatibility locus antigen (HLA) B27. Other joints outside the spine can be affected and enthesopathy (inflammation where tendons attach to bone) is common. There may also be extra-articular features such as eye inflammation and skin involvement.

Patients on long-term corticosteroids or who are known to have osteoporosis may develop ALBP due to vertebral fracture.

Back pain from extraspinal sources

Pathology arising outside of the spine may present as LBP. Retroperitoneal and pelvic sites of pathology such as pancreatic, renal, aortic dissection, retroperitoneal bleeding and some gynaecological issues may present as LBP. Patients, particularly those over the age of 50 presenting for the first time with LBP and without restrictions in spinal movements, should alert the clinician to the possibility of an extra-spinal cause.

Case 4.3 Malignancy: 1

Case history

SM is a 72-year-old woman who presents with her first episode of low back pain on the background of a previous history of carcinoma of breast 12 years ago treated with a right-sided mastectomy. The pain onset was slow without any traumatic precedent but the pain was now waking her at night. The pain had not improved despite NSAIDs and paracetamol. She has also felt tired and generally unwell. On examination she has pain on all movements of the lumbar spine with palpation of the spinous processes for L2 and L3 being painful. A low T1 signal and hyperintense STIR signal on MRI suggested tumour and soft tissue swelling involving the vertebral body of L2 and spinous and transverse processes of L3. SM had a normocytic normochromic anaemia.

This story is highly suggestive of malignancy as the cause of her low back pain. SM has the 'red flags' of a history of malignancy, weight loss and anaemia. Her pain has failed to improve and wakes her at night, all signifying a red flag condition causing acute low back pain.

Any assessment of the lumbar spine is not complete without an examination of the hip. Although hip pain is classically described as being felt in the groin, some people experience buttock pain from hip disease. Suspected hip joint pain can usually be confirmed by the clinical examination findings of irritability or restricted range of hip movements. The hip–spine syndrome refers to disorder where dual pathologies coexist. Hip irritability with lateral hip pain associated with gluteus medius pain may also accompany long standing lumbar pain.

Treatment of low back pain

Acute low back pain

Patient education

This is vital and should be the foundational to the treatment of LBP. For some patients, the onset of LBP may trigger concerns about having serious disease or the fear that it may threaten their independence, work capacity or long-term mobility. Based upon the natural history and following the above triage approach, reassurance can be given as to the benign and self-limiting nature of acute back pain. Avoid bed rest and encouragement to the patient to pursue normal activities, including work and physical activities should be imparted early in the therapeutic relationship. Encourage being active and staying at work is a proven strategy for the prevention of future disability. The language used within the consultation is vital. Ensure negative, non-evidence-based concepts regarding back pain are avoided. Explanation about the pain followed by a treatment strategy and support until the pain has resolved is needed.

In the sub-acute phase (i.e. 6 weeks to 3 months), a long consultation with a medical clinician has been shown to decrease by 50% the rate of work disability over a control group of 'usual treatment with no additional consultation' at both 12 months and 5 years.

Exercise

Systematic reviews of the literature have shown that rest, beyond reducing a specific inciting or aggravating factor, does not lead to improvement but rather is likely to prolong the recovery from an episode of LBP. It is recommended that exercise programs should take into account each person current situation and capabilities for the exercise prescribed. But generally progressive addition of exercise as improvements occurs produces the best outcomes.

Case 4.1 — Low back pain: 2

Case note: Management

Mr CK was most worried about his back, and he was asked to complete a STarTBack questionnaire (see suggested reading). This disclosed that he thought his pain would never get better, and also that he had worrying thoughts as since his injury he had stopped enjoying all the things he usually enjoyed. These worries were discussed with his physiotherapist and he gradually became aware that his movements were improving and were no longer painful. He had 10 days of naproxen (500 mg twice daily) with orphenadrine (100 mg twice a day) for 3 days at the beginning of his treatment. Over 4 weeks his pain settled to a dull background ache, and he returned to full time work, taking care to avoid lifting and twisting simultaneously.

Pharmacological treatments

The use of simple analgesics such as paracetamol/acetaminophen is a safe initial option, although a recent study has shed doubt on the efficacy of paracetamol in ALBP. However, confirmatory studies are awaited before this recommendation is changed. Non-steroidal anti-inflammatory drugs (NSAIDs) can be used for pain relief, although they offer small benefits. The limiting factor for their use is gastrointestinal adverse effects such as gastritis, ulceration and bleeding and impaired renal function, discussed in Chapter 1. Skeletal muscle relaxants have also been shown to have short-term benefit. Diazepam has not been shown to be effective. The use of pregabalin for radicular pain was not effective in a recent study. Opiates should be used prudently for short periods of time with the minimum dose required and review of opiate efficacy is needed every 5 days. Adverse events associated with opiates can be serious and should also be monitored.

All patients should be reassessed and reviewed until resolution of their symptoms. If improvement is slow and you are concerned that yellow flag issues may be barriers to recovery, then the use of Orebro or STarT Back Questionnaires are able to be used to identify such obstacles. In such cases, the use of cognitive behavioural approaches is required.

Intra-spinal injections

A recent Cochrane systematic review concluded that lumbar epidural corticosteroid injections slightly reduce pain and disability at the short-term, in people with radicular pain. Whether computed tomography (CT)-guided perineural injections have an advantage over inter laminar epidural injections has not yet been determined. There is no evidence that ZA joint injections give long-term benefit.

Non-pharmacological therapies

Manipulation

This may be considered a second line option and with potential short-term benefit for ALBP. It is not suggested for long-term therapy.

Acupuncture

There is moderate strength of evidence to support the short-term benefits of acupuncture in ALBP and some short-term reduction in the pain intensity of CLP.

Mindfulness

Moderate effects have been shown with mindfulness and with multi-disciplinary rehabilitation programs

Interesting facts

Patients with nerve root compression will often have both back pain as well as leg pain. When patients are considering spinal surgery, they should be aware that only the leg pain will be improved with a decompressive procedure.

Chronic low back pain

When assessing a patient with CLP for the first time the focus should be on identifying nociceptive factors, including possible red flags, and establishing any psychosocial factors that may delay recovery.

Treatments

Education, weight loss and exercise still form the foundational treatment for all low back pain. Systematic reviews of the empirical treatment of CLP attest to the efficacy of intensive, inpatient structured exercise programmes with behavioural elements. Movement towards a self-management program has rendered better long-term results. The use of cognitive behavioural techniques, often in the setting of multidisciplinary pain clinics, has been shown to help certain parameters such as the behavioural expression of pain and specific coping skills. As such, the use of passive physical modalities is ineffective.

The use of NSAIDs for short periods of time can be helpful but avoidance of constant long-term use is best avoided. Opiates should be avoided in chronic non-cancer pain. The use of tricyclic antidepressants or selective serotonin reuptake inhibitors may help when there is superimposed depression and are sometimes used to treat sleep disturbances.

Combinations of cognitive behavioural therapy-infused exercise program within a multi-disciplinary setting have shown greater benefit than a purely pharmacological approach. The American College of Physicians have published guidelines and there are also National Institute for Clinical Excellence (NICE) guidelines.

Target-specific treatments

Those people with CLP represent a heterogeneous group with pathologies ranging from those with pain that is driven by central sensitization factors to those who have severe degenerative changes with chronic radicular pain such as occurs in spinal canal stenosis.

Target-specific treatments are those which are directed against pain arising from specific structures. If a painful lumbar zygapophyseal joint is identified, radiofrequency denervation can provide pain relief, typically for around 12 months. As in ALBP, perineural injections are of limited benefit for demonstrated root compression which is often bony hypertrophy-induced compression in the older patient compared to disc herniation as the cause in the younger patient.

Surgery

In the context of non-red flag spinal conditions, two spinal surgery options are available: spinal decompression and spinal fusion. Spinal decompression may be achieved by performing a laminectomy/laminotomy (removal of part of the laminae) or discectomy or sometimes a combination of both. This is indicated in cases of nerve root compression from herniated disc or from canal stenosis where non-operative measures have not eased pain or where there is progressive loss of neurological function. There is conflicting evidence supporting the effectiveness of decompression surgery compared to non-surgical treatments.

Spinal fusion is a procedure to permanently join two or more vertebrae in order to prevent movement between those structures. The commonly used indication is in the context of degenerative lumbar disc disease is to treat symptomatic spinal instabilities. The role of fusion in treating CLP is not established. There is evidence that undertaking spinal fusion in addition to decompression for the treatment of lumbar canal stenosis offers no benefit compared to decompression alone.

Acknowledgements

Les Barnsley, BMed (Hons), Grad Dip Epi, PhD, FRACP, FAFRM (RACP), Associate Professor, Department of Medicine, Sydney Medical School, Head of Department of Rheumatology, Concord Hospital, Sydney, Australia

Further reading

Bogduk, N. 2005. Clinical Anatomy of the Lumbar Spine and Sacrum, (fourth ed. Churchill Livingstone, Melbourne.

Clark, S., Horton, R., 2018. Low back pain: a major global challenge. The Lancet 391, 2302.

Foster, N.E., Anema, J.R., Cherkin, D., et al, 2018. Prevention and treatment of low back pain: evidence, challenges, and promising directions. The Lancet 391, 2368–2383.

Hartvigsen, J., Hancock, M.J., Kongsted, A., et al., 2018. What low back pain is and why we need to pay attention. The Lancet 391, 2356–2367.

Hill, J.C., Fritz, J.M., 2011. Psychosocial influences on low back pain, disability, and response to treatment. Physical Therapy 91, 712–721.

Qaseem, A., Wilt, T.J., McLean, R.M., Forciea, M.A., 2017. Noninvasive treatments for acute, subacute, and chronic low back pain: a clinical practice guideline from the American College of Physicians. Annals of Internal Medicine 166, 514–530. https://startback.hfac.keele.ac.uk/.

BONE STRUCTURE AND FUNCTION IN NORMAL AND DISEASE STATES

5

Chapter objectives

After studying this chapter, you should be able to:

1. Understand normal bone structure, function and biology including bone remodelling and the different hormones that affect calcium metabolism.

2. Appreciate the aetiopathogenesis of the most common metabolic bone diseases.

3. Understand the epidemiology of osteoporosis and its clinical importance.

4. Assess the risk factors commonly associated with osteoporosis.

5. Describe the essential anatomy of the hip joint relevant to femoral neck fractures and some other common diseases affecting the hip.

6. Understand the general principles of management of osteoporosis.

7. Understand the general principles of surgical treatment of hip fractures and their complications.

Lyn March, Roderick Clifton-Bligh and Andrew Ellis

This chapter is dedicated to our colleague and friend Professor Phillip Sambrook.

Introduction

The principal functions of the skeleton are mechanical support, maintenance of calcium and mineral homeostasis and haematopoiesis in the bone marrow. These can be disturbed in a variety of conditions encompassed by the general term, metabolic bone disease. Osteoporosis, characterized by low bone mineral density (BMD) is the commonest metabolic bone disease. In 2019, the global burden of disease (GBD) estimates identified that 25% and 7% of DALYs (disability adjusted life years) for falls and road injuries, respectively, could be attributed to the risk factor low BMD. It is an important public health problem in all developed countries and is becoming one in most developing countries. Osteoporosis means skeletal fragility leading to an increased risk of fracture. Hip fractures are the most important type of osteoporotic fracture, both in terms of direct health costs and social effects on the patient. Men and women aged 60 years and over who sustain an osteoporotic fracture, including hip, vertebral, humeral and pelvic fractures, have significant deterioration in quality of life and independence and increased risk of dying over the next 5 years when compared with other men and women of similar age (Chen et al., 2018). In Western countries, up to one in two women and one in three men will sustain an osteoporotic fracture during their lifetime. The direct annual cost of treating osteoporotic fractures is reported to be as high as USD 6500 billion in Canada, Europe and the USA alone (Kemmak et al., 2020). The indirect costs related to the disability and productivity loss that can follow for many have not been included so total costs are even greater. Prolonged loss of quality of life has been highlighted globally and in Australia where additional costs of almost USD 3 billion are reported (Tatangelo et al., 2019). Early diagnosis is now possible using precise methods such as bone density measurement.

This chapter will review normal bone structure and function as well as the major metabolic bone diseases. Since this topic will be illustrated by a case in which an osteoporotic hip fracture has occurred, the key anatomy of the hip joint will also be reviewed.

Normal skeletal structure and function

Bones are extremely dense connective tissue that, in various shapes, constitute the skeleton. Although one of the hardest structures in the body, the bone maintains a degree of elasticity owing to its structure and composition. Bone is enclosed, except where it is coated with articular cartilage within a joint, in a fibrous outer membrane called the periosteum. Periosteum is composed of two layers, an outer fibrous layer and a deeper elastic layer containing osteoblasts that are capable of proliferating rapidly when a fracture occurs, as will be discussed further in Chapter 10. In the interior of the long bones is a cylindrical cavity (called the medullary cavity) filled with bone marrow and lined with a membrane composed of highly vascular tissue called the endosteum.

Case 5.1   Osteoporosis: 1

Case history

Mrs Jones, a 74-year-old woman living independently in the community, has suffered several recent falls. Today, while out walking, she fell backwards onto her left hip. Her general practitioner (GP) has been treating her for cardiac failure, obstructive airways disease, intermittent low back pain and gastro-oesophageal reflux. Because of the back pain, she has been sleeping poorly, and her GP recently started her on a sedative, to be taken before retiring to bed. On admission to hospital, it is found she is taking 10 different medications. Mrs Jones is uncertain of what these were all for but is able to remember that she is on 'fluid tablets for her heart', 'a cortisone puffer for her lungs' and 'an anti-inflammatory for her back pain'. Her past medical history reveals several risk factors for osteoporosis. These include an early menopause at the age of 44, a family history of osteoporosis with her mother sustaining a hip fracture in her 80s, smoking and poor nutrition.

On examination in hospital, her left leg is noted to be shortened and externally rotated. Mrs Jones is also tender over the lateral aspect of the right hip but without bruising there. X-rays reveal a fracture through the neck of her left femur (Fig. 5.1).

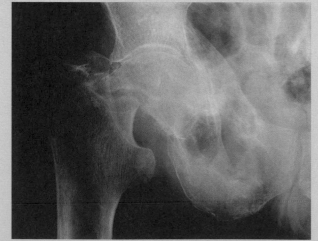

Fig. 5.1 X-ray showing fracture of left femoral neck.

We can see from the details of this case that Mrs Jones has suffered a hip fracture due to osteoporosis. In deciding what investigations are appropriate and how best to manage her, an understanding of calcium metabolism and bone structure and function is necessary.

Types of bone: cortical and cancellous

There are two types of bone: (1) compact or cortical bone and (2) trabecular or cancellous bone. Cortical bone is found principally in the shafts (diaphysis) of long bones. It consists of a number of irregularly spaced overlapping cylindrical units termed Haversian systems. Each consists of a central Haversian canal surrounded by concentric lamellae of bony tissue (Fig. 5.2A). Trabecular bone is found principally at the ends of long bones, and in vertebral bodies and flat bones. It is composed of a meshwork of trabeculae within which are intercommunicating spaces (Fig. 5.2B).

The skeleton consists of approximately 80% cortical bone, largely in peripheral bones, and 20% trabecular bone, mainly in the axial skeleton. These amounts vary according to site and relate to the need for mechanical support. While trabecular bone accounts for the minority of total skeletal tissue, it is the site of greater bone turnover because of its different structure and because its total surface area is greater than that of cortical bone.

Blood supply of bone

Bones are generally richly supplied with blood, via periosteal vessels, vessels that enter close to the articular surfaces and nutrient arteries passing obliquely through the cortex before dividing into longitudinally directed branches. Loss of the arterial supply to parts of a bone can result in death of bone tissue, usually called avascular necrosis or osteonecrosis. Certain bones in the body are prone to this complication, usually after injury, including the head of the femur (discussed later in this chapter), the scaphoid bone in the wrist, the navicular in the foot and the tibial plateau. Nutrient arteries to the scaphoid bone are large and numerous at the distal end but become sparse and finer as the proximal pole is approached. Fractures of the scaphoid, especially of the waist or proximal pole, may be associated with inadequate blood supply resulting in necrosis and later secondary osteoarthritis in the wrist. In the foot, the navicular bone is the last tarsal bone to ossify and its ossification centre may be dependent on a single nutrient artery. Compressive forces on weight bearing are thought to be the cause of avascular necrosis of the ossification centre, which usually presents as a painful limp in a child. This condition is also known as Köhler's disease.

Calcium homeostasis and hormonal control

In addition to its role as a support structure, the bone's other primary function is mineral homeostasis. More than 99.9% of the total body calcium and 85% of total body phosphate resides in the skeleton. The maintenance of normal serum calcium depends on the interplay of intestinal calcium absorption, renal reabsorption and skeletal mobilization or uptake of calcium. Serum calcium represents less than 1% of total body calcium but the serum level is extremely important for maintenance of normal cellular functions. Serum calcium regulates and is regulated by three major hormones: parathyroid hormone (PTH), 1,25-dihydroxyvitamin D and calcitonin (Fig. 5.3). PTH is an 84-amino acid peptide secreted by the four parathyroid glands located adjacent to the thyroid gland in the neck. Calcitonin is a 32-amino acid peptide secreted by the parafollicular cells of the thyroid gland. Vitamin D, from dietary sources (D_3) or synthesized in skin (D_2), is converted to 25-hydroxyvitamin D in the liver and then to 1,25-dihydroxyvitamin D in the kidney.

PTH and 1,25-dihydroxyvitamin D are the major regulators of calcium and bone homeostasis. Although calcitonin can directly inhibit osteoclastic bone resorption, it appears to play a relatively minor role in calcium homeostasis in normal adults. PTH acts on the kidney to increase calcium reabsorption, phosphate excretion and 1,25-dihydroxyvitamin D production. It acts on bone to increase bone resorption. 1,25-dihydroxyvitamin D is a potent stimulator of bone resorption and an even more potent stimulator of intestinal calcium (and phosphate) absorption. It is also necessary for bone mineralization. Intestinal calcium absorption is probably the most important calcium homeostatic pathway.

A number of feedback loops operate to control the level of serum calcium and the two major calcium homeostatic hormones. The calcium-sensing receptor (CaSR), identified in parathyroid and kidney cells but also found in other tissues, which senses extracellular calcium levels plays a critical role in calcium homeostasis. Low serum calcium levels stimulate 1,25-dihydroxyvitamin D synthesis via stimulation of PTH release (and synthesis). The physiological response to increasing levels of PTH and 1,25-dihydroxyvitamin D is a gradual rise in serum calcium level. To prevent an elevated level of serum calcium, a second set of feedback loops operate to decrease PTH and 1,25-dihydroxyvitamin D levels. These feedback loops maintain serum calcium within a narrow physiological range. Disturbances in these control mechanisms or over/underproduction of these three major hormones can lead to various clinical states, discussed in more detail below. A PTH-related peptide (PTHrP) also plays a role in calcium homeostasis, especially in the foetus and in the growing skeleton.

Circulating phosphate concentration depends upon intestinal absorption, renal reabsorption and skeletal storage and is regulated by PTH, 1,25 dihydroxyvitamin D and fibroblast growth factor-23 (FGF-23). Internal cellular redistribution is also important and results in hypophosphataemia under specific circumstances.

Cellular basis of bone remodelling

The structural components of bone consist of extracellular matrix (largely mineralized), collagen and cells. The collagen fibres are of type I, comprise 90% of the total protein in bone and are oriented in a preferential direction giving lamellar bone its structure. Spindle- or plate-shaped crystals of hydroxyapatite $[3Ca_3(PO_4)_2] \cdot (OH)_2$

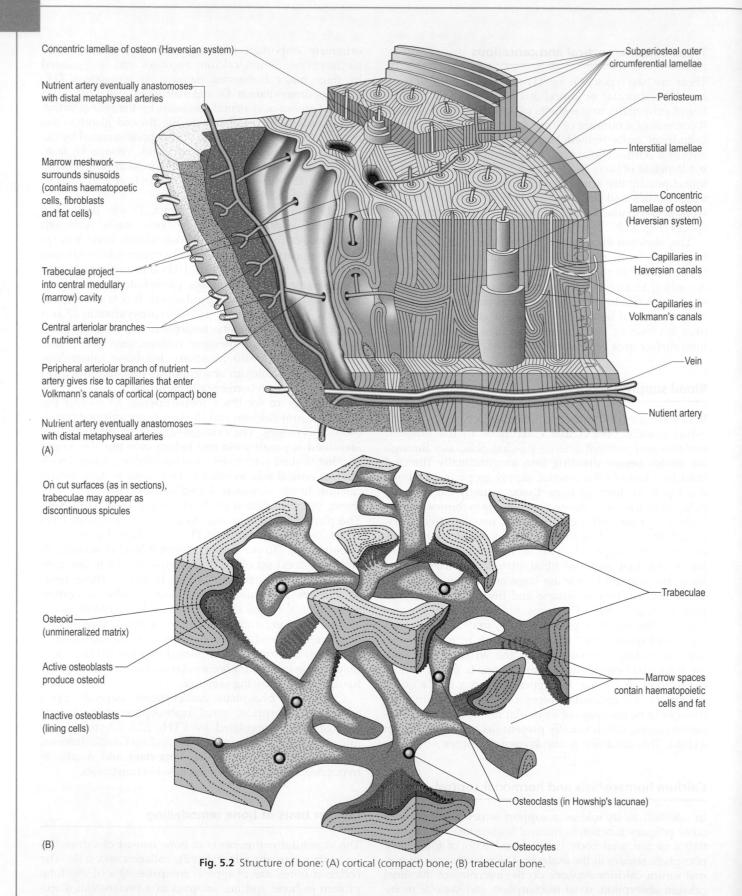

Concentric lamellae of osteon (Haversian system)

Nutrient artery eventually anastomoses with distal metaphyseal arteries

Marrow meshwork surrounds sinusoids (contains haematopoetic cells, fibroblasts and fat cells)

Trabeculae project into central medullary (marrow) cavity

Central arteriolar branches of nutrient artery

Peripheral arteriolar branch of nutrient artery gives rise to capillaries that enter Volkmann's canals of cortical (compact) bone

Nutrient artery eventually anastomoses with distal metaphyseal arteries

(A)

Subperiosteal outer circumferential lamellae

Periosteum

Interstitial lamellae

Concentric lamellae of osteon (Haversian system)

Capillaries in Haversian canals

Capillaries in Volkmann's canals

Vein

Nutient artery

On cut surfaces (as in sections), trabeculae may appear as discontinuous spicules

Osteoid (unmineralized matrix)

Active osteoblasts produce osteoid

Inactive osteoblasts (lining cells)

Trabeculae

Marrow spaces contain haematopoietic cells and fat

Osteoclasts (in Howship's lacunae)

Osteocytes

(B)

Fig. 5.2 Structure of bone: (A) cortical (compact) bone; (B) trabecular bone.

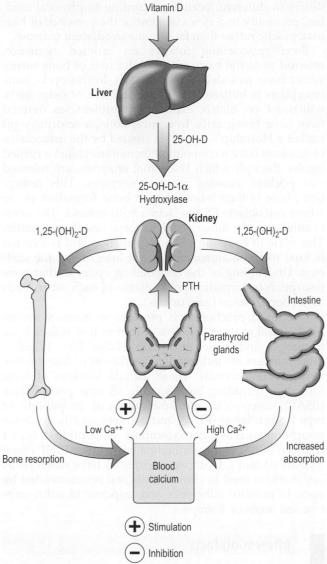

Fig. 5.3 Schematic diagram of the hormonal control loop for calcium metabolism.

are found on the collagen fibres, within them, and in the ground substance. The ground substance is primarily composed of glycoproteins and proteoglycans. These highly anionic complexes have a high ion-binding capacity and are thought to play an important role in the calcification process. Numerous non-collagenous proteins have been identified in bone matrix, such as osteocalcin synthesized by the osteoblasts, but their role is unclear.

The principal cells in bone are the osteoclasts, osteoblasts and osteocytes. Osteoclasts, the cells responsible for resorption of bone, are derived from haematopoietic stem cells. Osteoblasts are derived from local mesenchymal cells. They are responsible directly for bone formation and indirectly, via paracrine factors, for regulating osteoclastic bone resorption. Osteocytes are formed when osteoblasts become entombed within the hard mineralized matrix. More than 90% of all cells within the adult

skeleton are osteocytes. Osteocytes are thought to sense mechanical loads on the skeleton and have a dendritic structure that allows communications with other cells via gap junctions so that bone fluid flow shear stress can be translated into biochemical signals that direct bone modelling and remodelling. Once thought to be relatively inert, osteocytes are now recognized to express genes encoding proteins important for bone turnover such as sclerostin, also expressed by osteoblasts and other osteocyte specific genes related to bone mineralization and phosphorous metabolism such as fibroblast growth factor (FGF) 23 and dense matrix protein (DMP).

Various cytokines control osteoclast recruitment and activity, including interleukin-1β (IL-1β) and IL-6. A transmembrane protein belonging to the tumour necrosis factor superfamily plays an important role in osteoclast differentiation and activity (Fig. 5.4A). Its receptor is called RANK (receptor activator of NFκB) since, after binding, a transcription factor known as NFκB translocates to the nucleus and appears responsible for expression of genes that lead to the osteoclast phenotype. This process is inhibited by a soluble receptor, osteoprotegerin (OPG), which competes for binding of RANK ligand to produce an inactive complex. Control of osteoblast differentiation and function is achieved by integration of a number of pathways. Bone morphogenetic proteins and the Wnt signalling pathway are important modulators of osteoblast function and hence bone formation. Sclerostin, a product of the osteocyte, antagonizes the Wnt signalling pathway, which can inhibit osteoblast generation.

Interesting facts

Sclerostin is expressed by the *SOST* gene. Mutations in this gene leading to increased expression are associated with a low bone mass state whereas mutations that lead to decreased expression of the *SOST* gene lead to a high bone mass phenotype, first described in Dutch people and called Van Buchem disease. Van Buchem disease is characterized by overgrowth of bones, especially of the jaw, and enlargement of the skull, ribs, diaphysis of long bones, as well as tubular bones of the hands and feet. A similar phenotype is observed in hyperosteosis associated with activating mutations in *LRP5* that disrupt sclerostin binding. Newly developed anti-sclerostin antibody therapy leads to a significant increase in bone formation.

Bone is continually undergoing turnover and renewal called remodelling (Fig. 5.4B). In the normal adult skeleton, new bone laid down by osteoblasts exactly matches osteoclastic bone resorption, i.e. formation and resorption are closely 'coupled'. Although there is a lesser amount of trabecular bone than cortical bone in the skeleton, because trabecular bone 'turns over' between 3 and 10 times more rapidly than cortical bone, it is more sensitive to changes in bone resorption and formation. Most bone turnover occurs on bone surfaces, especially at endosteal surfaces. Moreover, the rate of remodelling

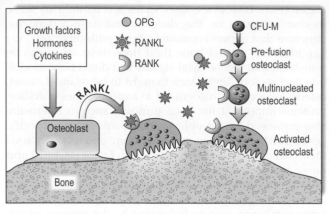

(A)

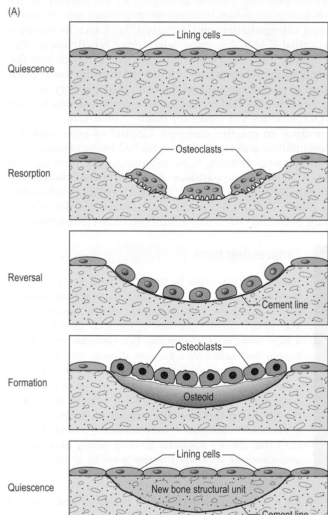

(B)

Fig. 5.4 (A) Osteoblasts and stromal cells produce RANKL. Binding of RANKL to its receptor (RANK) on osteoclast precursor cells results in their differentiation and activation. This process is regulated by an inhibitor of RANKL, osteoprotegerin (OPG), which competes with RANK for binding of RANKL to produce an inactive complex. (B) The bone remodelling sequence is initiated by osteoclasts. Subsequently, osteoblasts appear within the resorption bay and synthesize matrix, which is mineralized later.

differs in different locations according to physical loading, proximity to a synovial joint or the presence of haematopoietic rather than fatty tissue in adjacent marrow.

Bone remodelling follows an ordered sequence, referred to as the basic multicellular unit of bone turnover or bone remodelling unit (BMU). In this cycle, bone resorption is initiated by the recruitment of osteoclasts, which act on matrix exposed by proteinases derived from bone lining cells. In cortical bone, a resorptive pit (called a Howship's lacuna) is created by the osteoclasts. Osteoclasts have a convoluted membrane called a ruffled border through which lysosomal enzymes are released into pockets, causing matrix resorption. This resorptive phase is then followed by a bone formation phase where osteoblasts fill the lacuna with osteoid. The latter is subsequently mineralized to form new bone matrix. This cycle of coupling of bone formation and resorption is vital to the maintenance of the integrity of the skeleton. Uncoupling of the remodelling cycle, so that bone resorption or formation are in excess of each other, leads to net bone change (gain or loss).

In clinical practice, it is possible to measure serum biochemical markers of bone turnover that reflect bone formation and bone resorption (Table 5.1). Whether these markers are independent predictors of fracture risk remains controversial. These include markers of bone formation including bone specific alkaline phosphatase (BSAP), osteocalcin and aminoterminal propeptide of type I procollagen (PINP) and markers specific for bone resorption such as carboxyterminal telopeptide of type I collagen (CTX) and pyridinoline cross-links. PINP (bone formation) and CTX (bone resorption) have emerged as key markers used in clinical trials and recommended by some to monitor adherence and response to antiresorptive and anabolic therapies.

Interesting facts

Julius Wolff first postulated in 1892 that bone models 'In certain mathematical ways...as a consequence of primary changes in the shape or stresses on the bones'. In a paraphrased way this means that remodelling is influenced by mechanical load, and that bone is laid down where it is needed. It will change its internal and external architecture according to forces acting across it, and will do this in predictable ways. This is evident in response to deformity and fractures.

Table 5.1   Serum biochemical markers of bone turnover

Bone formation	Bone resorption
Aminoterminal propeptide of type I procollagen (PINP)	Tartrate-resistant acid phosphatase
Bone-specific alkaline phosphatase	Carboxyterminal telopeptide of type I collagen (CTX)

Skeletal development

Bones develop by one of two processes, either:

1. From a preformed cartilaginous structure (endochondral ossification), or

2. De novo at specific sites in the skeleton (intramembranous ossification).

Subsequent skeletal growth involves remodelling of bone. In the growing skeleton, the long bones consist of a diaphysis (or shaft) separated from the ends of the bone (called the epiphyses) by cartilage. The part of the diaphysis immediately adjacent to the epiphysial cartilage is the site of advancing ossification and is known as the metaphysis. Endochondral ossification is a complex process in which the growth plate cartilage is progressively replaced by bone. The growth plate (physis) and bone front steadily advance away from the bone centre, resulting in progressive elongation of bone. Longitudinal growth continues while the growth plate remains open.

Growth plates start to close after puberty in response to the surge in circulating oestrogen. Several hormones including growth hormone, insulin-like growth factor-1 (IGF-1) and PTHrP play a role in bone growth. With growth throughout early childhood, bone size and mass gradually increase in a linear fashion. Then between the onset of puberty and young adulthood, skeletal mass approximately doubles. Most of the increase in bone mass in early puberty is due to increases in bone size. In cortical bone, both the inner (endocortical) and outer (periosteal) diameters increase, owing to enhanced resorption and apposition on these surfaces respectively. Gains in BMD during puberty are dependent on the pubertal stage.

Growth ceases when closure of the growth plate occurs, but bone mass and density may continue to increase beyond this time by a process called consolidation. The maximum skeletal mass achieved is termed the peak bone mass (PBM). The age at which this is attained varies in different skeletal sites. Non-modifiable factors of PBM are genetic factors and gender but potentially modifiable factors can also play a role during childhood and adolescence including physical activity, calcium and vitamin D intake, weight, smoking and alcohol consumption, socioeconomic status, age at menarche, malabsorption and some medications.

The adult skeleton

In both men and women, bone mineral loss from the skeleton starts from age 40 to 50, again depending upon the skeletal site. In addition, in women bone loss can be rapid immediately after the menopause. Bone size also contributes to bone strength. Men have higher BMD (and lower fracture risk) than women in part because they have larger bones. In clinical practice, osteoporosis is usually defined in relation to the degree to which BMD is reduced. BMD can be measured by dual energy X-ray absorptiometry (DEXA), ultrasound or quantitative computed tomography (QCT) and is usually expressed as a T score (number of standard deviations from the young adult mean) or Z score (number of standard deviations from the age-matched mean). Osteoporosis is defined as a BMD T score below –2.5 measured by DXA (Fig. 5.5). An osteoporotic fracture or fragility fracture is defined as a fracture occurring from either no trauma (such as can occur with vertebral body fractures) or minimal trauma (such as occurs from fall from a standing height or less) and in this setting BMD T score criteria does not need to be met for a diagnosis of osteoporosis.

Metabolic bone disease

Metabolic bone disease is an overarching term encompassing diseases of bone in which abnormal bone remodelling results in a reduced volume of mineralized bone and/or abnormal bone architecture. These processes in turn give rise to bone pain and usually an increased risk of fracture. The commonest metabolic bone diseases are osteoporosis, osteomalacia, Paget's disease, hyperparathyroidism and bone disease associated with renal failure (renal osteodystrophy). There is a growing recognition that medications can contribute to abnormalities in bone mineralization and structure including glucocorticoids, anti-convulsants, proton-pump inhibitors, aromatase inhibitors used for breast cancer and androgen deprivation therapy for prostate cancer.

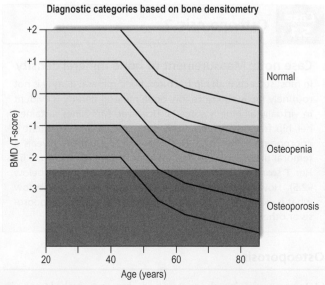

Fig. 5.5 Diagnostic categories based upon bone densitometry according to the number of standard deviations from the young normal mean (a T score of zero). T scores between -1 and -2.5 are called low bone mass or osteopenia. T scores below -2.5 are called osteoporosis.

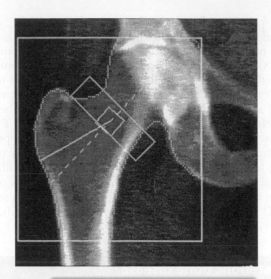

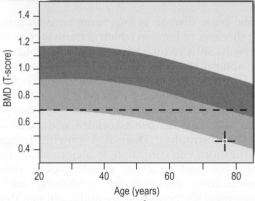

Fig. 5.6 Mrs Jones' right hip scan measured by dual energy X-ray absorptiometry showing her values plotted against the age-related normal range.

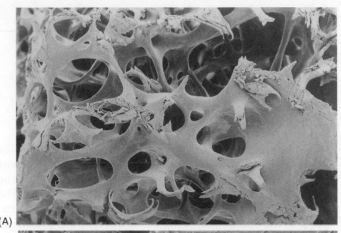

(A)

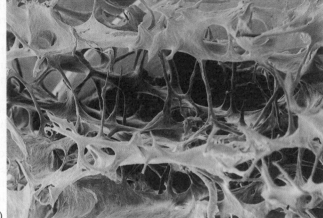

(B)

Fig. 5.7 Scanning electron micrographs of (A) normal and (B) osteoporotic bone. (Courtesy Lis Mosekilde, Institute of Anatomy, University of Aarhus, Denmark.)

Case 5.1 — Osteoporosis: 2

Case note: Measurement of bone mineral density

In most subjects with hip fractures, bone mineral density is not routinely measured since low bone mineral density is evident in virtually all elderly subjects. However, Mrs Jones sustained her hip fracture at a relatively early age, so measurement is appropriate in her case. Her bone mineral density reveals a femoral neck T score of –4.0 and her Z score is –2.3 (Fig. 5.6). Her T score confirms that she has osteoporosis (being below –2.5). However, since her Z score is also considerably below what is expected for her age, secondary causes for osteoporosis or other metabolic bone disease should be sought.

Osteoporosis

Osteoporosis is characterized by an imbalance in remodelling – a relative increase in resorption that is not matched by a concomitant increase in formation. The bone matrix is normally mineralized but there is simply less bone. In most forms of osteoporosis the loss of bone is not evenly distributed throughout the skeleton. For example, some struts of trabecular bone are resorbed completely, resulting in a loss of connectivity between adjacent bone plates (Fig. 5.7). This contributes to markedly decreased bone strength and fracture risk. Because the remodelling surface-to-volume ratio of trabecular bone is high, bone loss tends to affect this type of bone, in the spine and hip, to a greater extent.

An imbalance between resorption and formation occurs with ageing but also in several other circumstances. These include the following:

1. When bone is subject to reduced mechanical loading as a result of bed rest or immobilization.
2. In the presence of reduced sex hormone concentrations such as after the menopause in females.
3. In the presence of excess corticosteroids usually given as treatment for a variety of conditions such as arthritis or asthma.

Loss of bone mineral has no clinical effect itself, unless a fracture occurs. Common sites of fracture due

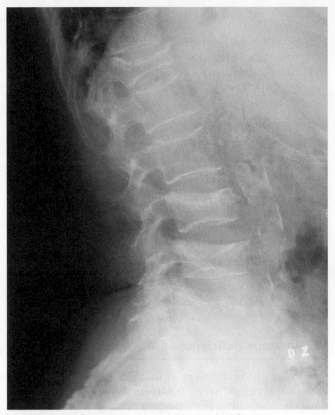

Fig. 5.8 X-ray of a patient with multiple vertebral fractures.

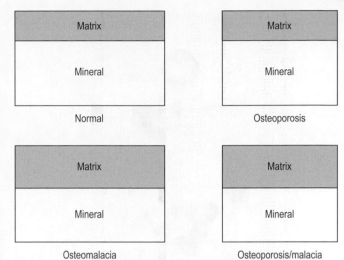

Fig. 5.9 Illustration of the difference between osteoporosis and osteomalacia. In osteoporosis, the amount of bone is decreased but the ratio of matrix to bone mineral is normal. In osteomalacia, the amount of bone is normal but the ratio of matrix to bone mineral is decreased.

to osteoporosis include the spine (Fig. 5.8), wrist, hip or pelvis after minor trauma, but almost any bone can be affected. Vertebral fractures can manifest as loss of anterior height (wedge fractures), loss of mid-vertebral height (called codfish vertebrae) or loss of anterior, middle and posterior height (called compression or crush fractures). Vertebral fractures may present with an acute self-limiting episode of back pain or sub clinically (i.e. asymptomatically) as height loss and increasing thoracic kyphosis (forward bending of the spine).

Osteomalacia

Osteomalacia occurs when there is insufficient calcium and phosphate to mineralize newly formed osteoid. Since bone mineral – hydroxyapatite – gives bone its compressive strength, osteomalacic bones are softer and more liable to bend, become deformed, or fracture. Rickets is essentially the same problem – impaired mineral deposition in bone – when it occurs in children or adolescents. Rickets is only seen before the growth plate disappears. Osteomalacia and rickets most commonly occur as a result of vitamin D deficiency, such as in institutionalized patients, those with reduced sun exposure and in patients with gut malabsorption or poor nutrition. Rarely, an inability of the kidney to reabsorb phosphate results in phosphate wasting and chronic hypophosphataemia and osteomalacia/rickets (Fig. 5.9).

This can occur in inherited conditions, most commonly X-linked hypophosphataemic rickets (XLH) due to *PHEX* mutations or acquired disorders such tumour-induced osteomalacia (TIO). In both these conditions, elevated circulating FGF23 causes renal phosphate wasting and inappropriately low 1,25-dihydroxyvitamin D which over time leads to rickets/osteomalacia. In XLH, elevated FGF23 is due to impaired catabolism of this hormone whereas in TIO the source of FGF23 is a tumour, typically mesenchymal, resection of which is curative.

Paget's disease

Paget's disease is a condition in which localized areas of bone show markedly increased bone turnover. There is gross disorganization of newly reformed bone, triggered by overactive osteoclasts. These local areas of increased remodelling may cause deformity such as bowing of a limb or enlargement (Fig. 5.10), bone pain, increased fracture risk and, rarely, neoplastic transformation to osteosarcoma. The X-ray appearance often shows a complex pattern of radiolucency (owing to early osteolysis) and bone expansion and sclerosis (generally later). Paget's disease is treated most effectively by drugs called bisphosphonates, which are discussed later in this chapter.

Hyperparathyroidism and renal osteodystrophy

Overproduction of PTH, usually by a benign tumour (adenoma) of one of the four parathyroid glands, leads to increased bone resorption and elevation of the serum calcium level. Hyperparathyroidism can occur as a discrete condition (primary hyperparathyroidism)

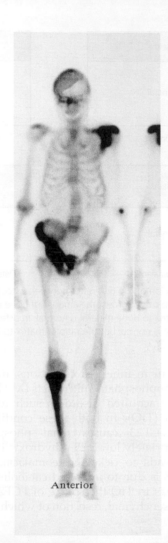

(A)

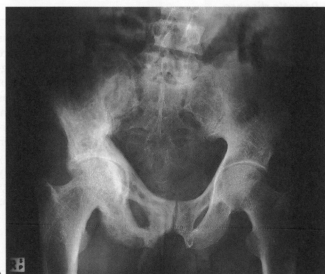

(B)

Fig. 5.10 (A) Bone scan showing increased uptake due to Paget's disease involving the right hemipelvis, right tibia, left scapula, skull and 11th thoracic vertebra. (B) X-ray of the same patient showing Paget's disease characterized by expansion of the right hemipelvis with cortical thickening and coarse trabecular pattern.

or may be secondary to conditions such as renal failure (owing to decreased production of 1,25-dihydroxyvitamin D by the kidney). In patients with renal failure, the mixed picture of secondary hyperparathyroidism and osteomalacia is commonly called renal osteodystrophy.

Osteoporosis: pathophysiology and risk factors

BMD is an important predictor of fracture risk. BMD at any age is the result of the PBM achieved and subsequent bone loss (postmenopausal and age-related). Other important and potentially modifiable factors, such as lower limb strength and balance and prior history of low trauma fracture independently contribute to fracture risk. This section will discuss factors contributing to bone loss that are considered important in the aetiology of osteoporosis.

Sex hormone deficiency

Since Albright first observed that the majority of women with osteoporosis were postmenopausal, sex hormone deficiency, resulting from natural or surgical menopause, has been recognized to cause bone loss. Replacement of oestrogen following the menopause prevents bone loss and fractures. In men, testosterone deficiency is similarly associated with bone loss and can be reversed with testosterone replacement.

Menopausal status is probably the most important risk factor for osteoporosis. Women with an early menopause (generally considered to be present in women who become menopausal before 45 years of age) or having bilateral oophorectomy have lower BMD and increased risk of subsequent fracture. The earlier the menopause, the greater the risk appears to be.

Genetic influences

It is well established that BMD at both the appendicular and axial skeleton is strongly genetically influenced. A family history of a relative sustaining a fracture after age 50, particularly a hip fracture in a parent or grandparent, is an independent risk factor for fragility fracture and is included in individual risk calculator algorithms such as FRAX®. Genetic factors are also inferred from certain racial factors influencing BMD and fracture risk. For example, black people in Africa or in the USA, appear to have higher bone density than white people of the same age and sustain fewer fragility fractures. People of Asian origin often have lower bone densities which may result in higher fracture rates than white people although other factors such as exercise levels which can influence falls risk can also alter this risk.

Case 5.1 Osteoporosis: 3

Case note: Screening for metabolic bone disease

We recall that Mrs Jones had poor nutrition, so vitamin D deficiency should be checked for by measuring serum 25-hydroxyvitamin D. A simple screen for metabolic bone disease can be performed (Table 5.2). The usual tests to exclude a metabolic bone disease include measuring serum calcium, phosphate, creatinine, alkaline phosphatase and PTH. Serum calcium will be elevated in hyperparathyroidism and often low in osteomalacia or renal failure. If the serum calcium is elevated in renal failure, this may be due to so-called tertiary hyperparathyroidism. Phosphorous is the most abundant intracellular anion in the body and 85% is located in the skeleton. Serum phosphate generally has an inverse effect on serum calcium concentration. Serum creatinine will be elevated in renal impairment. Alkaline phosphatase is an enzyme found in human serum, mainly produced by the liver or osteoblasts. Bone-specific isoenzymes can be measured but automated biochemical screens mostly measure total serum alkaline phosphatase (i.e. enzyme from both sources) and it is usually modestly elevated in osteomalacia but much higher in Paget's disease. Serum PTH should be measured when the serum calcium is elevated, to confirm hyperparathyroidism.

Table 5.2 Differential diagnosis of common metabolic bone disorders

Disorder			Blood		
	Ca++	P	Alkaline phosphatase	PTH	25-OH-vitamin D
Primary hyperparathyroidism	↑	↓	↑, normal	↑	Normal
Osteomalacia	↓	↓	↑	↑	↓
Paget's disease	Normal	Normal	↑↑	Normal	Normal
Osteoporosis	Normal	Normal	Normal	Normal	Normal

Physical activity and muscle strength

Bone is responsive to physical strain. Changes in the forces applied to bone produce effects in bone. For example, weightlessness and immobilization induce marked degrees of bone loss. On the other hand, athletes tend to have greater BMD, although this effect is often site specific. For example, tennis players have increased bone density in their dominant but not non-dominant arm and weightlifters have greater femoral bone density than other athletes. This is consistent with a local effect of exercise on bone. By contrast, some athletes can train to a level of low body mass index that is associated with amenorrhoea leading to loss of BMD placing them at risk of stress fractures.

Nutrition

Although the majority of body calcium is stored in the skeleton, there is controversy about the role of dietary calcium intake in the aetiology and prevention of osteoporosis. However, there appears to be a role for dietary calcium intake in the attainment of peak adult bone density. Moreover, a daily dietary calcium intake of around 800 mg/day in premenopausal women and 1200 mg/day in postmenopausal women is generally considered appropriate to avoid negative calcium balance. All guidelines recommend getting adequate dietary calcium and only suggest calcium supplements when this cannot be achieved due to a suggestion that excess calcium intake may increase cardiovascular event risk in older people.

Other dietary factors have been postulated to play a role in skeletal homeostasis. Sodium intake may have important effects on bone and calcium metabolism. Sodium loading results in increased renal calcium excretion, which has led to the suggestion that lowering dietary sodium intake diminishes age-related bone loss. Excessive protein and caffeine intakes are associated with bone loss.

Glucocorticoids

Glucocorticoids or corticosteroids are commonly used to treat inflammatory diseases, including arthritis and asthma. Corticosteroids affect calcium metabolism deleteriously in a variety of ways. The most important effect is to inhibit osteoblastic bone formation directly. They also decrease calcium absorption in the intestine, increase urinary calcium excretion and enhance osteoclast activity by inhibiting OPG. These mechanisms cause rapid bone loss when corticosteroids are used in high doses for prolonged periods. Adequate dietary calcium intake and safe sunlight exposure to maintain normal vitamin D levels are recommended with prolonged

Case 5.1 Osteoporosis: 4

Case note: Risk factors

We recall that on admission to hospital, Mrs Jones' past medical history revealed several risk factors for osteoporosis. These include an early menopause, a positive family history, smoking, poor nutrition and lack of weight-bearing or strengthening physical activity.

- An early menopause is one that occurs before 45 years of age.
- A positive family history could include a mother who sustained any fracture after age 50 or early height loss due to kyphosis.
- Smoking exposure can be quantified in terms of pack years. One pack year is smoking 20 cigarettes per day for 1 year. Someone who smokes 10 cigarettes per day for 10 years thus has 5 pack years of exposure.
- Poor nutrition includes avoidance of dairy products, and thus a low dietary intake of calcium, or a poor diet overall.

Mrs Jones' medications also include corticosteroid therapy. Although corticosteroid-induced osteoporosis is dose dependent, even inhaled corticosteroids can cause bone loss if used in excessive doses. Given her Z score being <−2.0 other factors should also have been screened for such as by serum protein electrophoretogram (EPG) to screen for myeloma, thyroid stimulating hormone (TSH), parathyroid hormone (PTH), vitamin D level, calcium level and coeliac antibodies.

Case 5.1 Osteoporosis: 5

Case note: Preoperative management of hip fracture

After admission to hospital, Mrs Jones is transferred to the Orthopaedic Ward, 24 of whose 30 beds are occupied by elderly subjects recovering from hip fractures. These fractures all occurred following a fall or minimal trauma. Like many older subjects, Mrs Jones is on a large number of drugs (polypharmacy) and her 10 current medications should be critically reviewed to determine if they are all necessary. Her sleeping tablets should be stopped, as these types of medications are commonly associated with falls. Since she also takes diuretics, postural hypotension should be checked for as a cause of her falls. To reduce the risk of morbidity or mortality, she must be assessed by her anaesthetist prior to surgery for co-morbid conditions, and her cardiopulmonary and fluid–electrolyte state should be evaluated. Fluid and electrolyte imbalance is common in an elderly patient taking diuretics and anti-inflammatory drugs and with poor nutrition. Any imbalance must be corrected before surgery.

glucocorticoid use and in older people antiresorptive medication may be recommended to prevent corticosteroid-induced osteoporosis.

Epidemiology of fractured hip

Hip fractures, or fractures of the neck of the femur, are a frequent and serious fragility fracture type in older people, at both an individual and population level. Their economic cost is enormous because of the need for hospitalization, surgery and rehabilitation. The annual cost of treatment in the European Union and the United States reported in 2017 as ∈32 billion and $20 billion, respectively (International Osteoporosis Foundation, 2017). The recognition of the size of the burden of hip fracture on patients, families and health systems has led to a global call for action to improve the care of people with fragility fractures (Dreinhöfer et al., 2018).

The incidence of hip fracture rises dramatically with increasing age in most countries. Hip fractures are more common in women than in men: epidemiological studies suggest a White woman has a 16% lifetime risk of suffering a hip fracture and a White man has a 5% lifetime risk. While age specific incidence rates of hip fractures have shown slight decline in high-income countries, likely related in part to availability of antiresorptive medications over the past 2 decades, the total numbers of hip fractures will continue to rise with the ageing and growing population, particularly in the low and middle-income countries globally.

Risk factors for falls

The high rate of hip fracture in older people is due not only to their lower bone strength and but also to their increased risk of falling. Established risk factors for falls and hence hip fracture include impaired balance, muscle weakness, poor vitamin D status and use of psychotropic medication. Although physical activity levels are related to bone density, the benefits of exercise in the elderly may relate more to reduced risk of falling than increases in bone strength.

Essential anatomy of the hip

The hip joint, like most of the lower limb joints, is a synovial joint. Synovial joints are characterized by the following features:

1. hyaline articular cartilage covering the bony surfaces (allowing low friction movement)
2. a joint cavity containing viscous synovial fluid (providing lubrication and nutrition)
3. a surrounding joint capsule that consists of outer fibrous tissue and an inner lining called a synovial membrane (forming an envelope for the joint)

4. fibrocartilaginous structures such as the hip labrum or knee meniscus that add to joint stability joints and improve joint lubrication (tribology)

The hip joint is a deep ball-and-socket joint, formed by the articulation of the rounded head of the femur within the cup-shaped acetabulum of the pelvis. The primary stability of the hip joint is provided by its bony anatomy. The acetabulum is formed by fusion of three pelvic bones: the ischium, ilium and pubis (Fig. 5.11).

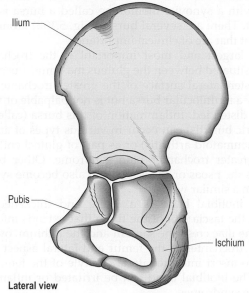

Lateral view

Fig. 5.11 Anterior view of bones of the hip joint showing three main sites of fracture: high in the femoral neck (subcapital), across the neck itself (cervical) or in the trochanteric region (pertrochanteric).

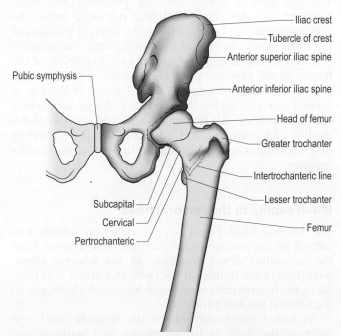

Fig. 5.12 Lateral view of the right hip of a child showing the three bones that form the acetabulum before fusion occurs.

Antero-inferiorly within the rim of the acetabulum is a notch which allows blood vessels and an intracapsular ligament (ligamentum teres) to pass into the acetabular floor to provide some blood supply and stability to the femoral head from within the joint.

The ball-and-socket structure allows a wide range of motion with great stability. This is possible because of the deep containment of the femoral head into the acetabulum, the strong articular capsule (condensed parts to form ligaments, resisting dislocation) and the muscles that pass over the joint and insert at a distance below the head of the femur.

The fibrocartilaginous acetabular labrum completely surrounds the rim, helping to seal synovial fluid and helps hip stability through a suction effect, especially as the joint moves. These anatomical features provide leverage for the femur and stabilization for the joint, especially in moving from seating to standing. The hip joint has the important function of being the main weight-bearing articulation between the axial and appendicular skeleton. The hip joint capsule is strong and thick over the upper and anterior portions of the joint (pubofemoral and iliofemoral ligaments) providing stability in the erect position. The hip joint structure is well suited to its function, especially in bipedal gait. One consequence of its unique anatomy is that the entire femoral head, and most of the femoral neck is intracapsular. There are three main sites of hip fracture; high in the femoral neck, across the neck itself or in the trochanteric region (Fig. 5.12).

Important structures around the hip joint

Ligaments

Ligaments are organized, dense and slightly elastic fibrous bands which connect bones across joints to provide secondary stability during movement (Fig. 5.13A). There are a number of important extracapsular ligaments around the hip joint named according to the bones they join. The pubofemoral ligament prevents excess abduction and extension, the ischiofemoral prevents excess extension, and the iliofemoral prevents hyperextension. The iliofemoral ligament is the strongest of these. Crossing the front of the capsule, it extends from the ilium to the anterior portion of the base of the neck. Its lower portion divides into two bands, forming an inverted Y shape. It is relaxed in flexion and taut in extension of the thigh and prevents excessive extension of the hip. In the upright position, the iliofemoral ligament stabilizes the hip by resisting subluxation of the femoral head anteriorly.

The ligamentum teres is an intracapsular ligament that loosely attaches the femoral head to the lower portion of the acetabulum and adjacent ligaments. It has little effect on the normal motion or stability of the joint but is a channel for blood vessels to the head of the femur.

The acetabular labrum

The acetabular labrum is a ring of fibrocartilage that sits on the edge of the bony rim of the acetabulum and is

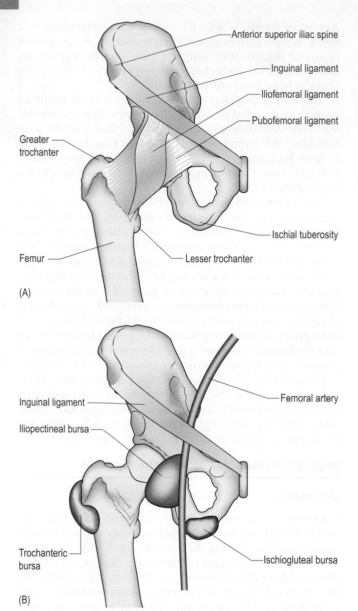

Fig. 5.13 Anterior view of the right hip joint showing: (A) the main ligaments; (B) the key bursae.

formed separately to the capsule. It is tough and flexible and acts to seal synovial fluid in the articulation between the hyaline cartilage surfaces where the femoral head meets the acetabulum. The ball-shaped head will rotate a long way in movement and the labrum acts as to contain synovial fluid at this interface. Additionally, it contributes to the biomechanics of the hip through load distribution and stabilization.

In injury and degeneration, the labrum can separate from the bony rim of the acetabulum.

Tears of the labrum have been credited to a variety of causes such as excessive force or movement, traumatic hip dislocation, capsular hip hypermobility, hip dysplasia and hip degeneration. Most 'tears' however remain uncertain in their aetiology.

Synovial membrane

A synovial membrane lines the deep surface of the articular capsule. It is a common site of pathology in septic arthritis in children (see Ch. 11) and chronic inflammatory diseases in adults such as rheumatoid arthritis and ankylosing spondylarthritis (see Ch. 1).

Bursae and other structures

In areas of the skeleton where movement between soft tissue structures such as tendons occurs, a definite sac lined with a synovial membrane called a bursa is often present. There are several bursae (Fig. 5.13B) around the hip joint that are of clinical importance.

The largest and most important is the trochanteric bursa, situated between the gluteus maximus muscle and the posterolateral surface of the greater trochanter. It is usually a multilocular bursa but is not palpable or visible unless distended. Inflammation of this bursa (called trochanteric bursitis) can occur in various types of arthritis (e.g. rheumatoid arthritis) or as part of gluteal enthesopathy/greater trochanter pain syndrome. Other bursae, such as the psoas or the ischial can also become symptomatic in a similar way.

The iliotibial band is a dense and thickened portion of the fascia lata of the thigh that extends inferiorly from the iliac crest, the sacrum and the ischium, over the greater trochanter of the femur and lateral aspect of the thigh to insert into the lateral condyle of the femur and tibia. The iliotibial band can be irritated or inflamed in overuse syndromes.

Muscles

The hip joint is surrounded by powerful and well-balanced muscles (Fig. 5.14) that not only move the extremity but also help maintain the upright position of the trunk. They are critical for maintaining core stability and conserving energy in bipedal gait. Extension of the femur on the pelvis is performed largely by the gluteus maximus and hamstring muscles. Flexion of the hip is carried out mainly by the iliopsoas, iliacus and rectus femoris muscles. Abduction is achieved by the glutei medius and minimus, and adduction by the adductors magnus, longus and brevis, the pectineus and the gracilis muscles.

Blood supply to the femoral head

The femoral head blood supply relies on vessels that ascend on the surface of the femoral neck derived from the circumflex artery branches of the femoral artery. Surprisingly the branch of the obturator artery that travels in the ligamentum teres provides very little supply to the femoral head in adults.

As noted previously all of the femoral head and most of the neck is intracapsular, and without any

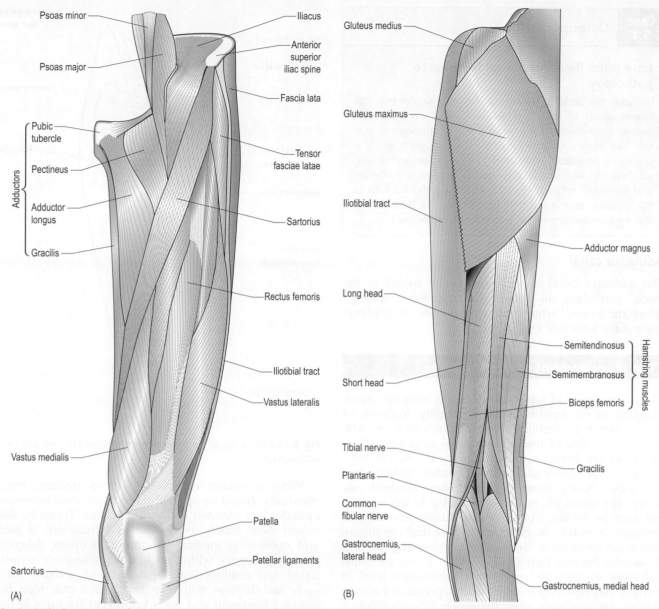

Fig. 5.14 The key muscles of the hip joint: (A) anterior view of the left hip joint; (B) posterior view of the left hip joint.

attachment (e.g. muscles or capsule); therefore any fracture through the neck or below the head will threaten the blood supply of the head. The more displaced such a fracture is the higher the risk of infarction of the bone of the head (osteonecrosis/avascular necrosis).

Femoral triangle

The femoral triangle is a clinically important subfascial space whose main contents are the femoral artery and vein, and branches of the femoral nerve. It is located in the superomedial third of the thigh and appears as a depression below the inguinal ligament when the leg is actively flexed at the hip joint. The boundaries of the femoral triangle are shown in Figure 5.15.

Interesting facts

Of clinical importance, the femoral artery is easily exposed and cannulated in the femoral triangle. Moreover, the superficial position of the femoral artery in the triangle makes it vulnerable to lacerations and puncture from trauma.

The femoral nerve is the largest branch of the lumbar plexus (L2–L4) and passes lateral to the femoral vessels in the triangle.

Case 5.1 Osteoporosis: 6

Case note: Relating clinical features to pathology

We can now understand why Mrs Jones is tender over the lateral aspect of the right hip. Tenderness over the right greater trochanter is likely to be a sign of trochanteric bursitis. Her history includes recurrent low back pain, which is commonly associated with altered gait and trochanteric bursitis. We can also appreciate why her left leg is shortened and externally rotated. Key muscles around the hip such as the iliopsoas muscle are de-functioned by the fracture and the normal lever arm of the femoral neck is disrupted.

Adductor canal

The adductor canal is a narrow fascial tunnel in the thigh, providing an intramuscular passage through which the femoral artery and vein pass into the popliteal fossa of the knee (see Fig. 5.15).

The management of hip fractures

The management of hip fractures begins with the understanding of the epidemiology of fragility fractures, of the frequency of significant comorbidities in those who sustain them and of the significant risk of complications and mortality during surgery and recovery. Additionally, loss of independence and financial burden are important issues that these patients face. The in-hospital death rate is typically about 5% in high-functioning health systems but may be higher. Complications during recovery are frequent, especially in those with co-morbid conditions, which are common in these patients. More than 20% of those who fracture their hip die within 1 year and most survivors struggle to regain their pre-fracture level of physical function. Hip fractures lead to permanent admission to a nursing home in approximately 20% of patients.

The care of patients with hip fractures is therefore multidisciplinary and coordinated. Integrated and driven care is the cornerstone of successful treatment. Hip fracture registries (nationally), the Fragility Facture Network (internationally) and engaged clinicians have led to the implementation of agreed care standards for hip fractures in many health services. The principles espoused by the Fragility Facture Network for treatment include:

I. Multidisciplinary care of the acute fracture episode along orthogeriatric lines
II. Excellent rehabilitation to recover function, independence and quality of life, starting immediately but continued long term
III. Reliable secondary prevention after every fragility fracture, addressing falls risk as well as bone health
IV. Formation of multidisciplinary national alliances to promote policy change that enables the above three.

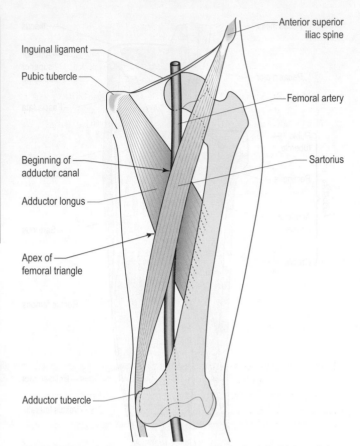

Fig. 5.15 Boundaries of the femoral triangle in the left thigh and the adductor canal.

When a patient experiences a hip fracture, these standards should be applied throughout their treatment episode, in a planned and systemic way. Typically, this would mean timely assessment and treatment of pain and optimizing medical conditions (without delaying surgery); surgery within 48 hours (or sooner); coordinated and combined orthopaedics and geriatric care; early mobilization within a day; and a care plan for ongoing treatment and ways to prevent fractures in the future after discharge.

Timely surgical management that allows prompt early full weight bearing and mobilization is the treatment of choice for hip fractures.

Surgical management varies according to the type of fracture and can be broadly divided into two types: fixation or prosthetic replacement.

Femoral neck fractures

When a hip fracture occurs, it is either within the hip joint (intracapsular) or distal to the capsule insertion (extracapsular). Intracapsular fractures are most often described by their anatomical position: those beneath the head (subcapital) or through the neck (cervical), with the importance of this classification relating to the blood supply. The more displaced, in intracapsular fractures, the more the perfusion supply to the femoral head is threatened. In extracapsular fractures this issue of vascularity is not so significant because of the rich alternate supply afforded by multiple alternate arterial inflows through muscle and other attachments.

Undisplaced femoral neck fractures are most commonly treated operatively by internal fixation, using multiple screws or short plates/screw combinations. The treatment of displaced femoral neck fractures depends on the patient's age and activity level: young active patients should undergo open reduction and internal fixation; older, less active patients, are usually treated with prosthetic partial or total hip replacement The ultimate goal is to return patients to their pre-fracture level of function by rapid rehabilitation and to avoid treatment failure by choosing wisely the index operative procedure so as to avoid complications (e.g. failure of fixation, non-union or avascular necrosis).

Trochanteric fractures

Trochanteric and subtrochanteric fractures are usually treated by open reduction and internal fixation, aimed at restoring the bony anatomy and allowing bony union to occur. Two main types of fixations are used. A sliding hip screw and plate construct applies a plate to the lateral cortex of the femur and a screw within the femoral head. Intramedullary nailing uses a device place through smaller incisions and within the shaft of the bone, but with a screw within the head. Increasingly intramedullary nailing seems more used, especially with unstable (comminuted and displaced) fractures. A longer nail is used typically in subtrochanteric fractures. Either type of device can fail and complication rates of up to 30% have been reported through breakage, loss of fixation or infection.

Medical management of osteoporotic hip fracture, including refracture prevention.

Please refer to Figure 5.16 for Hip Fracture Care Standards

After initial surgical management, diagnostic approaches should be directed at a general medical assessment. Elderly patients often have significant unrecognized multisystem disease that may impair the rehabilitation process. Investigations to exclude different types of underlying metabolic bone disease should include looking for the possibility of subclinical vitamin D deficiency as a contributing factor to falls (due to muscle weakness) and fracture (due to osteomalacia), especially in institutionalized patients.

Measurement of BMD is the best method for confirming the diagnosis of osteoporosis and is commonly used for monitoring the response to therapy. Bone density is usually measured at two sites, most commonly the spine and hip, using the technique of dual energy X-ray absorptiometry (DEXA). A relatively new DEXA-derived trabecular bone score (TBS) can assess internal texture of the vertebral bodies and is emerging as an additional independent predictor of fracture risk. Bone density can also be assessed by QCT and peripheral QCT (pQCT). The ability of bone density to predict fracture is at least as good as cholesterol level to predict heart disease and blood pressure to predict stroke. Bone biopsy may rarely be performed to exclude diseases like osteomalacia. Ultrasound measurements, usually of the heel (calcaneus), can also be used to provide an assessment of bone density and structure. Spinal X-rays may be appropriate to examine for vertebral wedge or compression fractures. These fractures may be associated with pain but often occur silently and result in height loss and increased kyphosis.

Treatment of osteoporosis is aimed at preventing further fractures. It is important to select treatment individually for each patient. Treatment options for osteoporosis will differ depending on whether it is for primary or secondary prevention and include calcium, vitamin D, oestrogen, selective oestrogen-receptor modulators (SERMS), bisphosphonates, monoclonal antibodies that affect the RANKL and sclerostin pathways, PTH and calcitonin.

Calcium

Calcium is weakly antiresorptive (i.e. a weak inhibitor of bone resorption) and supplementation may reduce negative calcium balance and so reduce bone resorption, particularly in older age. Controlled trials have demonstrated calcium supplementation can prevent bone loss in postmenopausal women and this appears to be associated with a mild reduction in fracture risk. There is also evidence that calcium supplementation augments the effect of oestrogen on bone density.

Vitamin D

Since a substantial proportion of institutionalized (or house-bound) elderly may be vitamin D deficient, vitamin D supplementation is recommended in institutionalized or house-bound elderly subjects.

Oestrogen and selective oestrogen-receptor modulators

In the past, oestrogen replacement therapy was the treatment of first choice in most perimenopausal women. Oestrogen reduces osteoclastogenesis by decreasing production of cytokines such as IL-1 and RANK (Fig. 5.4) and despite just small gains in BMD has been shown to reduce the risk of hip and other fractures. However, because oestrogen therapy has been linked to adverse effects including thromboembolism and an increased risk of breast cancer, its long-term use for treating osteoporosis is not advocated. SERMS act to decrease bone resorption, like oestrogen, while not stimulating the estrogen receptor in breast or uterus. Controlled clinical

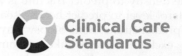

Clinical Care Standards

Clinician Fact Sheet:

Hip Fracture Care

The goal of the Hip Fracture Care Clinical Care Standard is to improve the assessment and management of patients with a hip fracture to optimize outcomes and reduce their risk of another fracture.

Clinicians and health services can use this Clinical Care Standard to support the delivery of high-quality care.

Under this clinical care standard

Care at presentation

A patient presenting to hospital with a suspected hip fracture receives care guided by timely assessment and management of medical conditions, including diagnostic imaging, pain assessment and cognitive assessment.

Pain management

A patient with a hip fracture is assessed for pain at the time of presentation and regularly throughout their hospital stay, and receives pain management including the use of multimodal analgesia, if clinically appropriate.

Orthogeriatric model of care

A patient with a hip fracture is offered treatment based on an orthogeriatric model of care as defined in the *Australian and New Zealand Guideline for Hip Fracture Care*.

Timing of surgery

A patient presenting to hospital with a hip fracture, or sustaining a hip fracture while in hospital, receives surgery within 48 hours, if no clinical contraindication exists and the patient prefers surgery.

Mobilization and weight-bearing

A patient with a hip fracture is offered mobilization without restrictions on weight-bearing the day after surgery and at least once a day thereafter, depending on the patient's clinical condition and agreed goals of care.

Minimizing risk of another fracture

Before a patient with a hip fracture leaves hospital, they are offered a falls and bone health assessment, and a management plan based on this assessment, to reduce the risk of another fracture.

Transition from hospital care

Before a patient leaves hospital, the patient and their carer are involved in the development of an individualized care plan that describes the patient's ongoing care and goals of care after they leave hospital. The plan is developed collaboratively with the patient's general practitioner. The plan identifies any changes in medicines, any new medicines and equipment and contact details for rehabilitation services they may require. It also describes mobilization activities, wound care and function post-injury. This plan is provided to the patient before discharge and their general practitioner and other ongoing clinical providers within 48 hours of discharge.

More information on the Clinical Care Standards programme is available from the Australian Commission on Safety and Quality in Health Care website at **www.safetyandquality.gov.au/ccs**.

AUSTRALIAN COMMISSION
ON **SAFETY** AND **QUALITY** IN **HEALTH CARE**

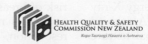

HEALTH QUALITY & SAFETY
COMMISSION NEW ZEALAND
Kupu Taurangi Hauora o Aotearoa

Hip Fracture Care Clinical Care Standard
Clinician Fact Sheet, September 2016.

Fig. 5.16 Hip fracture care clinical care standards (Australian Commission on Safety and Quality in Health Care. Hip Fracture Care).

Case 5.1	Osteoporosis: 7

Case note: Postoperative management of hip fracture

A multidisciplinary team comprising her orthopaedic surgeon, a physician, a physiotherapist, an occupational therapist and a social worker were all involved in Mrs Jones' postoperative progress. In the acute perioperative period, many hip fracture services aim to offer an orthogeriatric model of care to manage the delirium, fluid balance and pain management that can be difficult to balance in this group of patients. The main goals were re-establishing her independence and early mobilization to avoid pressure sores, infections and thromboembolism.

As falls were involved in Mrs Jones' case, a general medical assessment that included her visual function, and neuromuscular and cardiovascular systems was made. A key component of the hip fracture standards of care is to ensure there is adequate management with antiresorptive agents to reduce the risk of a future osteoporotic fracture by commencing, or ensuring commencement of soon after discharge, of antiresorptive therapy in addition to calcium and vitamin D supplements. She was transferred to a rehabilitation unit on day 8 after her surgery where a focus of ongoing strength and balance exercises will be critical.

trials have shown modest increases in bone density and significant reductions in spine but not hip fractures with SERM.

Antiresorptive agents

Bisphosphonates

Bisphosphonates are potent inhibitors of bone resorption, acting through the inhibition of osteoclast function (see Fig. 5.4). Treatment with these agents can significantly increase bone density and reduce further fracture risk at both spine and non-spine sites.

Interesting facts

Because bisphosphonates are retained in the skeleton for prolonged periods, the usual plasma pharmacokinetics do not apply to dosing. Rather, differences between bisphosphonates in binding affinity to hydroxyapatite and their potency of inhibition of the key enzyme, FPPS, mean that regimens can vary from daily oral, to weekly oral, monthly oral, 3 monthly intravenous or once yearly intravenous.

Denosumab

Denosumab is a human monoclonal antibody to the RANKL-ligand receptor that is required for osteoclast formation and activation. Hence it is a powerful inhibi-

tor of bone resorption. Like bisphosphonates it can lead to significant increases in BMD and reduction in further fracture risk at both spine and non-spine sites including hip. Unlike bisphosphonates, it is given as a subcutaneous injection every 6 months, does not accumulate in bone tissue and treatment should not be ceased without an exit strategy and shift to other agents.

Anabolic agents

Teriparatide

Teriparatide is a form of PTH made up of the first (N-terminus) bio-active part of the hormone. When given as a daily injection it promotes osteoblast activation and stimulates new bone formation. While it has a greater impact on increasing BMD when compared with the antiresorptive agents it has a similar impact on significantly reducing the risk for further vertebral and non-vertebral fractures. Treatment is only given for 18–24 months.

Romosozumab

Romosozumab is the most recent treatment to be approved for osteoporosis treatment and fracture reduction. It is a monoclonal antibody that binds to sclerostin produced by osteocytes and blocking it results in markedly increased bone formation accompanied (paradoxically) by reduced bone resorption. It is the only example of a drug that uncouples bone formation and resorption. It is given as a monthly injection for 12 months and shown to significantly increase BMD and reduce further vertebral and hip fractures.

Other considerations

Weight-bearing and strengthening exercise programmes are most useful in relation to preventing further falls and possibly useful for preventing the falls-related fractures, even though quite intense impact and strengthening programmes are required to have any effect on bone density. Serum biochemical markers of bone turnover may be used to monitor response and adherence to therapy.

Interesting fact

Non-weight-bearing states such as space travel or spinal cord injury leads to rapid bone loss and osteoporosis. Up to 1%–2% of BMD is lost per month in the microgravity of space. Exercise is encouraged during long space missions as a countermeasure.

A period of weeks to months in a specialist rehabilitation unit may be necessary to improve coordination and gradually strengthen muscle power. However, functional impairment in activities of daily living because of poor mobility will be present in many of these patients. For example, about 50% of hip fracture survivors are discharged to nursing homes. Rehabilitation will enable many patients to regain independence. Prior to discharge, a home visit by the occupational therapist may be necessary to ensure that the home environment is safe. In addition, a variety of aids may be recommended by the occupational therapist to promote independent living.

Further reading

Bilezikian, J.P., Bouillon, R., Clemens, T., et al. (Eds.), 2018. Primer on the Metabolic Bone Diseases and Disorders of Mineral Metabolism, ninth ed. American Society for Bone and Mineral Research, Washington DC.

Dempster, D., Cauley, J., Bouxsein, M., Cosman, F. (Eds.), 2020. Marcus and Feldman's Osteoporosis, fifth ed. Elsevier Philadelphia.

Moore, K.L., Dalley, A.F. 2017. Clinically Oriented Anatomy, eight ed. Williams & Wilkins, Baltimore.

References

Chen, W., Simpson, J.M., March, L.M., et al., 2018. Comorbidities only account for a small proportion of excess mortality after fracture: A record linkage study of individual fracture types. Journal of Bone and Mineral Research 33 (5), 795–802. https://doi.org/10.1002/jbmr.3374.

Dreinhöfer, K.E., Mitchell, P.J., Bégué, T. et al., 2018. A global call to action to improve the care of people with fragility fractures. Injury, 49 (8), 1393–1397.

International Osteoporosis Foundation, 2017. Health Economics: Capture the Fracture. Available from http://www.capturethefracture.org/health-economics.

Economic burden of osteoporosis in the world: A systematic review. Medical Journal of the Islamic Republic of Iran, 34, 154. https://doi.org/10.34171/mjiri.34.154.

Kemmak, A.R., Rezapour, A., Jahangiri, R., et al. 2020.

Tatangelo, G., Watts, J., Lim, K., et al., 2019. The cost of osteoporosis, osteopenia, and associated fractures in Australia in 2017, 34 (4), 616–625. https://doi.org/10.1002/jbmr.3640. Epub 2019 Jan 7.

THE SYNOVIAL JOINT IN HEALTH AND DISEASE: OSTEOARTHRITIS

6

Chapter objectives

After studying this chapter you should be able to:

1. Understand normal joint tissue structure and function.

2. Appreciate the essential structure and anatomy of the knee joint.

3. Understand the joint-wide pathological processes of osteoarthritis, including articular and meniscal cartilage degeneration, subchondral bone remodelling and synovial inflammation.

4. Understand the clinical symptoms and signs of osteoarthritis.

5. Understand the epidemiology of osteoarthritis, including risk factors for development and progression.

6. Understand the general principles of medical and surgical management of the osteoarthritic knee.

Christopher B. Little, David J. Hunter and Lyn March

Introduction

The principal function of appendicular synovial joints is to allow the low-friction articulation between the rigid (bony) skeletal elements essential for routine ambulation (legs) and manual tasks (arms and hands). This normal mechanical functioning requires the health and coordinate action of multiple different tissues and tissue-compartments that make up the synovial joint-organ, including: articular cartilage, subchondral bone, menisci, synovial tissues and intra- and extrasynovial ligaments. Osteoarthritis involves pathological change in all of these tissues to a greater or lesser extent in different individuals and stages of disease, which contribute to biomechanical dysfunction, pain and disability. Osteoarthritis affects 10%–15% of the population of the Western world and is the leading cause of chronic disability in these communities. It increases dramatically with age, with as many as 50% of those over 65 years suffering from musculoskeletal symptoms, the majority of which will be due to osteoarthritis. No 'cure' presently exists for osteoarthritis, but much is now known about the biomolecular mechanisms and risk factors that could contribute to disease onset and progression, and thus may be targets for prevention and treatment in addition to numerous interventions, including non-pharmacological ones, having proven benefits for symptom relief.

This chapter will review normal anatomy, structure and function of the synovial joint with a focus on the knee as an exemplar. The changes in joint tissues occurring in osteoarthritis will be described, and a case used to demonstrate the clinical symptoms and signs, risk factors and treatment.

Anatomy

The knee is a synovial joint. It is formed by three articulations:

- that between the lateral femoral and tibial condyles with its corresponding meniscus
- that between the medial femoral and tibial condyles with its corresponding meniscus
- that between the patella and the femur.

All of these articulations share the same articular (joint) cavity (Fig. 6.1). Magnetic resonance imaging (MRI) of the normal knee in Fig. 6.2 outlines clearly the structures that would be seen on anatomical dissection. Both menisci and articular cartilage can be visualized with MRI, which is not possible with plain radiography. The knee is predominantly a hinge joint, with the main movements being extension and flexion. A small amount of rotation is required to allow the full extension. The knee should normally extend to a straight line (0 degrees) and flex to 130–150 degrees.

As a typical synovial joint, the knee has a surrounding capsule, an internal synovial lining that produces the lubricant joint fluid and articular cartilage covering the surface of the bones. The knee has additional specialized anatomical features that enable its complex biomechanical function, particularly the menisci and internal stabilizing ligaments. In the pathogenesis of osteoarthritis, changes occur in all structures, including the synovial tissues, the synovial fluid, the ligaments and menisci, the articular cartilage and the subchondral bone (Fig. 6.3). Debate exists as to the earliest changes and/or tissues affected in osteoarthritis, and it is likely that this may differ depending on different risk- and initiating-factors and the particular joint affected. Furthermore, with the intimate mechanical and chemical cross-talk that occurs between joint tissues, pathology in one can initiate and/or worsen change in another (Fig. 6.4). Ultimately it is disease in a combination of joint tissues that signifies progressive osteoarthritis and eventually results in joint-organ failure. This first part of this chapter will summarize the key features of the different joint tissues in homeostasis and the mechanisms and consequences of their breakdown in disease. In each section, interesting facts and suggested additional reading and references are provided.

Case 6.1 — Osteoarthritis: 1

Case history

Mrs C is a 64-year-old retired teacher, living independently with her husband in their own home. She is in good health but, although always on the larger side, has become more overweight in recent years. For the past 5 years she has had gradually increasing right knee pain. This initially troubled her after her weekly tennis, with aching felt on the inside aspect of the knee. This has progressed to the point where she no longer wants to play, she is experiencing pain during the games and some low-grade swelling after. She is also having trouble kneeling down to do her gardening and is particularly concerned that she cannot keep up with her grandchildren. The knee has not been catching, locking or giving way but she is now also having trouble getting out of low lounge chairs and feels lack of confidence in the knee when going down stairs and slopes.

She has a strong family history of osteoarthritis with her 88-year-old mother having knobbly arthritic fingers and her father requiring a total knee replacement when he was 70 years of age. Mrs C had played a lot of sport in her youth and recalled numerous knee injuries when playing hockey. She has taken the occasional paracetamol/acetaminophen tablet for pain but generally does not like to take medications. She is on no other regular prescription or non-prescription medications. A provisional diagnosis of osteoarthritis of the knee is made.

In taking a history, it's important to pay attention to psychosocial factors that can influence behaviour change, exposure to previous treatments and success with those, appetite for exercise, increasing physical activity and dietary intervention.

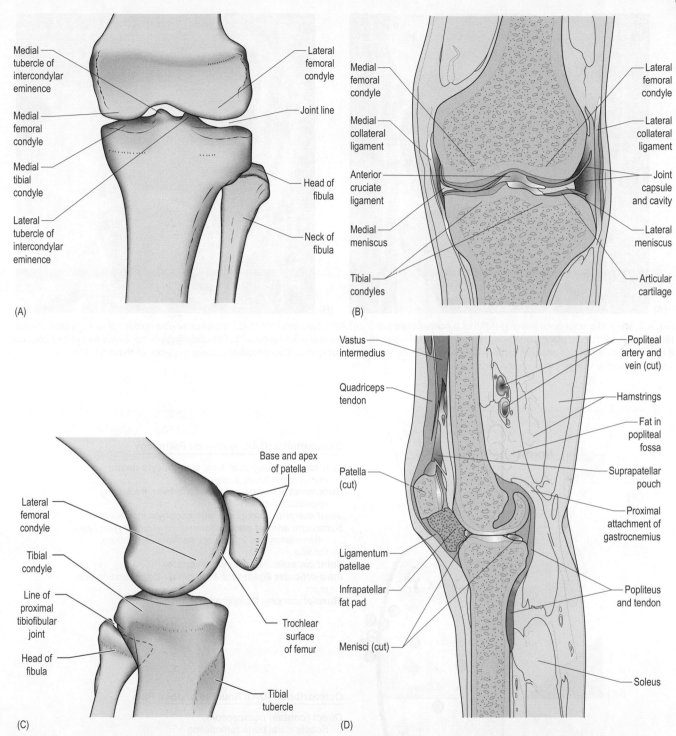

Fig. 6.1 The normal knee. (A) Anatomical bony landmarks (anteroposterior view); (B) soft-tissue structures, showing articular cartilage, menisci, synovial membrane and main knee ligaments (coronal section); (C) bony landmarks (lateral view); (D) soft-tissue structures (sagittal section).

Articular cartilage

Articular cartilage is a specialized form of connective tissue that covers and protects the ends of the bones in synovial joints. For the knee joint, this makes up the surfaces covering the femoral and tibial condyles and the under surface of the patella. The surface is smooth with an extraordinarily low coefficient of friction, while the deeper layer merges with a calcified layer that interlocks with the subchondral bone (Fig. 6.5).

Non-calcified cartilage is an elastic, resilient polymeric structure that acts as a shock absorber to protect the underlying bone and allow almost frictionless movement between the bony elements of the joint. The ability

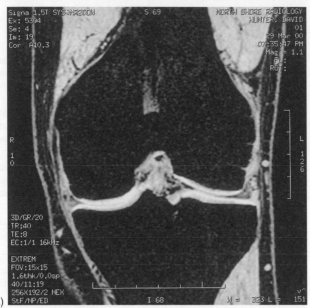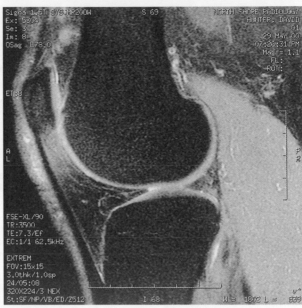

Fig. 6.2 Magnetic resonance imaging (MRI) of a normal knee joint. (A) Anteroposterior view; (B) lateral view. The epidermal layer, subcutaneous fatty tissue and muscle planes are clearly delineated. No effusion or soft-tissue swelling is evident. The underlying bone shows no cysts or oedema. It is covered by a layer of articular cartilage (appears white on these films) of normal thickness without any evidence of thinning. The menisci appear as wedge shapes between the joint surfaces.

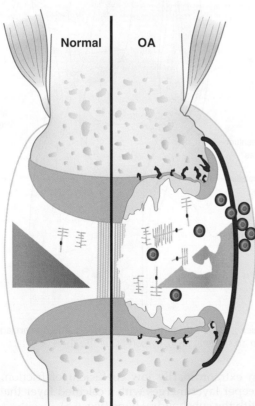

Osteoarthritis (OA): Joint-wide Pathology

Cartilage: proteoglycan loss, chondrocyte death, matrix breakdown, erosion
Subchondral bone: increased turnover, thickening, neovascularization
Joint margin: osteophyte, enthesophyte formation
Synovium and fat pad: inflammation (lining hyperplasia, inflammatory cell infiltration, neovascularization), fibrosis
Joint capsule: fibrosis, enthesopathy
Intra-articular ligaments & menisci: degeneration and tears
Muscle: atrophy, fat infiltration

Osteoarthritis (OA): Sources of Joint Pain

Direct (contain nociceptors):
    Subchondral bone remodeling
    Synovitis (including fat pad)
    ⊥ outer meniscus, ligament insertion, joint capsule, osteophytes
Indirect (source of inflammatory catabolites, cytokines, chemokines, neuropeptides):
    Cartilage, inner meniscus, ligamnt

Fig. 6.3 Schematic showing normal knee joint anatomy (left side) and changes in all joint tissues that occurs in osteoarthritis (right side) and their direct and indirect contribution to joint pain.

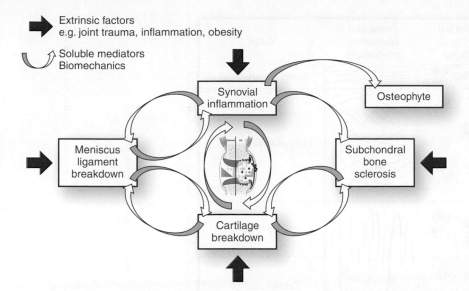

Extrinsic factors
e.g. joint trauma, inflammation, obesity

Soluble mediators
Biomechanics

Fig. 6.4 There is extensive cross-talk and interaction between joint tissues via biomechanical and soluble signals, that is important for normal joint function but can also contribute to a vicious cycle of osteoarthritic joint-wide pathology and disease progression.

of articular cartilage to resist the compressive deformation associated with joint loading is largely due to the entrapment of high concentrations of the polyanionic large proteoglycan, aggrecan within the collagen fibrillar network. In articular cartilage, collagen types II, IX and XI predominate and are arranged in heterofibrils, with small amounts of other collagens in distinct locations such as type VI in the pericellular lacuna and type X in calcified cartilage. The osmotic pressure provided by the highly sulphated glycosaminoglycan (GAG) chains on the aggregated aggrecan molecules draws in water and is resisted by and constrained within the insoluble collagenous meshwork. While the major proteoglycan by mass in articular cartilage is aggrecan, numerous other proteoglycans such as biglycan, decorin fibromodulin, lumican and perlecan are found, and together with other glycoproteins (e.g. cartilage oligomeric matrix protein (COMP)) and non-collagenous proteins (e.g. thrombospondin, fibronectin) that play key roles in regulating collagen fibrillogenesis and cross-linking, and growth factor binding and activity.

Interesting facts

Normal articular cartilage is made up of 80% water. There are 28 different types of collagen throughout the body. The main one in articular cartilage is collagen type II. Proteoglycans have a very strong negative charge that helps trap the water in the cartilage as well as to repel each other when the cartilage is compressed which gives cartilage its resilience and ability to maintain its shape.

The functional integrity of articular cartilage in a healthy joint depends on its specialized cells, chondrocytes, synthesizing the many different matrix components in the appropriate amounts and in the right sequence. Since cartilage lacks blood and lymphatic

vessels, the survival and synthetic activity of the chondrocyte depends on diffusion and transport of nutrients and metabolites predominantly from the synovial fluid through the matrix. Chondrocyte metabolism and biosynthesis are regulated by mechanical loading, osmotic pressure and numerous growth factors (e.g. transforming growth factor-beta (TFG-β), fibroblast growth factor (FGF)-2 and -18, insulin-like growth factor (IGF)) and cytokines (e.g. interleukin (IL)-1 and -6, tumour necrosis factor-alpha (TNF-α)). Thus a fine balance exists between anabolism (synthesis) and catabolism (tissue breakdown), with ongoing tissue remodelling as part of the normal healthy process and response to mechanical requirements.

Interesting facts

The chondrocyte has a unique role in both the synthesis and degradation of its surrounding extracellular matrix and shows diurnal regulation by clock genes. The chondrocyte can turnover, that is, divide, but the rate is very slow in adult life and decreases with age.

Subchondral bone

The deepest calcified layer of articular cartilage represents an intermediate/transitional zone between the overlying elastic and compressible non-calcified cartilage and the rigid subchondral bone plate (Fig. 6.6). Collagen fibres in the non-calcified zone penetrate the tidemark (the demarcation between calcified and non-calcified zones) anchoring it to the calcified cartilage layer but it is unclear if these also cross the cement line at the osteochondral junction. Nevertheless, the close association and undulating pattern of the osteochondral interface anchors the cartilage to the bone, and provides

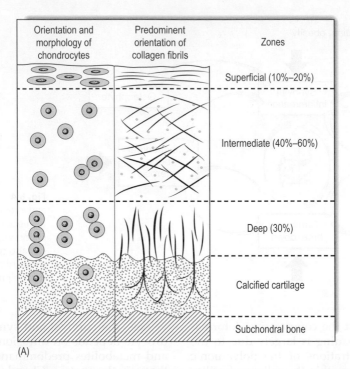

(A)

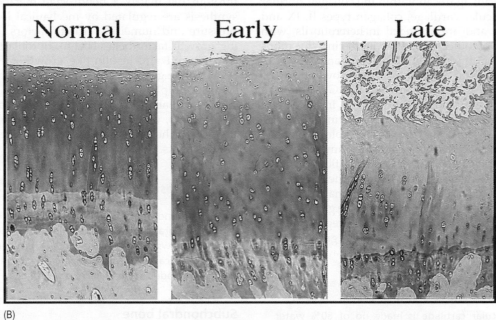

(B)

Fig. 6.5 Articular cartilage. (A) Schematic illustrating the zonal variability in density and orientation of the chondrocytes and collagen network in different layers. (B) histologic image showing normal cartilage and progressive changes occurring on osteoarthritis. (A, Based on a drawing by Professor Peter Ghosh, Raymond Purves Laboratory, Institute of Bone and Joint Disease, University of Sydney.)

a large surface area for load transmission and resistance to shearing forces experienced with joint movement. A cortical lamellar subchondral bone plate separates the calcified cartilage from the deeper vascularized epiphyseal trabecular bone and associated marrow spaces. Originally thought to be a relatively quiescent and impenetrable barrier, the osteochondral interface made up of the subchondal bone plate and calcified cartilage,

is metabolically active and undergoes remodelling in response to changing mechanical loads. Recent studies have also suggested that while slower than from the cartilage surface, diffusion of fluid and small molecules can occur across the cement line and tidemark, permitting not only nutritional flow from, but molecular cross-talk between, the vascularized bone and the avascular noncalcified cartilage.

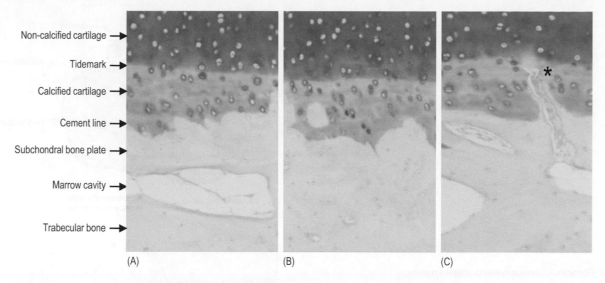

Non-calcified cartilage →
Tidemark →
Calcified cartilage →
Cement line →
Subchondral bone plate →
Marrow cavity →
Trabecular bone →

(A)   (B)   (C)

Fig. 6.6 The articular cartilage is separated from the deeper vascularized trabecular bone by a layer cortical bone called the subchondral bone plate (A). The subchondral bone plate may thicken (B) or thin (C) in response to altered loading, and may even be breached by blood vessels (C, asterisk).

Interesting facts

The deepest zone of articular cartilage contains as much mineral as the underlying bone. The subchondral bone plate supports the overlying cartilage allowing transfer and absorption of load to the deeper trabecular bone. Small molecules can diffuse through the subchondral bone plate and calcified cartilage to access chondrocytes in the deep non-calcified cartilage.

The predominant collagen in bone is type 1 (~30% of bone wet-weight; in heterofibrils with types III and V), which forms a rigid composite with the mineral component, largely hydroxyapatite (>60% of bone wet-weight). Other non-collagenous proteins make up ~5% of the bone extracellular matrix including: small proteoglycans (e.g. decorin, biglycan, asporin), Gla-containing proteins (e.g. osteocalcin, matrix-Gla-protein, periostin), glycoproteins (e.g. osteocalcin thrombospondins) and small integrin-binding ligand N-linked glycoproteins (SIBLINGs; e.g. bone sialoprotein, osteopontin, dentin matrix protein-1, matrix extracellular phosphoglycoprotein). These non-collagenous matrix proteins contribute to and regulate collagen fibrillogenesis, matrix mineralization, and growth factor and cytokine binding and activity. The integrity of the subchondral bone plate and underlying trabeculae is maintained through a balance of bone formation by surface lining osteoblasts and bone remodelling/removal by osteoclasts. Osteocytes, the predominant cell type in bone, are embedded in the bone matrix but have an extensive canalicular network. This network enables osteocytes to sense mechanical load and regulate both osteoblast and octeoclast activity through secretion of signalling proteins (e.g. sclerostin, rank ligand (RANKL), osteoprotegerin (OPG), IL-6, TNF)

to maintain the appropriate bone material properties to resist the loads that are experienced.

Interesting facts

While predominantly mineral, over a third of bone is made up of protein, the major one being type I collagen. Subchondral bone is highly metabolically active and is constantly remodelled in response to mechanical loading sensed by the osteocytes.

Menisci

The knee joint contains specialized crescent-shaped fibrocartilaginous menisci that sit between the femoral condyles and tibial plateau in both the medial and lateral compartments (Fig. 6.7). They are colloquially referred to somewhat misleadingly as the knee 'cartilages' and are often injured, which in the past has led to their surgical debridement or removal, although this is no longer recommended. The menisci provide congruity between the curved femoral and flat tibial articulating surfaces, contributing to force distribution and dissipation during weight bearing, and knee stability, especially in anterior–posterior translation and rotation. These complex biomechanical functions are made possible by anchoring of the anterior and posterior poles of the menisci to bone and the wedge shaped cross section of the more mobile meniscal body. Thereby, compressive forces from the curved femoral condyles are transformed into hoopstress in and absorption by the meniscus, while allowing some anterior–posterior and medial–lateral movement but constraining excessive motion. As the menisci therefore experience both compressive loading, especially

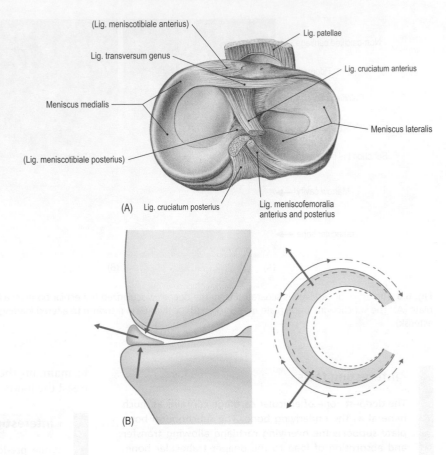

Fig. 6.7 Fibrocartilagenous crescent-shaped menisci are interposed between the medial and lateral femoral condyles and their respective tibial plateau (A). The wedge-shaped cross-section and anterior and posterior anchoring to the bone, enable the menisci to transform and absorb compressive loading as hoop-stress (B). (A, reprinted with permission from Paulsen, F., Waschke, J., (Eds). 2018. Sobotta Atlas of Anatomy, vol. 1, sixteenth ed., pp. 291–434.; B, reprinted with permission from Susan, S., (Ed.), 2021. Gray's Anatomy, pp. 1395–1429.e2.).

in the inner third, and tensile forces, particularly in the outer regions, they show zonal compositional and structural heterogeneity. The inner third of the meniscus and the articulating surfaces have higher levels of cartilage-like matrix proteins (e.g. collagen type II, aggrecan, biglycan). The outer third of the meniscus in contrast, is more fibrous (e.g. collagens type I and III, decorin), with the collagen fibres predominantly arranged circumferentially with intermittent radial tie-fibres crossing into the middle and inner zones. At its periphery, the meniscus is intimately associated with the synovium allowing the outer third along with the bony attachments to be vascularized and contain nerves, while the inner zone, like articular cartilage, is avascular and aneural.

Interesting facts

The menisci are biologically active tissues that show zonal heterogeneity in composition and structure synthesized in response to mechanical loading. The inner third of the meniscus is avascular and cartilage-like, while the outer third is fibrous with circumferentially arranged collagen fibres that participate in dissipation of knee loads, and contains blood vessels and nerves.

While originally considered inert fibrocartilaginous structures, it is now recognized that menisci and are biologically active tissues. Meniscal fibrochondrocytes maintain the heterogeneous matrix composition in response to both mechanical and molecular signals. Importantly, meniscal cells are also a source of these soluble bioactive molecules that can play a role in cross-talk with and homeostasis of other joint tissues including: growth factors (e.g. TGF-β, IGF), cytokines (e.g. IL-1β, IL-6, TNF), chemokines (e.g. C-C motif ligand (CCL) 3 and 20, C-X-C motif ligand (CXCL) 1 and 3), and matrix degrading enzymes (e.g. matrix metalloproteinase (MMP)-1, MMP-3, MMP-9 and MMP-13; a disintegrin and metalloproteinase with thrombospondin repeats (ADAMTS) 4 and 5).

Interesting facts

Beyond their biomechanical function, menisci play an important role in knee joint homeostasis through the secretion of soluble bioactive molecules that regulate the function of other joint tissues.

Synovial tissues, synovial fluid and ligaments

Synovial joints are so named because the bony and cartilaginous elements are fully enclosed within a distinct fibrous connective tissue structure that is filled with

Case 6.1 Osteoarthritis: 2

Case note: examination

When examining any joint, remember to *look, feel* and *move*.

On examination, with Mrs C first standing up with lower limbs exposed, *look* for:

- difficulty rising from a seated position
- deformity
- malalignment
- swelling (anteriorly and posteriorly because Baker's cysts are seen best from behind while the patient is standing)
- muscle wasting
- scars.

Mrs C has mild genu varum (bow-leggedness), which she says has been lifelong but has been more obvious in the right knee in recent years. This would be due to thinning of the articular cartilage in the medial tibiofemoral compartment. Her genu varum would have predisposed her to degenerative change initially and now would be increasing the wear and tear with increased weight bearing through the damaged compartment of the knee.

She had some difficulty rising from the chair and there was some wasting of the quadriceps muscle at the front of the thigh. This would also be associated with her loss of confidence on weight bearing, particularly when walking down stairs or slopes. The tendency is then to 'favour' the knee and not use it as much, thus contributing to further atrophy. Epidemiological studies suggest that quadriceps weakness predicts further deterioration or progression of the arthritis. This is manifested by more osteophytes and more joint space narrowing seen on X-ray, because of loss of articular cartilage. Management should include attention to building back the quadriceps strength.

When Mrs C turns around, a small 2-cm swelling is evident in her popliteal fossa.

With Mrs C lying on a couch, *feel* for:

- increased warmth
- effusion (patellar tap, bulge sign)
- bony swelling
- local tenderness.

Mrs C has some medial joint line tenderness in the right knee, suggestive of local periosteal reaction due to osteophyte formation, low-grade synovitis and/or local bursitis. There is a small positive bulge sign when fluid is 'milked' out of the supra-patellar pouch, consistent with a slight increase in synovial fluid but there is no increased warmth to suggest inflammation. The small swelling in the popliteal fossa is non-pulsatile and soft, consistent with a fluid-filled Baker's cyst.

Move for:

- crepitus
- pain
- restriction
- ligament instability
- locking, catching or meniscal tears.

Mrs C has retropatellar crepitus of both knees that is more marked on the right, reduced bulk on contraction of her quadriceps muscles on the right side compared with the left, particularly in the medial band, tightness in her hamstring muscles but no ligamentous instability, and McMurray's sign (discussed in Ch. 10) of meniscal damage is negative.

General examination shows that she has some asymptomatic bony osteophytic swelling of the distal and proximal inter-phalangeal joints in her hands consistent with Heberden's and Bouchard's nodes, respectively. Other joint and spinal movements are within normal limits. She weighs 70 kg and is 160 cm tall. Her body mass index (BMI 5 weight (kg)/height (m)^2) is 27.3, which puts her in the moderately overweight range.

In order to focus on what is happening in Mrs C's knee and what might be causing the pain, an understanding of the anatomy of the knee joint is required. When examining someone with knee osteoarthritis pay particular attention to modifiable factors, including muscle strength, malalignment and body mass index.

---

viscous synovial fluid. This encapsulating structure consists of three layers (Fig. 6.8). The intimal lining is found closest to the joint cavity and consists layer of specialized cells only 1–2 cells thick, and while often called the 'synovial membrane' there is no true underlying basement membrane. Rather, beneath the lining cells lies a vascularized subintimal layer, consisting of loosely arranged 'areolar' collagenous connective tissue and adipocytes. Finally, the outer most layer consists of a much denser fibrous joint capsule, which attaches circumferentially to the articulating bones where it is continuous with the periosteum but with proximal and distal reflections that allow for joint movement. These reflections can be quite extensive, for example, extending superiorly beneath the quadriceps muscle for as much as 6 cm above the superior pole of the patella. Outside the joint capsule although closely associated, lateral and medial collateral ligaments arise from their respective distal femoral epicondyles and attach to the proximal fibula head and medial tibial condyle and tibial shaft, respectively. Within the joint, the anterior and posterior cruciate ligaments arise in the intercondylar notch from the distal posterolateral and anteromedial femoral condyles and insert on the anterior and posterior aspects of the tibial intercondylar eminence, respectively. The knee also harbours several distinct adipose tissue deposits, including

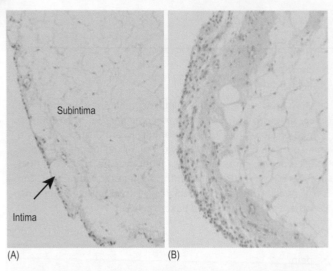

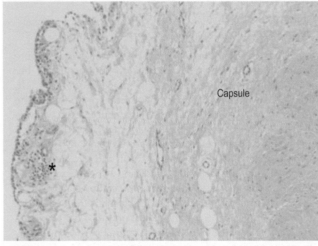

Fig. 6.8 The synovial intima or lining layer is 1–2 cells thick and has no basement membrane, but sits directly on the connective tissue layer subintimal layer containing adipocytes and blood vessels (A). In osteoarhritits there is hyperplasia and hypertrophy of the lining with increased fibrosis and vascularization of the subintima (B), along with accumulation of subintimal inflammatory cells (asterisk) and thickening and fibrosis of the joint capsule (C).

the infrapatellar (Hoffa's) and suprapatellar fat pads, that are located intra-articularly (i.e. inside the capsule) but extrasynovial.

The ligaments and joint capsule are rich in type I collagen but also contain up to 5% elastin (by dry weight) which enables these structures to provide stabilization but sufficient elasticity to allow the articulating bones to move relative to each other. The collateral ligaments provide medial-lateral stability, the anterior and posterior cruciate ligaments resist the femur moving posterior or anterior to the tibia, respectively, and all contribute to controlling rotation. The subintima, joint capsule and ligament osseous insertions are vascular and contain both nociceptive and proprioceptive nerves, thereby participating in pain perception and joint position and fine motor control. The fatpads are also vascularized and

innervated and in addition to adipocytes, have resident macrophage populations, and beyond filling the space in the joint cavity, they play a role absorbing shock and secreting cytokines, growth factors and adipokines that participate in joint homeostasis.

> ### Interesting facts
>
> The bones of the knee are stabilized by the articular capsule, the medial and collateral ligaments and the anterior and posterior cruciate ligaments. The overlying quadriceps femoris muscle and its distal insertion, the patella tendon, is another essential element for maintaining stability.

The cells of the synovial intima consist of macrophages ('type A cells') and fibroblasts ('type B cells'). While lacking a basement membrane, these lining cells form tight junctions with each other creating a semipermeable protective barrier that controls the molecular and cellular traffic in and out of the joint. This renders the synovial cavity relatively immune-privileged, and also contributes to the formation of synovial fluid, which is a dialysate of plasma combined with hyaluronic acid that is produced by the synovial lining cells. The large molecular weight of hyaluronic acid determines the elasticity and viscosity of the fluid and contributes to joint lubrication. In addition, lubricin (proteoglycan-4), a large glycoprotein of the mucin family, is produced by synovial lining cells as well as and superficial cartilage chondrocytes and meniscal cells. Lubricin concentrates on the synovial and cartilage surfaces and plays a critical role in their lubrication. At homeostasis, macrophages are virtually the only immune cells in the synovial membrane, and while the underlying subintima does harbour other lineages like mast cells and lymphocytes, macrophages still predominate. These normal tissue-resident macrophages are largely a self-renewing population receiving minimal if any input from circulating/systemic monocytes in the adult steady state. Synovial lining macrophages serve a protective function, acting as sentinels for molecular and cellular changes and clearing cartilage and bone debris shed due to mechanical shear stress.

> ### Interesting facts
>
> Synovial lining cells form a protective semi-permeable barrier to reduce cell and protein influx from the blood, generating synovial fluid as a dialysate into which they secrete hyaluronic acid and lubricin to enable joint lubrication.

Muscles nerves and bursae

While not strictly part of the joint itself, muscles, their tendon insertions and associated bursae and nerves are essential components of normal joint function, and show pathological change in association with osteoarthritis. The quadriceps femoris covers the anterior and lateral aspects of the thigh and is responsible for knee extension. The lateral portion is the vastus lateralis, the medial portion the vastus medialis and between these lies a double layer with rectus femoris superficially and vastus intermedius beneath. The four muscle bellies merge into a common tendon that encloses the patella and inserts on the proximal anterior tibial tuberosity as the patella tendon. The quadriceps femoris is essential for maintaining stability of the knee joint on weight bearing. The vastus medialis is often the first to waste in painful conditions of the knee and because this portion is responsible for the final 10 degrees of extension it is critical for normal weight bearing. The hamstring muscles make up the bulk of the posterior aspect of the thigh and are the main muscles responsible for knee flexion. They are formed by the biceps femoris, semitendinosus and semimembranosus. The gastrocnemius muscle forms the bulk of the calf muscle and helps to limit hyperextension of the knee.

Interesting facts

The hamstring muscles flex the knee and are formed by the biceps femoris, semitendinosus and semimembranosus. The quadriceps femoris extend the knee and are formed by the vastus lateralis, the vastus medialis, the rectus femoris and vastus intermedius.

The major nerves associated with the knee joint are the sciatic (arising from L4, 5 and S1, 2, 3 nerve roots) and femoral (arising from L2, 3, 4 nerve roots) nerves. These nerves carry motor and sympathetic efferents controlling muscle and vasodilator function respectively, and sensory and proprioceptive afferents involved respectively in pain and joint spatial position perception. The hamstrings controlling joint flexion are supplied by the sciatic nerve and its tibial and peroneal branches. The quadriceps is predominantly supplied by the femoral nerve and is responsible for knee joint extension. The majority of nerves innervating the knee joint itself are small diameter nociceptive fibres. The synovium has the greatest density of joint nociceptors but they are also found in the subchondral bone, the outer third of the menisci, the bony insertion and superficial layer of ligaments and the infrapatellar fat pad.

Interesting facts

Found in highest numbers in the synovial tissues and subchondral bone, most joint nerves are pain sensing. Proprioceptive nerves in the joint capsule, ligament insertions and outer menisci play a role in joint position sense and feedback.

There are multiple bursae surrounding the knee at sites where tendons and ligaments are required to glide over bony prominences. While almost all are extra-articular,

they may be a source of pain associated with knee osteoarthritis. The prepatellar bursa lies on the anterior aspect of the knee between the skin and the patella. The infrapatellar bursa has two components, a small superficial bursa between the skin and the proximal part of the patella tendon and a deep bursa that lies beneath the distal part of the tendon and the infrapatellar fat pad. The semimembranosus bursa is located posteriorly on the medial aspect of the knee and lies between the semimembranosus muscle and the medial head of the gastrocnemius muscle. It will usually communicate with the medial gastrocnemius bursa, which lies deep to it between the medial head of the gastrocnemius and the articular capsule. Posteriorly on the lateral aspect lies the other gastrocnemius bursa between the lateral head of the muscle and the joint capsule. The anserine bursa, so named for its 'goose-neck' shape, lies on the medial aspect of the knee between the medial collateral ligament and the common tendon insertions of the sartorius, gracilis and semitendinosus muscles as they attach to the medial tibial condyle and shaft. This bursa is felt to be the source of pain in many patients with early medial tibiofemoral joint involvement.

Interesting facts

While bursa contain synovial-like fluid, other than the medial gastrocnemius bursa they do not actually communicate with the knee joint cavity.

Pathophysiology of osteoarthritis

Osteoarthritis is a whole joint disease; involving structural alterations in hyaline articular cartilage, subchondral bone, menisci, ligaments, capsule, synovium and periarticular muscles (see Fig. 6.3). This complex process involves mechanical, inflammatory and metabolic factors, ultimately leading to the structural changes in individual tissues and failure of the synovial joint (see Fig. 6.4). It is an active dynamic alteration arising from an imbalance between repair and destruction of joint tissues and not, as inferred from commonly using terms such 'degenerative' or 'wear-and-tear', a passive disease. Similarly, inflammation is pervasive, so the 'I' is accurate and archaic terms like 'osteoarthrosis' are out of place. There is growing awareness that the language used to describe health conditions such as osteoarthritis and back pain can have important influences on behaviours and health outcomes. Recognition that osteoarthritis is an active biological pathological process is important, as it means there is potential for interventions that will halt the disease that is, it is treatable. The key changes that occur in different joint tissues in osteoarthritis and the pathophysiological mechanisms driving these are summarized below.

Articular cartilage

Macroscopically, cartilage shows varying levels of progressive pathology from surface fibrillation through cracking, clefts and partial thickness erosion, to full-thickness loss with exposure of the underlying subchondral bone (see Fig. 6.5). In the knee joint, the areas of cartilage damage are most apparent on the surfaces exposed to highest load bearing and may be quite focal in the early phases. Prior to and underlying the gross pathology are biomolecular cartilage changes, including decreased proteoglycan (aggrecan) concentration largely through ADAMTS-4 and -5 driven proteolysis. Paradoxically despite aggrecan loss cartilage water content increases as a result of enzymatic degradation of cross-linking molecules, such as decorin, fibromodulin and other glycoproteins, allowing the collagen network to loosen, which facilitates swelling. These changes leave the cartilage less able to resist compression, more permeable to tissue breakdown products and thus the matrix and chondrocytes more prone to damage from impact loading and catabolic signals. Ultimately the collagen network itself breaks down as enzymes, particularly the collagenases (MMP-1, -2, -9 and -13) and cathepsin K, are released from stressed chondrocytes, as well as synovial lining and infiltrating inflammatory cells, meniscal fibrochondrocytes and even fibroblasts in injured ligaments.

While there is chondrocyte loss (largely through apoptosis but also necrosis) there is also evidence of increased proliferation and attempted repair, with surviving chondrocytes increasing synthesis of aggrecan and collagen type II. However, the remaining chondrocytes also show evidence of senescence and abnormal differentiation similar to that of hypertrophic chondrocytes in growth cartilage. This is accompanied by changes in their expression profile, including increased synthesis of abnormal matrix components (e.g. collagen type I, III and X, versican), catabolic enzymes (e.g. MMP-13, ADAMTS-4 and -5), and cytokines and chemokines (e.g. IL6 and CCL2). This chondrocyte de-differentiation is driven by altered mechanical loading, osmotic pressure, and autocrine and paracrine soluble mediators (e.g. TGF-β, FGF-2 and -18, IL-1 and -6, TNF, hypoxia-inducible factors (HIF-2a), Wnt pathway activators, reactive oxygen species (ROS)). The increased fibrocartilaginous content offers less compressive resistance decreasing mechanical protection to the underlying bone, and is more susceptible to mechanical disruption with further release of matrix breakdown products acting as damage-associated molecular patterns (DAMPs) that activate toll-like receptors (TLRs) and exacerbate chondrocyte catabolic process as well as being pro-inflammatory.

Interesting facts

Chondrocytes play a central role in the breakdown of cartilage in osteoarthritis by secreting matrix degrading enzymes. Aggrecan is broken down by members of the ADAMTS family (*A Disintegrin And Metalloproteinases with ThromboSpondin*) motif, ADAMTS-4 and ADAMTS-5 appear to be the most important. Specific members of a family of enzymes called matrix metalloproteinases (MMPs) breakdown fibrillar collagen; MMP-13 appears to be the most important in cartilage.

Subchondral bone

Typically in osteoarthritis the subchondral bone plate thickens and there is increased bone volume relative to total epiphyseal volume (BV/TV; see Fig. 6.6). However, there is both elevated formation by activated osteoblasts and increased number and activity of osteoclasts accelerating bone removal. This increased rate of remodelling and turnover interrupts the normal slow process of mineral accumulation and deposition resulting in relatively hypomineralized bone. Thus despite the increased volume, osteoarthritic subchondral bone is less dense and has reduced stiffness compared with normal. Additionally, there is new blood vessel formation and vascular invasion from the deeper trabecular bone into the subchondral bone and through the cement line into the deeper zones of calcified cartilage zone and even crossing the tide mark and penetrating non-calcified cartilage (see Fig. 6.6). This process is driven and facilitated by increased deep zone chondrocyte synthesis and secretion of pro-angiogenic factors (e.g. vascular endothelial growth factor (VEGF)), and loss of anti-angiogenic proteins (e.g. aggrecan, chondromodulin). These invading blood vessels have accompanying nerves and may play a key role in osteoarthritic pain.

Subchondral bone changes may vary with osteoarthritis disease stage, with greater resorption often seen early while formation may predominate later. However, change can be quite focal with areas of increased loss and increased formation concurrent in the one joint. There is often a close association between areas of bone remodelling with regions of maximal cartilage pathology, supporting the strong interdependence of these tissues and both mechanical and biological cross-talk and communication. Changes in osteocyte canalicular networks and expression and activation of bioactive factors and pathways in these cells (e.g. MMP-13, sclerostin, IL-6, TGF-β) have been shown to play a central role in not only bone remodelling but overlying cartilage pathology. Focal areas of intense subchondral and trabecular bone remodelling, detected by MRI as areas of increased hydration, are known as 'bone marrow lesions' (BMLs). BMLs show evidence of bone microdamage, repair and inflammation histologically and have variably been shown to be associated with both pain and disease progression. The evolution of these lesions can lead to necrosis and the formation of focal subchondral cysts. At the joint margins, new bone formation occurs in the form of osteophytes and enthesophytes, the former developing within the joint at or near the transition between articular cartilage and bone/periosteum, while the latter develop within attachment zones of fibrous tissues (e.g. joint capsule, ligament) to bone. Osteophytes and enthesophytes form as a result of mesenchymal stem cell activation and endochondral ossification, in association with increased inflammation (predominantly macrophages), TGF-β signalling and abnormal joint kinematics. While osteophyte and enthesophyte presence is highly correlated, the latter may be particularly prevalent in a subset of patients with high bone mass.

Meniscus

Meniscal pathology includes tears of varying configuration (vertical longitudinal, oblique, transverse/radial, horizontal and complex/degenerate), maceration/loss particularly of the inner zone, ill-defined 'intra-substance degeneration' and root/ligament tears. While many of these pathologies can be seen as incidental findings in non-osteoarthritic joints, they are more common and their presence is associated with increased risk and progression of osteoarthritis. Playing a key role in load distribution, joint stability and proprioception, disruption of meniscal function leads to increased risk of osteoarthritis and pathology on cartilage and bone through abnormal biomechanical signalling. Meniscal pathology is also associated with altered gene expression profiles, including for a number secreted factors implicated in osteoarthritis pathology in other tissues and activation of nociceptors for example, MMP-1, MMP-9, MMP-13, ADAMTS-5, IL-1, TNF, CCL3, VEGF, S100A8 and A9. Furthermore the meniscus is a rich source of potential DAMPs that can activate catabolic response in cells in other joint tissues such as cartilage and ligament, as well as an inflammatory response in the synovium.

Synovial tissues and synovial fluid

Despite the name implying an inherent inflammatory process, osteoarthritis was historically considered a non-inflammatory primarily biomechanically driven disease. However, a consistent finding from studies in patients and preclinical animal models is the presence of synovial inflammation across multiple osteoarthritis phenotypes and disease stages, and its association not just with symptoms but structural disease severity and progression. While commonly thought to be a secondary response to joint tissue breakdown in later stages of disease, synovial inflammatory mediators are more elevated acutely after joint injury, and in early compared with late osteoarthritis. Further, the presence of synovitis/joint effusion is not only associated with faster progression of established osteoarthritis but also more incident disease.

Together, the data suggest that synovial inflammation plays a key role in the initiation and progression of structural and symptomatic osteoarthritis.

Osteoarthritic synovium is characterized by lining hyperplasia and hypertrophy with increased numbers of synovial lining cells and development of villi or folds (see Fig. 6.8). There is focal infiltration of inflammatory cells (macrophages, lymphocytes, plasma cells) and an increase in the vascularity in the subintimal layer, and the joint capsule becomes thickened and fibrotic, contributing to reduced joint range of motion. Inflammatory cell influx and fibrotic changes are also seen in the infrapatellar fat pad, although with some differences noted compared with other areas of the synovium. With increased vascularization and loss of the lining cell continuity, synovial fluid volume and protein content is increased while hyaluronic acid and lubricin are decreased. This results in a reduction in fluid viscosity and other mechanical properties of the fluid, including its lubricating function. The joint fluid is still usually clear with cell counts often only slightly higher than normal ($100–2000/mm^3$) with mononuclear cells predominating (mostly monocytes and macrophages with fewer and lymphocytes). This contrasts with rheumatoid arthritis where cell counts are much higher ($5000/mm^3$) and there is a higher percentage of polymorphonuclear cells.

Activation of the innate inflammatory/immune response has been well-described in osteoarthritis, with influx of systemically derived monocytes and macrophages and their secretion of cytokines, growth factors and enzymes (e.g. IL-1 and -6, TNF, TGF-β, MMP-1 and -13, ADAMTS-4 and -5). However, lymphocytes, particularly CD4+ and CD8+ T cells are also increased in osteoarthritic synovium from very early stages of disease, and produce cytokines, chemokines and enzymes implicated in driving pathology in other joint tissues (e.g. IL-8 and -17, TNF, CCL2, MMP-1, -3 and -9). synovial, subintimal and capsular fibroblast activation contributes to synthesis of pro-inflammatory cytokines and catabolic enzymes as well as fibrosis. Similarly fibroblasts in other joint tissues such as injured cruciate ligaments can contribute to the inflammatory and catabolic milieu of the joint. The inflammatory molecules along with neurokines, neuropeptides produced by the inflammatory and stromal cells, and DAMPs released from degrading tissues contribute to a complex cycle of cross-talk that perpetuates and progresses osteoarthritic joint-wide damage and pain (Fig. 6.9).

Clinical features of osteoarthritis

Symptoms and signs of osteoarthritis are summarized in Box 6.1.

Symptoms

The key clinical features of osteoarthritis are joint pain and disability associated with varying degrees of swelling, deformity and decreased range of motion. Osteoarthritis emerges as a clinical syndrome when there is sufficient joint damage to cause impairment of function. Importantly, it has become clear that with chronicity, osteoarthritis pain in many patients includes aspects of both peripheral and central sensitization. With the former, normally non-noxious peripheral mechanical and soluble stimuli lead to excessive firing of afferents which is interpreted as pain. Centrally, changes in brain areas responsible for processing and interpreting pain as well as descending inhibitory pathways not only enhance osteoarthritic pain but may also alter motor reflexes and motor deficits.

Symptom onset is usually very gradual over a number of years, with pain as the key feature. It is likely that the structural changes occurring in the synovial joint have been progressing for many years before pain develops. The pain is usually deep, aching and poorly localized. In the early phases, it is related to activity, often being worse at the end of the day. In more advanced stages of osteoarthritis there will be pain at rest. Osteoarthritis usually progresses very slowly and symptoms will fluctuate over many years. Not all patients will progress to advanced rest-associated pain and loss of function. Studies of osteoarthritic knee X-rays suggest that only a third will progress significantly over a 10-year period.

Osteoarthritis can affect any joint but most commonly affects the hands, knees, spine (where it is called spondylosis), feet and hips. Involvement of other joints such as shoulders, elbows and wrists does occur, but other causes of arthritis should always be considered.

The cause of the pain is usually multifactorial. Interestingly, the cartilage itself, has no nerve supply and therefore is not a direct source of pain, although damaged chondrocytes may secrete neuroactive peptides that can activate nociceptors in other joint tissues. Pain

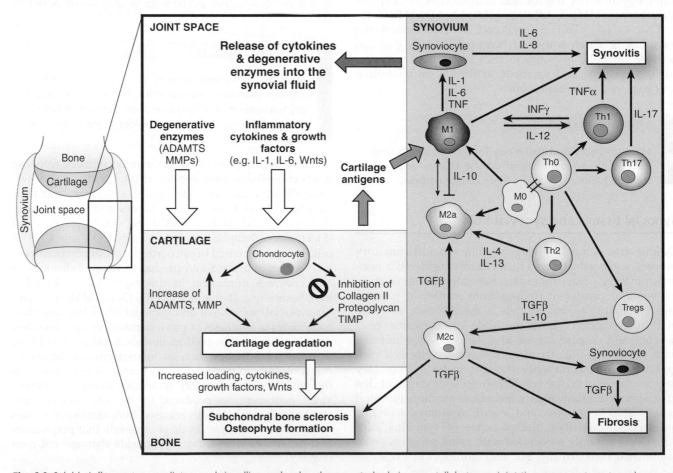

Fig. 6.9 Soluble inflammatory mediators and signalling molecules play a central role in cross-talk between joint tissue compartments and contribute to osteoarthritis propagation, progression and pain.

Box 6.1 Symptoms and signs of osteoarthritis

Symptoms

- Joint pain
  - gradual onset
  - deep, aching, poorly localized
  - activity related, worse at the end of day
  - later stages, pain at rest
- Joint stiffness
  - early feature
  - usually a few minutes, rarely exceeds 15–30 min
  - after inactivity ('gelling') and when first getting out of bed
- Crepitus
- Limitation of joint motion
- Loss of function
  - difficulty rising from chair, toilet
  - trouble turning taps

Signs

- Tenderness on palpation
- Pain on passive motion
- Crepitus on joint motion
- Joint enlargement—bony spurs and osteophytes, synovitis
- Limitation of range of motion
- Deformity

Box 6.2 Possible sources of pain in osteoarthritis

Intra-articular

- Periosteum, osteophyte formation
- Subchondral bone pressure, microfractures, engorgement
- Intra-articular ligament degeneration
- Capsule distension
- Synovitis

Periarticular

- Tendons, fasciae
- Bursitis
- Muscle spasm
- Nerve pressure

Psychosocial

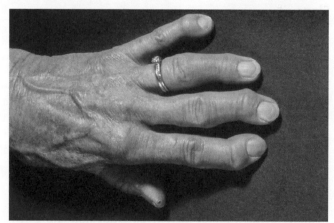

Fig. 6.10 An osteoarthritic hand with bony swelling and deformities at all the distal interphalangeal (DIP) joints (Heberden's nodes) and the third and fourth proximal interphalangeal (PIP) joints (Bouchard's nodes). Deformity is also present at the first carpometacarpal (CMC) joint at the base of the thumb.

comes from the activation of nerves both intra-articular and periarticular structures (Box 6.2). Intra-articular sources include periosteal stretching and elevation over remodelling bone and osteophyte formation, trabecular microfractures in subchondral bone, pressure on exposed subchondral bone in advanced stages, vascular engorgement of the bone, degenerative changes in intra-articular ligaments, inflammation of the synovial lining, pinching or abrasion of the synovial villi and distension of the synovial capsule.

Periarticular sources include the tissues, tendons and bursae around the joints, which become stretched and/or inflamed, spasm of the muscles around the joints or pressure on local nerves.

Joint stiffness is localized to the involved joints and usually of short duration, in contrast to the more prolonged and generalized stiffness of the inflammatory rheumatoid arthritis. It rarely lasts more than 15–30 min and is most notable when first mobilizing in the morning after waking, or after inactivity during the day (referred to as gelling), for example, long car trips, sitting in the waiting room, watching a movie.

Patients will often complain of crepitus or grating that they can feel and hear as they move the joints. Later in the course of the disease, they will notice limitation of joint movement and difficulty carrying out some activities such as turning on taps or opening jars for osteoarthritic hands; getting up from a chair or toilet seat, going

up and down stairs, bending and kneeling for osteoarthritic knees and hips. The loss of function may be quite marked early in osteoarthritic hands in the presence of pain due to inflammation and soft-tissue swelling. However, this tends to settle over months to years to leave a stiffened joint with bony enlargement (Fig. 6.10) but quite reasonable function. In osteoarthritic knees (Fig. 6.11), degenerative tears in the menisci or loose bodies of broken-off articular cartilage may lodge between other intra-articular structures during joint movement, causing locking and catching. Weakness of muscles around the joint may also cause a feeling of the joint 'giving way' in later-stage disease.

Systemic features with generalized morning stiffness, fevers, weight loss or anorexia are not features of osteoarthritis, and other causes for the pain should be considered.

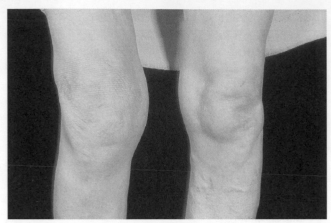

Fig. 6.11 Dilateral osteoarthritic knees with the right knee most affected. Bony swelling and low-grade soft-tissue swelling is evident, with probable effusion in the suprapatellar pouch on the right. There is some valgus deformity suggesting loss of articular cartilage from the lateral tibiofemoral joint.

Signs

The signs depend on the joints involved and the stage of the disease process, which could be at very different stages for different joints in one patient.

In the early stages, there may be very few signs. Later, joints may be tender to palpation along the joint line or surrounding tissues, particularly if synovitis is present. Pain may be present on passive motion, usually at the extremes of the joint range. Later, there is loss of full range of motion that may be due to a number of features, including change in joint surfaces, muscle spasms, and tendon and capsular fibrosis and contractures. Crepitus is often palpable on movement of the joint, and is particularly evident under the patella on flexion and extension of the knee. Crepitus appears to be due to cartilage loss and joint surface irregularity. Swelling may be palpable, both bony swelling as a result of osteophyte formation and soft-tissue swelling because of joint effusions and synovitis. In the hand, the hard swelling of the bony osteophytes classically involves the distal interphalangeal joints (called Heberden's nodes), the proximal interphalangeal joints (called Bouchard's nodes) and the first carpometacarpal joint at the base of the thumb. Ongoing joint destruction due to cartilage loss and subchondral bone collapse combined with proliferative bone overgrowth can lead to deformities, alteration in joint alignment and joint subluxation. Fusion or ankylosis of the joints is rare, apart from distal interphalangeal joints in the hands. Surrounding muscle atrophy is common, particularly at the knee, hip and thumb.

Epidemiology of osteoarthritis

Osteoarthritis, is the most common form of arthritis. It is a heterogeneous group of conditions with different parts of the skeleton being involved at different rates and hav-

ing variability in risk factors for development and progression of the disorder.

Classification

Classically, the diagnosis of osteoarthritis in epidemiological and clinical studies has been taken from the characteristic radiographic changes described in the *Atlas of Individual Radiographic Features in Osteoarthritis*. These features include (Fig. 6.12):

- formation of osteophytes on the joint margins or in ligamentous and joint-capsule attachments (enthesophytes)
- narrowing of the joint space sclerosis and/or cysts in the subchondral bone
- altered shape of the bone ends.

Prevalence estimates will vary depending on which criteria have been used to classify osteoarthritis. Prevalence of radiographic knee osteoarthritis is low before age 40 years (5%), and then increases with age, with females having greater frequency than males at each age group and at each joint site. Among 45- to 65-year-old women clinically symptomatic osteoarthritis would be expected with approximately 5% prevalence, while X-ray changes consistent with knee osteoarthritis may be present in up to 20%. Radiological estimates are higher than self-reported clinical osteoarthritis and the two are not always well correlated. Structural osteoarthritis assessed with MRI shows similar moderate associations with the presence of joint pain. With MRI we have learned that the presence and severity of pain are associated with specific osteoarthritis features such as BMLs and synovitis, and that an increase or decrease of pain within a person correlates with a change in synovitis or change in size or number of BMLs.

The diagnosis of osteoarthritis is a clinical one made based upon symptoms (pain, brief morning stiffness and functional limitations) and a limited physical examination (crepitus, restricted or painful movement, joint tenderness and bony enlargement). Appropriate use of diagnostic criteria (such as those from EULAR (EUropean League Against Rheumatism) and ACR (American College of Rheumatology)) is recommended. Plain radiographs are not needed for the diagnosis but like laboratory tests can be considered when the presentation is atypical or when other diagnoses are strongly suspected.

Risk factors for the development of osteoarthritis (Box 6.3)

Racial differences

Some racial differences have been shown in the distribution of the joints affected by osteoarthritis. For example, African-American females appear to have higher rates

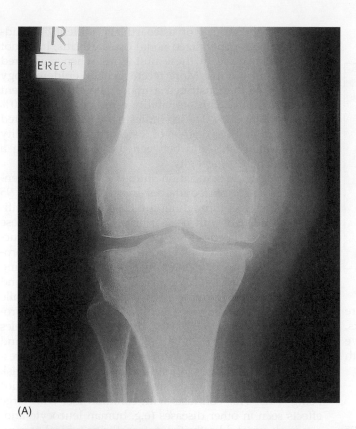

(A)

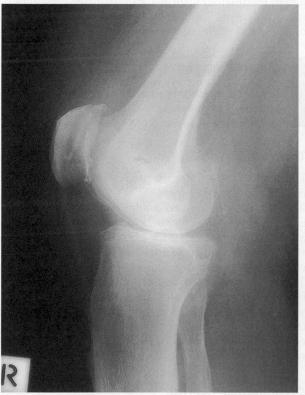

(B)

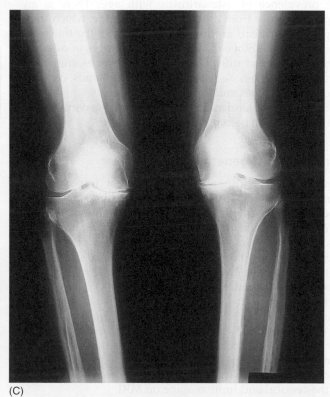

(C)

Fig. 6.12 Radiographic changes in osteoarthritis. (A) AP weight-bearing X-ray of a right knee showing moderate changes of osteoarthritis with joint space narrowing and osteophytes most marked at the medial tibiofemoral joint, and early joint space narrowing in the lateral compartment. (B) Lateral view of the same knee showing osteophytes representing moderate patellofemoral compartment osteoarthritis (C) AP weight-bearing X-ray showing typical advanced bilateral osteoarthritis most marked in the medial tibiofemoral compartments, with advanced joint space narrowing, subchondral sclerosis and varus deformity.

Box 6.3 Risk factors for the development of knee osteoarthritis

Unalterable

- Age
- Female sex
- Race
- Genetics, family history

Potentially modifiable

- Obesity
- Injury
- Muscle weakness
- Occupational overuse
- Malalignment

of knee osteoarthritis than Caucasian females but are less likely to have the Heberden's nodes; African-Blacks, Chinese and Asian-Indians have all been shown to have lower prevalence of hip osteoarthritis compared with European Caucasians.

Age

There is a dramatic increase in the incidence and thus the prevalence of osteoarthritis with age. There is an exponential rise from around 55 years of age, which then appears to plateau around 75–80 years. By the time our skeletons reach 80 years, radiological changes of osteoarthritis are almost universal in joints so far examined in large population-based studies, including hands, cervical and lumbar spines and knees.

Symptomatic and radiographic knee osteoarthritis is very uncommon before the age of 40 years.

Family history: genetic factors

Genetic factors appear to be the most important in generalized nodal (that is, accompanied by Heberden's nodes) osteoarthritis. Early studies found at least a two-fold increase in Heberden's nodes among mothers of people living with osteoarthritis and a three-fold increase among their sisters. There appears to be an autosomal dominant inheritance among females and a recessive inheritance in males.

More recently, twin studies have shown a clear genetic predisposition with a heritability of 65% for osteoarthritis of the hand, 50% for osteoarthritis of the hip and 45% for osteoarthritis of the knee when radiographs were compared between identical and non-identical twins, and a 70% heritability of degenerative disc changes seen in the cervical and lumbar spine on MRI.

Studies among rare clusters of multi-case families with early-onset, aggressive osteoarthritis have identified a number of different abnormalities/mutations in the gene for type II collagen, *COL2A1*. However, studies

among larger groups of osteoarthritic patients, including those with generalized nodal osteoarthritis, have not found an increase in these mutations when compared with control groups. More recent genetic epidemiology studies have demonstrated a major genetic component to osteoarthritis, with heritability estimates of over 50% for most joint sites. These studies have also highlighted differences in the degree of osteoarthritis heritability between joint sites and between the sexes, implying a high level of heterogeneity.

Genome wide association studies (GWAS) have identified 124 single nucleotide polymorphisms (SNPs) in 95 independent loci throughout the genome that are significantly associated with osteoarthritis risk. Many of these SNPs are associated with genes encoding cartilage structural proteins (e.g. *COL9A1*, *COL11A1*, *COMP*), and proteins involved in cytokine and growth factor signalling (e.g. *GDF5*, *TGFB1*, *TGFA*, *SMAD3*, *BMP5*, *FGF18*), and cell growth and differentiation (e.g. *SOX9*, *NF1*). While some variants affect the structural properties of the protein, the majority (~90%) of osteoarthritis risk alleles reside in non-protein coding regions of the genome and likely function through regulating nearby gene expression. The effect sizes of individual osteoarthritis risk alleles are generally quite small, with most odds ratios being <-1.5. This contrasts with common loci with large effects seen in other diseases (e.g. human leucocyte antigen in rheumatoid arthritis), osteoarthritis typical of common, polygenic diseases associated with inheritance of multiple risk alleles of modest individual impact.

Interesting facts

Numerous osteoarthritis susceptibility genetic mutations have been identified, all with low individual effect sizes and the majority in non-protein coding regions.

Trauma/injury

Joint injury is a well-documented risk factor for subsequent osteoarthritis development. This is shown for major ligamentous damage around a joint or damage to the bones and growth plates within joints. Injury is particularly apparent as a risk factor for knee osteoarthritis in the setting of a damaged or removed meniscus, or derangement of the supportive anterior cruciate or collateral ligaments. The time lag between significant injury and development of clinically apparent osteoarthritis in the order of 10–15 years in human studies. In experimental animal models of osteoarthritis, however, the articular cartilage damage occurs very early following anterior cruciate ligament disruption or removal of the medial meniscus.

Occupational 'overuse'

Certain occupations that involve repeated heavy use of particular joints over long periods of time have been associated with the development of osteoarthritis. Occupations that require repeated knee bending, heavy lifting, climbing and carrying have shown an increase in knee osteoarthritis, particularly for males, while farmers appear to be at particular risk for hip osteoarthritis.

Obesity

Obesity is associated with the development of knee osteoarthritis in both sexes but the association is strongest for women. Initial epidemiological evidence was cross-sectional but the association has now been confirmed in a number of prospective studies. Mean body mass index is significantly higher among those with knee osteoarthritis than those without. The risk of osteoarthritis is increased at least two-fold when those in the heaviest groups are compared with individuals in the lightest groups. In addition, obesity is a predictor of disability related to radiographic changes and also appears to be related to the radiological progression of osteoarthritis once identified. At a population level, obesity represents one of the most important potentially modifiable risk factors for osteoarthritis of the knee, along with prevention of joint injury. The association is not as strong with osteoarthritis of hips or hands but numerous studies have demonstrated a significant risk of incident and worsening osteoarthritis in these joints with higher body mass index. The association in non-load-bearing joints (hand) is consistent with data from preclinical animal models that soluble mediators from and pro-inflammatory metabolic effects of adipose tissue may be more important than mechanical body mass and mechanical loading in the obesity-associated osteoarthritis risk.

> ### Interesting facts
>
> Obesity is a major modifiable risk factor for osteoarthritis of the knee, particularly in women.

Sport and recreational activities

There is consensus that extreme levels of physical activity among elite competitive sportsmen and women may lead to a greater risk of osteoarthritis of the knees and hips. However, although epidemiological studies have shown conflicting results, a moderate level of activity, in the absence of joint injury or anatomical malalignment, is unlikely to be a risk factor for the development of osteoarthritis.

These factors and other secondary causes of osteoarthritis may predispose to the development of osteoarthritis, as shown in Fig. 6.13.

Risk factors for progression

Epidemiological studies have identified female gender, obesity, quadriceps strength, malalignment and having nodal hand osteoarthritis as strong predictors of radiological progression of knee osteoarthritis. In addition, some preliminary reports have shown associations with

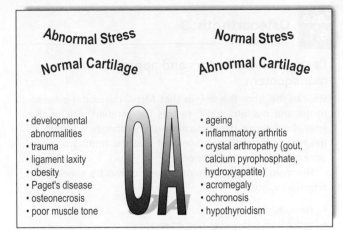

Fig. 6.13 The factors contributing to secondary osteoarthritis. Factors are divided into two groups: those that place abnormal stress on baseline normal cartilage; and those that have abnormalities in biochemistry or structure of the articular cartilage but are not subject to abnormal stresses. It is recognized that some individuals will have contribution from multiple factors covering both groupings.

other factors that warrant further study. These include a raised C-reactive protein and positive technetium bone scan suggestive of inflammation, a diet low in vitamin C and other antioxidants, and low vitamin D.

Management of osteoarthritis

Management of osteoarthritis has focused on symptom modification, predominantly characterized by pain relief. As the mechanisms surrounding joint failure are likely to be multivariate in nature, it is likely that strategies to modify disease progression will also need to target multiple mechanisms. Despite many promising *in vitro* and *in vivo* animal experiments, to date no disease or structure-modifying drug for osteoarthritis has been approved by regulatory bodies for this indication. The main candidates that have shown some promise in trials include those slowing the rate of cartilage degeneration (e.g. FGF-18, Wnt pathway inhibitors), modifying bone turnover (e.g. bisphosphonates, cathepsin K inhibition) and targeting inflammation/synovitis (e.g. IL-1 inhibition).

Nevertheless, there is now considerable scientific evidence about what can be done to help prevent osteoarthritis from getting worse. The myths that 'nothing can be done about it' and that 'it is just something to be put up with' need to be dispelled. The knowledge that the disease progresses only *very* slowly over 10 years in the majority of knee osteoarthritis patients and that most will not need joint replacement surgery can make a big difference to the patient's outlook.

All patients presenting with symptomatic osteoarthritis of the knee should be given education, an exercise prescription, guidance for weight loss if above a healthy weight and suggestions for pain relief. Management should start with these principles and continue with

THE SYNOVIAL JOINT IN HEALTH AND DISEASE: OSTEOARTHRITIS

Case 6.1 Osteoarthritis: 3

Case note: risk factors and approach to management

We can see from the details that Mrs C has nodal osteoarthritis and numerous risk factors for osteoarthritis of the knee, including a strong family history, obesity, a history of trauma, anatomical malalignment and the finding of more generalized joint involvement.

The main features of management of Mrs C's knee osteoarthritis include:

- pain reduction
- reduction and prevention of disability
- modification of risk factors
- prevention of progression

them throughout. Thus, at whatever stage in the disease process a patient is seen, education and discussion about the disease and these core treatment measures should be undertaken. Treatments supported by randomized controlled trial evidence are listed in Box 6.4.

The typical management approach to symptomatic osteoarthritis of the knee is shown in Box 6.5 and discussed further below.

Patient education and support

Patient education and self-help courses have been shown in randomized trials to be modestly effective and associated with reduced pain, increased wellbeing, increased knowledge, reduced use of healthcare services and increased compliance with exercises. The effect sizes are small for these types of interventions, however, all osteoarthritis guidelines and chronic disease management programmes strongly recommend education about the disease and active self-management strategies to explain the importance of exercise and weight loss in particular. Clinical status and symptoms have also been shown in small randomized trials to be improved if patients are contacted regularly by telephone.

Exercise

Exercise is also important at all stages of knee osteoarthritis. The quadriceps muscle wastes early and quickly when there is pain and even more so when there is swelling as well. Maintaining quadriceps strength, which is the main support mechanism for the knee, may help prevent radiological progression and disability. Regular aerobic exercises have been shown in elderly men and women with established osteoarthritis to be safe and effective in reducing pain and improving wellbeing. Exercises to improve aerobic fitness, muscle strength and range of motion are

Box 6.4 Treatments with randomized controlled trial evidence for symptomatic benefit in knee osteoarthritis

Non-pharmacological

- Patient education and self-management
- Exercise—aerobic, muscle strengthening, range of motion, Tai Chi
- Knee braces for varus or valgus instability
- Weight loss—reduced kilojoule intake and exercise
- TENs
- Regular telephone contact

Topical/injectable

- Capsaicin
- Anti-inflammatory gels
- Intra-/periarticular corticosteroids

Oral

- Non-steroidal anti-inflammatory drugs
- COX-2 selective NSAIDs
- Duloxetine

Box 6.5 Key steps in management

Step 1

Education, reassurance, exercises, intermittent or regular analgesics, topical preparations

- *Non-pharmacological intervention:* patient education, reassurance, strengthening exercises, weight reduction counselling, orthotics, walking aid
- *Topical treatment:* anti-inflammatory (e.g. diclofenac, ketoprofen, piroxicam, methylsalicylate) or analgesic capsaicin-based creams (which act by depleting substance P in nociceptors) used up to four times daily

Step 2

Step 1 + trial of NSAIDs, ± intra-articular steroids

- Lowest dose of least toxic NSAIDs, e.g. ibuprofen 400–800 mg b.d. or diclofenac 50 mg b.d.
- In high-risk patients (elderly, previous ulcer history), consider prophylaxis with misoprostol or proton pump inhibitors (e.g. omeprazole, lansoprazole) or use of the COX-2 selective NSAIDs (celecoxib).
- Consider intra-articular or periarticular corticosteroids if there are elements of inflammation clinically.

Step 3

Consider surgery

all highly recommended for osteoarthritis management at all stages of the disease. The psychosocial benefits of exercise should also not be underestimated. Exercise and increased physical activity when combined with weight loss strategies have the greatest chance of reducing the pain and disability associated with knee osteoarthritis in those who are overweight. Referral to a physiotherapist may aid the process and encourage ongoing adherence to exercise recommendations.

Weight reduction

The majority of patients with knee and/or hip osteoarthritis are overweight. Sound epidemiological evidence has shown that being overweight is strongly associated with radiological progression and disability of knee osteoarthritis. Recent randomized trials combining weight loss and exercise strategies have resulted in improvement in symptoms with a reduction in pain and an increase in mobility and physical function. It has yet to be proven in prospective randomized studies whether weight reduction can help prevent progression of the arthritis.

TENS

TENS (transcutaneous electrical nerve stimulation) machines has been shown in randomized placebo-controlled trials to reduce pain associated with osteoarthritis of the knee.

Other non-pharmacological interventions

Walking aids, knee braces in the presence of varus or valgus instability and thermotherapy (both hot and cold) have been shown to provide small improvements in symptomatic knee osteoarthritis.

Analgesics

Pharmacologic modalities most often recommended in the guidelines include paracetamol/acetaminophen and non-steroid anti-inflammatory drugs (NSAIDs). Acetaminophen was historically the first-line pain medication for osteoarthritis, however, a recent meta-analysis [da Costa 2017] concluded that given the very small effect sizes (below 0.2) when compared with placebo, along with safety concerns, it has little role as a single agent for the treatment of osteoarthritis.

Non-steroidal anti-inflammatory drugs

These agents have been discussed in Chapter 1. Individual patient variability in response to both efficacy and toxicity has been documented and it may be worth trying several different NSAID regimens. One systematic review was unable to detect a significant difference in efficacy between different NSAIDs for osteoarthritis of the knee, while another meta-analysis observed a hierarchy for toxicity, with ibuprofen and diclofenac consistently showing the lowest peptic ulcer risk and longer-acting

NSAIDs such as piroxicam and ketoprofen the highest risk. NSAIDs are often preferred over paracetamol for short-term symptom relief but side-effects from NSAIDs are common, particularly in the elderly, in patients with reduced renal function or in those who are taking anti-hypertensives so their long-term use is not recommended. All guidelines suggest these agents should be used at the lowest dose for the shortest duration possible to provide symptom relief.

Several NSAID compounds (celecoxib, meloxicam) have been developed that have selectivity for blocking the cyclooxygenase 2 (COX-2) enzyme responsible for the production of prostaglandins at sites of inflammation, without blocking cyclooxygenase 1 (COX-1), which is expressed constitutively and is responsible for the production of prostaglandins in the gastric mucosa where it has a protective effect. These NSAIDs appear to have equivalent efficacy to available NSAIDs but with reduced propensity to cause gastric irritation. They appear not to have any effect on thromboxane and platelet activity, so do not confer any anticoagulant or anti-platelet risk or benefit. They still have the potential to exacerbate fluid retention, renal insufficiency, hypertension and congestive cardiac failure and must be used with caution in patients with these co-morbidities.

Topical therapies

Topical anti-inflammatory gels and creams can provide small improvements in pain and stiffness.

> **Interesting facts**
>
> Management of osteoarthritis should include a combination of non-pharmacological and pharmacological interventions.

Corticosteroids

Intra-articular corticosteroids are recommended for hip and knee osteoarthritis for patients who have not responded to oral or topical analgesics. However, the most recent Cochrane review concluded that the evidence for clinically important benefits of intra-articular corticosteroids for knee osteoarthritis up to six weeks (effect size 0.41) remains unclear in view of the overall low quality of trials. Controversy about this treatment has been raised recently because a randomized study indicated that a three monthly intra-articular injection with corticosteroids in knee osteoarthritis patients over two years resulted in slightly more loss of cartilage volume over this period than the placebo treatment did; it however is unknown whether such slight differences have an impact on long-term clinical outcomes.

Duloxetine, mentioned in some guidelines to consider for refractory pain, is a serotonin and norepinephrine reuptake inhibitor with antidepressant, central pain inhibitory and anxiolytic activities.

There are a large number of treatments that are widely used in the management of osteoarthritis that are not recommended in a variety of guidelines, including acupuncture, intra-articular hyaluronic acid injections, glucosamine/chondroitin, opioids. Their lack of endorsement in guidelines in part relates to either lack of effect over and above placebo or alternatively considerable harm or both.

Surgery

The main principles of surgical treatment for osteoarthritis are:

- to improve pain
- to correct deformity.

For knee osteoarthritis, the types of surgery available include arthroscopy, osteotomy, arthroplasty and arthrodesis.

Arthroscopy

Arthroscopic knee surgery, the most common elective orthopaedic procedure, continues to be widely used for the management of knee osteoarthritis despite lacking evidence of efficacy. Arthroscopy may be useful in the setting of a joint that is locked because this may be due to a degenerative meniscal tear or loose body. In the absence of this pathology, there is good evidence that arthroscopy will not benefit the diffusely arthritic knee.

Osteotomy

This involves the cutting of a wedge of bone and pinning to realign the weight-bearing surfaces of the knee. It is most useful in younger patients (under 55 years) in whom the osteoarthritis is limited to the medial tibiofemoral compartment and significant genu varum has developed. It does not alter the joint surfaces but redistributes the weight bearing more evenly through the medial and lateral compartments. It has a modest success rate.

Arthroplasty

Joint replacement involves the cutting away of the diseased surfaces of the joint and its replacement with artificial components of metal and special plastic. This usually involves a complete resurfacing of the femoral and tibial condyles, with or without a button on the back of the patella. Pain relief is usually dramatic but range of motion rarely goes back to normal. Recently, partial or hemi-arthroplasty has had a revival in which just one compartment of the joint is replaced (usually the medial tibiofemoral compartment). This is only successful in the setting of osteoarthritis limited to that one compartment and in the absence of significant malalignment.

Case 6.1 **Osteoarthritis: 4**

Case note: management

Mrs C was referred to a self-management programme, given advice on weight reduction and an exercise programme that included daily quadriceps straight-leg raising exercises, walking 2–3 times a week for 20 min and attending a weekly Tai Chi class. She massages her knee with a topical anti-inflammatory gel when needed. Her symptoms are reasonably controlled with this and to date she does not require NSAIDs and is unlikely to require surgery for many years.

Arthrodesis

Joint fusion is considered, rarely, for knee osteoarthritis in the setting of a joint that has failed because of repeated infection. Although it achieves pain relief, it is very disabling to live with a stiff leg.

When to have surgery?

Referral of patients with end-stage osteoarthritis to a surgeon should be considered when all appropriate conservative options, delivered for a reasonable period, have failed. The decision to refer to an orthopaedic surgeon should occur when there is a significant decline in quality of life because of end-stage osteoarthritis. The characteristics of end-stage osteoarthritis include joint pain which disrupts normal sleep patterns, causes a severe reduction in walking distance, and marked restriction of activities of daily living.

The choice of surgical management is dependent on a number of patient-related factors, including age, anatomical alignment and mechanical stability of the knee, and the level of pain and disability. Total knee joint replacement is a highly cost-effective operation resulting in a significant reduction in pain and disability and improvement in quality of life in the majority, with benefits being sustained for up to 10 years in more than 80% of patients.

Further reading

Alliston T, Hernandez CJ, Findlay DM, et al. Bone marrow lesions in osteoarthritis: What lies beneath. *Journal of Orthopaedic Research* 36(7):1818 1825, 2018, https://doi.org/10.1002/jor.23844 [published Online First: 2017/12/22].

Altman R, Asch E, Bloch D, et al. Development of criteria for the classification and reporting of osteoarthritis. Classification of osteoarthritis of the knee. Diagnostic and Therapeutic Criteria Committee of the American Rheumatism Association. *Arthritis & Rheumatism* 29(8):1039–1049, 1986.

Altman RD, Hochberg M, Murphy Jr WA, et al. Atlas of individual radiographic features in osteoarthritis. *Osteoarthritis Cartilage* 3(Suppl A):3–70, 1995, [published Online First: 1995/09/01].

Altman, R.D., Jr., Hochberg, M., Murphy, W.A., et al. (1995). Atlas of individual radiographic features in osteoarthritis. Osteoarthritis and Cartilage 33 (Suppl A), 3–70.

Andrews SHJ, Adesida AB, Abusara Z, et al. Current concepts on structure-function relationships in the menisci. *Connective Tissue Research* 58(3-4):271–281, 2017, https://doi.org/10.1080/03008207.2017.1303489 [published Online First: 2017/03/08].

Ashraf S, Mapp PI, Walsh DA: Contributions of angiogenesis to inflammation, joint damage, and pain in a rat model of osteoarthritis. *Arthritis & Rheumatology* 63(9):2700–2710, 2011, https://doi.org/10.1002/art.30422 [published Online First: 2011/05/04].

Aso K, Shahtaheri SM, Hill R, et al. Contribution of nerves within osteochondral channels to osteoarthritis knee pain in humans and rats. *Osteoarthritis Cartilage* 28(9):1245–1254, 2020, https://doi.org/10.1016/j.joca.2020.05.010 [published Online First: 2020/05/30].

Atukorala I, Kwoh CK, Guermazi A, et al. Synovitis in knee osteoarthritis: a precursor of disease?. *Annals of Rheumatic Diseases* 75(2):390–395, 2016, https://doi.org/10.1136/annrheumdis-2014-205894 [published Online First: 2014/12/10].

Aubourg G, Rice SJ, Bruce-Wootton P, et al. Genetics of osteoarthritis. *Osteoarthritis Cartilage*, 2021 https://doi.org/10.1016/j.joca.2021.03.002 [published Online First: 2021/03/17].

Ayral X, Pickering EH, Woodworth TG, et al. Synovitis: a potential predictive factor of structural progression of medial tibiofemoral knee osteoarthritis - results of a 1 year longitudinal arthroscopic study in 422 patients. *Osteoarthritis Cartilage* 13(5):361–367, 2005, https://doi.org/10.1016/j.joca.2005.01.005 [published Online First: 2005/05/11].

Bailey KN, Nguyen J, Yee CS, et al. Mechanosensitive Control of Articular Cartilage and Subchondral Bone Homeostasis in Mice Requires Osteocytic Transforming Growth Factor β Signaling. *Arthritis & Rheumatology (Hoboken, NJ)* 73(3):414–425, 2021, https://doi.org/10.1002/art.41548 [published Online First: 2020/10/07].

Bannuru, R. R., et al. (2019). OARSI guidelines for the non-surgical management of hip, knee and polyarticular osteoarthritis. *Osteoarthritis and Cartilage*, 27(11), 1578–1589.

Belluzzi E, Stocco E, Pozzuoli A, et al. Contribution of Infrapatellar Fat Pad and Synovial Membrane to Knee Osteoarthritis Pain. *Biomed Research International* 2019:6390182, 2019, https://doi.org/10.1155/2019/6390182 [published Online First: 2019/05/03].

Benito MJ, Veale DJ, FitzGerald O, et al. Synovial tissue inflammation in early and late osteoarthritis. *Annals of Rheumatic Diseases* 64(9):1263–1267, 2005, doi: ard.2004.025270 [pii] 10.1136/ard.2004.025270 [doi] [published Online First: 2005/02/26].

Blaker CL, Little CB, Clarke EC: Joint loads resulting in ACL rupture: Effects of age, sex, and body mass on injury load and mode of failure in a mouse model. *Journal of Orthopaedic Research* 35(8):1754–1763, 2017, https://doi.org/10.1002/jor.23418 [published Online First: 2016/09/08].

Blaker CL, Ashton DM, Doran N, et al. Sex- and injury-based differences in knee biomechanics in mouse models of post-traumatic osteoarthritis. *Journal of Biomechanics* 114:110152, 2021, https://doi.org/10.1016/j.jbiomech.2020.110152 [published Online First: 2020/12/08].

Block JA: Osteoarthritis: OA guidelines: improving care or merely codifying practice?, *Nature Reviews Rheumatology* 10(6):324–326, 2014, doi: nrrheum.2014.61 [pii] 10.1038/nrrheum.2014.61 [published Online First: 2014/04/23].

Bonnet CS, Walsh DA: Osteoarthritis, angiogenesis and inflammation. *Rheumatology (Oxford)* 44(1):7–16, 2005, https://doi.org/10.1093/rheumatology/keh344 [published Online First: 2004/08/05].

Boyde A: The Bone Cartilage Interface and Osteoarthritis. *Calcified Tissue International*, 2021https://doi.org/10.1007/s00223-021-00866-9 [published Online First: 2021/06/05].

Brandt K, Radin E, Dieppe P, et al. *Yet more evidence that osteoarthritis is not a cartilage disease*. BMJ Publishing Group Ltd and European League Against Rheumatism, 2006.

Brignardello-Petersen R, Guyatt GH, Buchbinder R, et al. Knee arthroscopy versus conservative management in patients with degenerative knee disease: a systematic review. *BMJ Open* 7(5), 2017https://doi.org/10.1136/bmjopen-2017-016114 e016114.

Brophy RH, Rai MF, Zhang Z, et al. Molecular analysis of age and sex-related gene expression in meniscal tears with and without a concomitant anterior cruciate ligament tear. *Journal of Bone and Joint Surgery, American* 94(5):385–393, 2012, https://doi.org/10.2106/jbjs.K.00919 [published Online First: 2012/03/01].

Brophy RH, Tycksen ED, Sandell LJ, et al. Changes in Transcriptome-Wide Gene Expression of Anterior Cruciate Ligament Tears Based on Time From Injury. *American Journal of Sports Medicine* 44(8):2064–2075, 2016, https://doi.org/10.1177/0363546516643810 [published Online First: 2016/05/10].

Brophy RH, Sandell LJ, Cheverud JM, et al. Gene expression in human meniscal tears has limited association with early degenerative changes in knee articular cartilage. *Connective Tissue Research* 58(3-4):295–304, 2017, https://doi.org/10.1080/03008207.2016.1211114 [published Online First: 2016/07/21].

Brophy RH, Sandell LJ, Rai MF: Traumatic and Degenerative Meniscus Tears Have Different Gene Expression Signatures. *American Journal of Sports Medicine* 45(1):114–120, 2017, https://doi.org/10.1177/0363546516664889 [published Online First: 2016/09/09].

Brophy RH, Rothermich MA, Tycksen ED, et al. Presence of meniscus tear alters gene expression profile of anterior cruciate ligament tears. *Journal of Orthopaedic Research* 36(10):2612–2621, 2018, https://doi.org/10.1002/jor.24025 [published Online First: 2018/04/19].

Brophy RH, Zhang B, Cai L, et al. Transcriptome comparison of meniscus from patients with and without osteoarthritis. *Osteoarthritis Cartilage* 26(3):422–432, 2018, https://doi.org/10.1016/j.joca.2017.12.004 [published Online First: 2017/12/21].

Carballo CB, Nakagawa Y, Sekiya I, et al.: Basic Science of Articular Cartilage, *Clinics in Sports Medicine* 36(3):413–425, 2017, https://doi.org/10.1016/j.csm.2017.02.001 [published Online First: 2017/06/05].

Chang PS, Brophy RH: As Goes the Meniscus Goes the Knee: Early, Intermediate, and Late Evidence for the Detrimental Effect of Meniscus Tears. *Clinics in Sports Medicine* 39(1):29–36, 2020, https://doi.org/10.1016/j.csm.2019.08.001 [published Online First: 2019/11/27].

Chen Z, Ma Y, Li X, et al. The Immune Cell Landscape in Different Anatomical Structures of Knee in Osteoarthritis: A Gene Expression-Based Study. *Biomed Research International* 2020:9647072, 2020, https://doi.org/10.1155/2020/9647072 [published Online First: 2020/04/08].

Chinzei N, Brophy RH, Duan X, et al. Molecular influence of anterior cruciate ligament tear remnants on chondrocytes: a biologic connection between injury and osteoarthritis. *Osteoarthritis Cartilage* 26(4):588–599, 2018, https://doi.org/10.1016/j.joca.2018.01.017 [published Online First: 2018/02/03].

Chou CH, Jain V, Gibson J, et al. Synovial cell cross-talk with cartilage plays a major role in the pathogenesis of osteoarthritis.

Scientific Reports 10(1):10868, 2020, https://doi.org/10.1038/s41598-020-67730-y [published Online First: 2020/07/04].

Clockaerts S, Bastiaansen-Jenniskens YM, Runhaar J, et al. The infrapatellar fat pad should be considered as an active osteoarthritic joint tissue: a narrative review. *Osteoarthritis Cartilage* 18(7):876–882, 2010, https://doi.org/10.1016/j.joca.2010.03.014 [published Online First: 2010/04/27].

Cook JL, Kuroki K, Stoker AM, et al. Meniscal biology in health and disease. *Connective Tissue Research* 58(3-4):225–237, 2017, https://doi.org/10.1080/03008207.2016.1243670 [published Online First: 2016/10/08].

Culemann S, Grüneboom A, Nicolás-Ávila J, et al. Locally renewing resident synovial macrophages provide a protective barrier for the joint. *Nature* 572(7771):670–675, 2019, https://doi.org/10.1038/s41586-019-1471-1 [published Online First: 2019/08/09].

Culliford DJ, Maskell J, Kiran A, et al. The lifetime risk of total hip and knee arthroplasty: results from the UK general practice research database. *Osteoarthritis Cartilage* 20(6):519–524, 2012, https://doi.org/10.1016/j.joca.2012.02.636 [published Online First: 2012/03/08].

da Costa BR, Reichenbach S, Keller N, et al. Effectiveness of non-steroidal anti-inflammatory drugs for the treatment of pain in knee and hip osteoarthritis: a network meta-analysis. *Lancet* 390(10090):e21–e33, 2017, doi: S0140-6736(17)31744-0 [pii] 10.1016/S0140-6736(17)31744-0 [published Online First: 2017/07/13].

de Lange-Brokaar BJ, Ioan-Facsinay A, Yusuf E, et al. Evolution of synovitis in osteoarthritic knees and its association with clinical features. *Osteoarthritis Cartilage* 24(11):1867–1874, 2016, https://doi.org/10.1016/j.joca.2016.05.021 [published Online First: 2016/10/21].

de Lange-Brokaar BJ, Ioan-Facsinay A, van Osch GJ, et al. Synovial inflammation, immune cells and their cytokines in osteoarthritis: a review. *Osteoarthritis Cartilage* 20(12):1484–1499, 2012, https://doi.org/10.1016/j.joca.2012.08.027 [published Online First: 2012/09/11].

Dole NS, Yee CS, Mazur CM, et al. TGFβ Regulation of Perilacunar/Canalicular Remodeling Is Sexually Dimorphic. *Journal of Bone and Mineral Research* 35(8):1549–1561, 2020, https://doi.org/10.1002/jbmr.4023 [published Online First: 2020/04/14].

Driban JB, Harkey MS, Barbe MF, et al. Risk factors and the natural history of accelerated knee osteoarthritis: a narrative review. *BMC Musculoskeletal Disorders* 21(1):332, 2020, https://doi.org/10.1186/s12891-020-03367-2 [published Online First: 2020/05/31].

Dudek M, Angelucci C, Pathiranage D, et al. Circadian time series proteomics reveals daily dynamics in cartilage physiology. *Osteoarthritis Cartilage* 29(5):739–749, 2021, https://doi.org/10.1016/j.joca.2021.02.008 [published Online First: 2021/02/22].

Englund M, Roemer FW, Hayashi D, et al. Meniscus pathology, osteoarthritis and the treatment controversy. *Nature Reviews Rheumatology* 8(7):412–419, 2012, https://doi.org/10.1038/nrrheum.2012.69 [published Online First: 2012/05/23].

Fan X, Wu X, Crawford R, et al. Macro, Micro, and Molecular. Changes of the Osteochondral Interface in Osteoarthritis Development. *Frontiers in Cell and Developmental Biology* 9:659654, 2021, https://doi.org/10.3389/fcell.2021.659654 [published Online First: 2021/05/28].

Felson DT, Niu J, Neogi T, et al. Synovitis and the risk of knee osteoarthritis: the MOST Study. *Osteoarthritis Cartilage* 24(3):458–464, 2016, https://doi.org/10.1016/j.joca.2015.09.013 [published Online First: 2015/10/04].

Ferrao Blanco MN, Bastiaansen-Jenniskens YM, Chambers MG, et al. Effect of Inflammatory Signaling on Human Articular Chondrocyte Hypertrophy: Potential Involvement of Tissue Repair Macrophages. *Cartilage*, 2021https://doi.org/10.1177/19476035211021907 19476035211021907. [published Online First: 2021/06/25].

Folkesson E, Turkiewicz A, Ali N, et al. Proteomic comparison of osteoarthritic and reference human menisci using data-independent acquisition mass spectrometry. *Osteoarthritis Cartilage* 28(8):1092–1101, 2020, https://doi.org/10.1016/j.joca.2020.05.001 [published Online First: 2020/05/15].

Folkesson E, Turkiewicz A, Rydén M, et al. Proteomic characterization of the normal human medial meniscus body using data-independent acquisition mass spectrometry. *Journal of Orthopaedic Research* 38(8):1735–1745, 2020, https://doi.org/10.1002/jor.24602 [published Online First: 2020/01/29].

Frank CB: Ligament structure, physiology and function. *Journal of Musculoskeletal Neuronal Interactions* 4(2):199–201, 2004, [published Online First: 2004/12/24].

Frank CB, Hart DA, Shrive NG: Molecular biology and biomechanics of normal and healing ligaments--a review. *Osteoarthritis Cartilage* 7(1):130–140, 1999, https://doi.org/10.1053/joca.1998.0168 [published Online First: 1999/06/15].

Fu K, Robbins SR, McDougall JJ: Osteoarthritis: the genesis of pain. *Rheumatology (Oxford)* 57(suppl_4):iv43–iv50, 2018, https://doi.org/10.1093/rheumatology/kex419 [published Online First: 2017/12/22].

Geraghty T, Winter DR, Miller RJ, et al. Neuroimmune interactions and osteoarthritis pain: focus on macrophages. *Pain Reports* 6(1):e892, 2021, https://doi.org/10.1097/pr9.0000000000000892 [published Online First: 2021/05/14].

Goldring SR, Goldring MB: Bone and cartilage in osteoarthritis: is what's best for one good or bad for the other?. *Arthritis Research & Therapy* 12(5):143, 2010, ar3135 [pii] 10.1186/ar3135 [doi] [published Online First: 2010/11/04].

Goldring SR, Goldring MB: Changes in the osteochondral unit during osteoarthritis: structure, function and cartilage-bone crosstalk. *Nature Reviews Rheumatology* 12(11):632–644, 2016, https://doi.org/10.1038/nrrheum.2016.148 [published Online First: 2016/10/21].

Griffin TM, Scanzello CR: Innate inflammation and synovial macrophages in osteoarthritis pathophysiology. *Clinical Experimental Rheumatology* 37(Suppl 120(5)):57–63, 2019, [published Online First: 2019/10/18].

Han D, Fang Y, Tan X, et al. The emerging role of fibroblast-like synoviocytes-mediated synovitis in osteoarthritis: An update. *Journal of Cellular and Molecular Medicine* 24(17):9518–9532, 2020, https://doi.org/10.1111/jcmm.15669 [published Online First: 2020/07/21].

Hardcastle SA, Dieppe P, Gregson CL, et al. Osteophytes, enthesophytes, and high bone mass: a bone-forming triad with potential relevance in osteoarthritis. *Arthritis & Rheumatology (Hoboken, NJ)* 66(9):2429–2439, 2014, https://doi.org/10.1002/art.38729 [published Online First: 2014/06/10].

Haywood L, McWilliams DF, Pearson CI, et al. Inflammation and angiogenesis in osteoarthritis. *Arthritis & Rheumatology* 48(8):2173–2177, 2003, https://doi.org/10.1002/art.11094 [published Online First: 2003/08/09].

Hsia AW, Emami AJ, Tarke FD, et al. Osteophytes and fracture calluses share developmental milestones and are diminished by unloading. *Journal of Orthopaedic Research* 36(2):699–710, 2018, https://doi.org/10.1002/jor.23779 [published Online First: 2017/10/24].

Hsueh MF, Khabut A, Kjellström S, et al. Elucidating the Molecular Composition of Cartilage by Proteomics. *Journal of Proteome Research* 15(2):374–388, 2016, https://doi.org/10.1021/acs.jproteome.5b00946 [published Online First: 2015/12/04].

Hu Y, Chen X, Wang S, et al. Subchondral bone microenvironment in osteoarthritis and pain. *Bone Res* 9(1):20, 2021, https://

doi.org/10.1038/s41413-021-00147-z [published Online First: 2021/03/19].

Hunter, D. J., & Bierma-Zeinstra, S. (2019). Osteoarthritis. *Lancet*, *393*(10182), 1745–1759.

Hunter D, Pietro-Alhambra D, Arden N: *Osteoarthritis*, Second ed., Oxford, 2014, Oxford University Press.

Ioan-Facsinay A, Kloppenburg M: An emerging player in knee osteoarthritis: the infrapatellar fat pad. *Arthritis Research & Therapy* 15(6):225, 2013, https://doi.org/10.1186/ar4422 [published Online First: 2013/12/26].

Juni P, Hari R, Rutjes AW, et al. Intra-articular corticosteroid for knee osteoarthritis. *Cochrane Database of Systematic Reviews*(10), 2015https://doi.org/10.1002/14651858.CD005328.pub3 CD005328. [published Online First: 2015/10/23].

Kawaguchi H: Endochondral ossification signals in cartilage degradation during osteoarthritis progression in experimental mouse models. *Molecules and Cells* 25(1):1–6, 2008, [published Online First: 2008/03/06].

Klein-Wieringa IR, de Lange-Brokaar BJ, Yusuf E, et al. Inflammatory Cells in Patients with Endstage Knee Osteoarthritis: A Comparison between the Synovium and the Infrapatellar Fat Pad. *Journal of Rheumatology* 43(4):771–778, 2016, https://doi.org/10.3899/jrheum.151068 [published Online First: 2016/03/17].

Klein-Wieringa IR, Kloppenburg M, Bastiaansen-Jenniskens YM, et al. The infrapatellar fat pad of patients with osteoarthritis has an inflammatory phenotype. *Annals of Rheumatic Diseases* 70(5):851–857, 2011, https://doi.org/10.1136/ard.2010.140046 [published Online First: 2011/01/19].

Kurowska-Stolarska M, Alivernini S: Synovial tissue macrophages: friend or foe?. *RMD open* 3(2), 2017:e000527 https://doi.org/10.1136/rmdopen-2017-000527 [published Online First: 2018/01/05].

Li L, Li Z, Li Y, et al. Profiling of inflammatory mediators in the synovial fluid related to pain in knee osteoarthritis. *BMC Musculoskeletal Disorders* 21(1):99, 2020, https://doi.org/10.1186/s12891-020-3120-0 [published Online First: 2020/02/16].

Li YS, Luo W, Zhu SA, et al. T Cells in Osteoarthritis: Alterations and Beyond. *Frontiers in Immunology* 8:356, 2017, https://doi.org/10.3389/fimmu.2017.00356 [published Online First: 2017/04/21].

Lieberthal J, Sambamurthy N, Scanzello CR: Inflammation in joint injury and post-traumatic osteoarthritis. *Osteoarthritis Cartilage* 23(11):1825–1834, 2015, https://doi.org/10.1016/j.joca.2015.08.015 [published Online First: 2015/11/03].

Lin X, Patil S, Gao YG, et al. The Bone Extracellular Matrix in Bone Formation and Regeneration. *Frontiers in Pharmacology* 11:757, 2020, https://doi.org/10.3389/fphar.2020.00757 [published Online First: 2020/06/13].

Little CB, Hunter DJ: Post-traumatic osteoarthritis: from mouse models to clinical trials. *Nature Reviews Rheumatology* 9(8):485–497, 2013.

Macchi V, Stocco E, Stecco C, et al. The infrapatellar fat pad and the synovial membrane: an anatomo-functional unit. *Journal of Anatomy* 233(2):146–154, 2018, https://doi.org/10.1111/joa.12820 [published Online First: 2018/05/16].

Madry H, Orth P, Cucchiarini M: Role of the Subchondral Bone in Articular Cartilage Degeneration and Repair. *Journal of the American Academy of Orthopaedic Surgeons* 24(4):e45–e46, 2016, https://doi.org/10.5435/jaaos-d-16-00096 [published Online First: 2016/03/19].

Madry H, van Dijk CN, Mueller-Gerbl M: The basic science of the subchondral bone. *Knee Surgery Sports Traumatology Arthroscopy* 18(4):419–433, 2010, https://doi.org/10.1007/s00167-010-1054-z [published Online First: 2010/02/02].

Malfait AM, Miller RE, Miller RJ: Basic Mechanisms of Pain in Osteoarthritis: Experimental Observations and New Perspectives. *Rheumatic Disease Clinics of North America* 47(2):165–180, 2021,

https://doi.org/10.1016/j.rdc.2020.12.002 [published Online First: 2021/03/31].

March, L.M. (1997). Osteoarthritis. In: Brooks, P.M. (Ed.), MJA Practice Essentials in Rheumatology. AMPCo, North Sydney, pp. 28–33.

Markes AR, Hodax JD, Ma CB: Meniscus Form and Function. *Clinics in Sports Medicine* 39(1):1–12, 2020, https://doi.org/10.1016/j.csm.2019.08.007 [published Online First: 2019/11/27].

Martel-Pelletier J, Barr AJ, Cicuttini FM, et al. Osteoarthritis. *Nature Reviews Disease Primers* 2, 2016, https://doi.org/10.1038/nrdp.2016.72.

Mathiessen A, Conaghan PG: Synovitis in osteoarthritis: current understanding with therapeutic implications. *Arthritis Research & Therapy* 19(1):18, 2017, https://doi.org/10.1186/s13075-017-1229-9 [published Online First: 2017/02/06].

Mazur CM, Woo JJ, Yee CS, et al. Osteocyte dysfunction promotes osteoarthritis through MMP13-dependent suppression of subchondral bone homeostasis. *Bone Research* 7:34, 2019, https://doi.org/10.1038/s41413-019-0070-y [published Online First: 2019/11/09].

McAlindon TE, LaValley MP, Harvey WF, et al. Effect of Intra-articular Triamcinolone vs Saline on Knee Cartilage Volume and Pain in Patients With Knee Osteoarthritis: A Randomized Clinical Trial. *Journal of the American Medical Association* 317(19):1967–1975, 2017, https://doi.org/10.1001/jama.2017.5283 [published Online First: 2017/05/17].

McDougall JJ: Osteoarthritis is a neurological disease – an hypothesis. *Osteoarthritis and Cartilage Open* 1(1-2), 2019.

Melrose J: The Importance of the Knee Joint Meniscal Fibrocartilages as Stabilizing Weight Bearing Structures Providing Global Protection to Human Knee-Joint Tissues. *Cells* 8(4), 2019, https://doi.org/10.3390/cells8040324 [published Online First: 2019/04/10].

Melrose J, Fuller ES, Little CB: The biology of meniscal pathology in osteoarthritis and its contribution to joint disease: beyond simple mechanics. *Connective Tissue Research* 58(3-4):282–294, 2017, https://doi.org/10.1080/03008207.2017.1284824 [published Online First: 2017/01/26].

Menarim BC, Gillis KH, Oliver A, et al. Macrophage Activation in the Synovium of Healthy and Osteoarthritic Equine Joints. *Frontiers in Veterinary Science* 7:568756, 2020, https://doi.org/10.3389/fvets.2020.568756 [published Online First: 2020/12/17].

Meneses SR, Goode AP, Nelson AE, et al. Clinical algorithms to aid osteoarthritis guideline dissemination. *Osteoarthritis Cartilage* 24(9):1487–1499, 2016, https://doi.org/10.1016/j.joca.2016.04.004.

Moore, K.L., Dalley, A.F. 1999. Clinically Oriented Anatomy, fourth ed. Williams & Wilkins, Baltimore.

Müller C, Khabut A, Dudhia J, et al. Quantitative proteomics at different depths in human articular cartilage reveals unique patterns of protein distribution. *Matrix Biology* 40:34–45, 2014, https://doi.org/10.1016/j.matbio.2014.08.013 [published Online First: 2014/09/07].

Nair A, Gan J, Bush-Joseph C, et al. Synovial chemokine expression and relationship with knee symptoms in patients with meniscal tears. *Osteoarthritis Cartilage* 23(7):1158–1164, 2015, https://doi.org/10.1016/j.joca.2015.02.016 [published Online First: 2015/03/01].

Nees TA, Rosshirt N, Zhang JA, et al. Synovial Cytokines Significantly Correlate with Osteoarthritis-Related Knee Pain and Disability: Inflammatory Mediators of Potential Clinical Relevance. *Journal of Clinical Medicine* 8(9), 2019https://doi.org/10.3390/jcm8091343 [published Online First: 2019/09/01].

Nees TA, Rosshirt N, Zhang JA, et al. T Helper Cell Infiltration in Osteoarthritis-Related Knee Pain and Disability. *Journal of Clinical*

Medicine 9(8), 2020https://doi.org/10.3390/jcm9082423 [published Online First: 2020/08/06].

Nelson AE, Allen KD, Golightly YM, et al. A systematic review of recommendations and guidelines for the management of osteoarthritis: The chronic osteoarthritis management initiative of the U.S. bone and joint initiative. *Seminars in Arthritis and Rheumatism* 43(6):701–712, 2014, doi: S0049-0172(13)00258-8 [pii] 10.1016/j.semarthrit.2013.11.012 [published Online First: 2014/01/07].

Neogi T, Guermazi A, Roemer F, et al. Association of Joint Inflammation With Pain Sensitization in Knee Osteoarthritis: The Multicenter Osteoarthritis Study. *Arthritis & Rheumatology (Hoboken, NJ)* 68(3):654–661, 2016, https://doi.org/10.1002/art.39488 [published Online First: 2015/11/12].

Oo WM, Little C, Duong V, et al. The Development of Disease-Modifying Therapies for Osteoarthritis (DMOADs): The Evidence to Date. *Drug Design, Development and Therapy* 15:2921–2945, 2021, https://doi.org/10.2147/dddt.S295224 [published Online First: 2021/07/16].

Önnerfjord P, Khabut A, Reinholt FP, et al. Quantitative proteomic analysis of eight cartilaginous tissues reveals characteristic differences as well as similarities between subgroups. *Journal Biological Chemistry* 287(23):18913–18924, 2012, https://doi.org/10.1074/jbc.M111.298968 [published Online First: 2012/04/12].

Pap T, Dankbar B, Wehmeyer C, et al. Synovial fibroblasts and articular tissue remodelling: Role and mechanisms. *Seminars in Cell and Developmental Biology* 101:140–145, 2020, https://doi.org/10.1016/j.semcdb.2019.12.006 [published Online First: 2020/01/21].

Platzer H, Nees TA, Reiner T, et al. Impact of Mononuclear Cell Infiltration on Chondrodestructive MMP/ADAMTS Production in Osteoarthritic Knee Joints-An Ex Vivo Study *Journal of Clinical Medicine* 9(5), 2020https://doi.org/10.3390/jcm9051279 [published Online First: 2020/05/02].

Rai MF, Brophy RH, Sandell LJ: Osteoarthritis following meniscus and ligament injury: insights from translational studies and animal models. *Current Opinion in Rheumatology* 31(1):70–79, 2019, https://doi.org/10.1097/bor.0000000000000566 [published Online First: 2018/11/06].

Rai MF, Patra D, Sandell LJ, et al. Transcriptome analysis of injured human meniscus reveals a distinct phenotype of meniscus degeneration with aging. *Arthritis & Rheumatology* 65(8):2090–2101, 2013, https://doi.org/10.1002/art.37984 [published Online First: 2013/05/10].

Reichenbach S, Rutjes AW, Nuesch E, et al. Joint lavage for osteoarthritis of the knee. *Cochrane Database of Systematic Reviews*(5), 2010https://doi.org/10.1002/14651858.CD007320.pub2 CD007320.

Rim YA, Nam Y, Ju JH: The Role of Chondrocyte Hypertrophy and Senescence in Osteoarthritis Initiation and Progression. *International Journal of Molecular Science* 21(7), 2020https://doi.org/10.3390/ijms21072358 [published Online First: 2020/04/03].

Ritter SY, Subbaiah R, Bebek G, et al. Proteomic analysis of synovial fluid from the osteoarthritic knee: comparison with transcriptome analyses of joint tissues. *Arthritis & Rheumatology* 65(4):981–992, 2013, https://doi.org/10.1002/art.37823 [published Online First: 2013/02/13].

Roelofs AJ, Kania K, Rafipay AJ, et al. Identification of the skeletal progenitor cells forming osteophytes in osteoarthritis. *Annals of Rheumatic Diseases* 79(12):1625–1634, 2020, https://doi.org/10.1136/annrheumdis-2020-218350 [published Online First: 2020/09/24].

Rosshirt N, Trauth R, Platzer H, et al. Proinflammatory T cell polarization is already present in patients with early knee osteoarthritis. *Arthritis Research & Therapy* 23(1):37, 2021, https://doi.org/10.1186/s13075-020-02410-w [published Online First: 2021/01/24].

Sakellariou G, Conaghan PG, Zhang W, et al. EULAR recommendations for the use of imaging in the clinical management of peripheral joint osteoarthritis. *Annals of Rheumatic Diseases* 76(9):1484–1494, 2017, https://doi.org/10.1136/annrheumdis-2016-210815.

Sakkas LI, Platsoucas CD: The role of T cells in the pathogenesis of osteoarthritis. *Arthritis & Rheumatology* 56(2):409–424, 2007, https://doi.org/10.1002/art.22369 [doi] [published Online First: 2007/02/01].

Scanzello CR: Role of low-grade inflammation in osteoarthritis. *Current Opinion in Rheumatology* 29(1):79–85, 2017, https://doi.org/10.1097/bor.0000000000000353 [published Online First: 2016/10/19].

Scanzello CR, Albert AS, DiCarlo E, et al. The influence of synovial inflammation and hyperplasia on symptomatic outcomes up to 2 years post-operatively in patients undergoing partial meniscectomy. *Osteoarthritis Cartilage* 21(9):1392–1399, 2013, https://doi.org/10.1016/j.joca.2013.05.011 [published Online First: 2013/08/27].

Scanzello CR, McKeon B, Swaim BH, et al. Synovial inflammation in patients undergoing arthroscopic meniscectomy: Molecular characterization and relationship to symptoms. *Arthritis & Rheumatology* 63(2):391–400, 2011.

Scanzello CR, Umoh E, Pessler F, et al. Local cytokine profiles in knee osteoarthritis: elevated synovial fluid interleukin-15 differentiates early from end-stage disease. *Osteoarthritis Cartilage* 17(8):1040–1048, 2009.

Schiphof D, Oei EH, Hofman A, et al. Sensitivity and associations with pain and body weight of an MRI definition of knee osteoarthritis compared with radiographic Kellgren and Lawrence criteria: a population-based study in middle-aged females. *Osteoarthritis Cartilage* 22(3):440–446, 2014, doi: S1063-4584(14)00007-7 [pii] 10.1016/j.joca.2013.12.017 [published Online First: 2014/01/15].

Schurman CA, Verbruggen SW, Alliston T: Disrupted osteocyte connectivity and pericellular fluid flow in bone with aging and defective TGF-β signaling. *Proceedings of the National Academy of Science of the United States of America* 118(25), 2021https://doi.org/10.1073/pnas.2023999118 [published Online First: 2021/06/24].

Siemieniuk RAC, Harris IA, Agoritsas T, et al. Arthroscopic surgery for degenerative knee arthritis and meniscal tears: a clinical practice guideline. *BMJ* 357, 2017https://doi.org/10.1136/bmj.j1982 j1982.

Silverwood V, Blagojevic-Bucknall M, Jinks C, et al. Current evidence on risk factors for knee osteoarthritis in older adults: a systematic review and meta-analysis. *Osteoarthritis Cartilage* 23(4):507–515, 2015, doi: S1063-4584(14)01342-9 [pii] 10.1016/j.joca.2014.11.019 [published Online First: 2014/12/03].

Singh P, Marcu KB, Goldring MB, et al. Phenotypic instability of chondrocytes in osteoarthritis: on a path to hypertrophy. *Annals of the New York Academy of Sciences* 1442(1):17–34, 2019, https://doi.org/10.1111/nyas.13930 [published Online First: 2018/07/17].

Smith MD, Barg E, Weedon H, et al. Microarchitecture and protective mechanisms in synovial tissue from clinically and arthroscopically normal knee joints. *Annals of Rheumatic Diseases* 62(4):303–307, 2003, https://doi.org/10.1136/ard.62.4.303 [published Online First: 2003/03/14].

Soul J, Barter MJ, Little CB, et al. OATargets: a knowledge base of genes associated with osteoarthritis joint damage in animals. *Annals of Rheumatic Diseases*, 2020https://doi.org/10.1136/annrheumdis-2020-218344 [published Online First: 2020/10/21].

Soul J, Dunn SL, Anand S, et al. Stratification of knee osteoarthritis: two major patient subgroups identified by genome-wide expression analysis of articular cartilage. *Annals of Rheumatic Diseases* 77(3):423, 2018, https://doi.org/10.1136/annrheumdis-2017-212603 [published Online First: 2017/12/24].

Thorlund JB, Juhl CB, Roos EM, et al. Arthroscopic surgery for degenerative knee: systematic review and meta-analysis of benefits and harms. *BMJ* 350, 2015https://doi.org/10.1136/bmj.h2747 h2747.

van der Kraan PM: The changing role of TGFβ in healthy, ageing and osteoarthritic joints. *Nature Reviews Rheumatology* 13(3):155–163, 2017, https://doi.org/10.1038/nrrheum.2016.219, [published Online First: 2017/02/06].

van der Kraan PM, van den Berg WB: Osteophytes: relevance and biology. *Osteoarthritis Cartilage* 15(3):237–244, 2007, https://doi.org/10.1016/j.joca.2006.11.006 [published Online First: 2007/01/06].

van der Kraan PM, van den Berg WB: Chondrocyte hypertrophy and osteoarthritis: role in initiation and progression of cartilage degeneration?, *Osteoarthritis Cartilage* 20(3):223–232, 2012, https://doi.org/10.1016/j.joca.2011.12.003 [published Online First: 2011/12/20].

van den Bosch MHJ: Inflammation in osteoarthritis: is it time to dampen the alarm(in) in this debilitating disease?, *Clinical and Experimental Immunology* 195(2):153–166, 2019, https://doi.org/10.1111/cei.13237, [published Online First: 2018/11/14].

Vincent TL: Peripheral pain mechanisms in osteoarthritis. *Pain* 161(Suppl 1(1)), 2020 https://doi.org/10.1097/j.pain.0000000000001923 S138-s46. [published Online First: 2020/10/23].

Walsh DA, McWilliams DF, Turley MJ, et al. Angiogenesis and nerve growth factor at the osteochondral junction in rheumatoid arthritis and osteoarthritis. *Rheumatology (Oxford)* 49(10):1852–1861, 2010.

Wang X, Hunter DJ, Jin X, et al. The importance of synovial inflammation in osteoarthritis: current evidence from imaging assessments and clinical trials. *Osteoarthritis Cartilage* 26(2):165–174, 2018, https://doi.org/10.1016/j.joca.2017.11.015 [published Online First: 2017/12/12].

Wei Y, Bai L: Recent advances in the understanding of molecular mechanisms of cartilage degeneration, synovitis and subchondral bone changes in osteoarthritis. *Connective Tissue Research* 57(4):245–261, 2016, https://doi.org/10.1080/03008207.2016.1177036 [published Online First: 2016/06/11].

Wilson R, Diseberg AF, Gordon L, et al. Comprehensive profiling of cartilage extracellular matrix formation and maturation using sequential extraction and label-free quantitative proteomics. *Molecular & Cellular Proteomics* 9(6):1296–1313, 2010, https://doi.org/10.1074/mcp.M000014-MCP201 [published Online First: 2010/03/02].

Woodell-May JE, Sommerfeld SD: Role of Inflammation and the Immune System in the Progression of Osteoarthritis. *Journal of Orthopaedic Research* 38(2):253–257, 2020, https://doi.org/10.1002/jor.24457 [published Online First: 2019/08/31].

Yusuf E, Kortekaas MC, Watt I, et al. Do knee abnormalities visualised on MRI explain knee pain in knee osteoarthritis? A systematic review. *Annals of Rheumatic Diseases* s 70(1):60–67, 2011, doi: ard.2010.131904 [pii] 10.1136/ard.2010.131904 [published Online First: 2010/09/11].

Zhang H, Cai D, Bai X: Macrophages regulate the progression of osteoarthritis. *Osteoarthritis Cartilage* 28(5):555–561, 2020, https://doi.org/10.1016/j.joca.2020.01.007 [published Online First: 2020/01/27].

Zhang W, Doherty M, Peat G, et al. EULAR evidence-based recommendations for the diagnosis of knee osteoarthritis. *Annals of Rheumatic Diseases* 69(3):483–489, 2010, doi: ard.2009.113100 [pii];10.1136/ard.2009.113100 [doi].

Zhang Y, Nevitt M, Niu J, et al. Fluctuation of knee pain and changes in bone marrow lesions, effusions, and synovitis on magnetic resonance imaging. *Arthritis & Rheumatology* 63(3):691–699, 2011, https://doi.org/10.1002/art.30148 [published Online First: 2011/03/02].

Zhang L, Wen C: Osteocyte Dysfunction in Joint Homeostasis and Osteoarthritis. *International Journal of Molecular Science* 22(12), 2021https://doi.org/10.3390/ijms22126522 [published Online First: 2021/07/03].

Zhang L, Xing R, Huang Z, et al. Synovial Fibrosis Involvement in Osteoarthritis. *Frontiers in Medicine (Lausanne)* 8:684389, 2021, https://doi.org/10.3389/fmed.2021.684389 [published Online First: 2021/06/15].

Zeng N, Yan ZP, Chen XY, et al. Infrapatellar Fat Pad and Knee Osteoarthritis. *Aging and Disease* 11(5):1317–1328, 2020, https://doi.org/10.14336/ad.2019.1116 [published Online First: 2020/10/06].

CRYSTAL ARTHROPATHIES AND THE ANKLE

Neil McGill

Chapter objectives

After studying this chapter, you should be able to:

1. Understand the possible causes of acute arthritis in a single joint and the approach to diagnosis.

2. Understand normal uric acid handling in the body, factors resulting in a high serum uric acid (hyperuricaemia) and how drug therapy can influence the production or excretion of uric acid.

3. Understand the principles of treatment of acute arthritis (a) when crystal arthritis is known to be the diagnosis and (b) when the diagnosis is unclear.

4. Appreciate joint aspiration technique using the ankle as an example.

5. Appreciate the indications and strategies for long-term prevention of gout, including avoidance of adverse drug interactions.

6. Be aware of the associations of gout and calcium pyrophosphate dihydrate deposition, with particular emphasis on those conditions that pose a threat to future health and are preventable/treatable.

7. Understand the principles of treatment of calcium crystal associated arthritis.

Introduction

Gout is the commonest inflammatory arthropathy and is a cause of severe joint pain. Clinicians in all areas of medicine can expect to be confronted with a patient with acute gout who requires prompt effective therapy. Septic arthritis can present in the same manner and needs prompt, but very different, therapy. The correct approach to assessment and diagnosis should allow the disorders that cause acute monoarthritis to be differentiated promptly so that the correct therapy is used. Gout is often accompanied by a range of other health problems such as obesity, hypertension, hyperlipidaemia (elevated serum lipids) and glucose intolerance. Although it may have been gout that led to the patient–doctor interaction, recognition and effective management of these other health problems may bring rewards greater than simply controlling gout.

Effective management for gout is available in the vast majority of cases. Achieving good compliance in the long term is the major practical problem and success in that aspect is based on the patient obtaining sufficient information to understand the need for lifelong therapy.

The calcium crystal associated arthropathies that occur with sufficient frequency to warrant consideration in this text can be divided into calcium pyrophosphate dihydrate (CPPD)- and basic calcium phosphate (BCP)-associated arthropathies. The presence of CPPD deposition in a person less than 55 years of age should prompt consideration of underlying causes such as haemochromatosis. Calcium crystal associated arthropathies can masquerade as other disorders and thus the correct identification is helpful in avoiding unnecessary treatment.

This chapter will review the principles of investigation of acute monarthritis, joint aspiration technique (using the ankle as an example), risks of hyperuricaemia, production and handling of uric acid in normal and disordered circumstances, and principles of the treatment of gout. Calcium crystal associated disorders will also be briefly reviewed with an emphasis on aspects with direct clinical relevance.

Differential diagnosis of acute monarthritis of the ankle

As discussed in Chapter 1, an acutely painful swollen joint can be explained by bacterial infection, crystal-induced inflammation (gout or acute calcium pyrophosphate arthritis), trauma, haemarthrosis (bleeding into the joint) and occasionally by disorders such as rheumatoid arthritis, psoriatic arthritis or reactive arthritis. The postoperative period is a time of increased risk for acute crystal-induced arthritis, particularly gout. Invasive procedures also have the potential to cause bacteraemia that could lead to septic arthritis, although the risk of that occurring at the time of a sterile

---

Case 7.1 Gout: 1

Case history

Mr Taufaao, a 43-year-old Polynesian man, awoke at 0400 h with pain in the left ankle. By 0800 h his ankle was swollen, red and warm. The previous day he had had an arthroscopy of his right knee because of a meniscal tear, suffered while playing touch football 2 months earlier. He had suffered several sprains of both ankles in the past as a result of rugby and had had one previous episode of right knee pain and swelling, also associated with a rugby injury. He had not previously experienced spontaneous joint pain. He worked as a security guard, enjoyed eating and would usually drink about four small bottles of full-strength beer each day.

He had not been aware of any other health problem. His elder brother and father had both had joint problems that he thought might have been gout. His father died at the age of 54 years of a heart attack and his mother remained well at the age of 68 years, although she was overweight.

On examination, he was overweight (120 kg, height 182 cm), afebrile and was barely able to walk owing to the combined effect of pain in the left ankle and post-arthroscopy discomfort in his right knee. The arthroscopic wounds were clean and there was no inflammation in that region. His left ankle was swollen, warm, tender and slightly red. His blood pressure was 180/95, there was no sign of liver disease and urinalysis was normal.

---

procedure such as arthroscopy is very low. One could consider the possibility of trauma (e.g. while anaesthetized) but for trauma to produce a red, swollen, warm joint, the injury needs to be substantial. Thus, the most likely diagnoses are crystal-induced arthritis or sepsis. They both typically produce an abrupt onset of marked joint inflammation.

Joint aspiration to allow examination of the synovial fluid is the best way of establishing the diagnosis. It should be performed promptly using correct aseptic technique and the fluid obtained should be promptly examined and processed for culture. Aspiration will require knowledge of the anatomy of the ankle region.

Essential anatomy

The ankle joints

The ankle region comprises three joints:

1. the true ankle (tibiotalar) joint between the tibia and the talus

2. the subtalar joint between the talus and calcaneus

3. the talonavicular joint between the talus and the navicular (Fig. 7.1A).

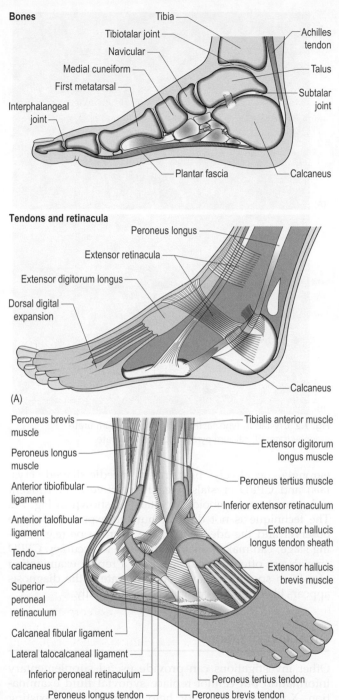

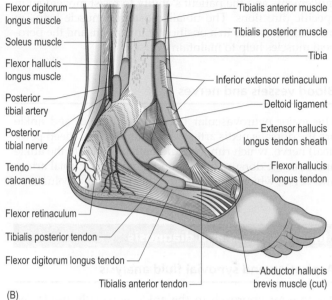

Fig. 7.1 Basic anatomy of the ankle. The relationships of (A) bones (upper; medial view), and tendons and retinacula (lower; lateral view); (B) tendons, ligaments and blood vessels (medial view); and (C) tendons and ligaments (lateral view).

Involvement of any of these three joints will cause 'ankle' pain. The tibiotalar joint is a true hinge joint whose movement is almost entirely limited to plantar flexion (downwards) and dorsiflexion (upwards). The fibula articulates on the lateral side of the tibia but does not bear weight. The subtalar joint allows the foot to be inverted or everted. The midtarsal joints, including the talonavicular joint, allow forefoot supination and pronation.

Articular capsule, ligaments and tendons

The articular capsule is lax on the anterior aspect but tightly bound on both sides by strong medial and lateral ligaments. All the tendons crossing the ankle joint lie superficial to the articular capsule and are partly enclosed in synovial sheaths (Fig. 7.1B). Disorders of the peroneal tendons (inferoposterior to the lateral malleolus), the tibialis posterior tendon (inferoposterior to the medial malleolus), the tendons that run anterior to the ankle joint (such as tibialis anterior, extensor hallucis longus and extensor digitorum longus) or the Achilles tendon can also cause 'ankle' pain. Which structure is responsible for the patient's pain can often be determined by testing specific movements and the patient's ability to resist movement in specific directions. The tibialis posterior muscle helps to maintain the ankle in a position of inversion, and the peroneal muscles help to maintain eversion.

Blood vessels and nerves

The major neurovascular bundles of the foot and ankle are the dorsalis pedis artery and anterior tibial (deep peroneal) nerve, which run longitudinally anterior to the ankle and over the dorsum of foot, and the posterior tibial artery and nerve, which course behind the medial malleolus.

Investigations and diagnosis

Aspiration and synovial fluid analysis

An anterior approach to the ankle is usually used. The joint line should be carefully palpated with the help of passive movement of the joint (if the patient actively moves the ankle, tendon movement obscures the joint line). The point at which the needle enters the skin is approximately 1 cm proximal to the tip of the medial malleolus. The needle is directed posteriorly.

Joint aspiration is usually performed as a clean (not sterile) procedure. Thus, palpation of the joint line and marking the site with an indentation of the skin needs to be performed prior to cleaning the skin. The solution used to clean the skin (e.g. chlorhexidine or iodine) should be allowed to dry. Gloves are worn to protect the person performing the aspiration against blood-borne viral infection. Unless the person performing the aspiration is very experienced and can confidently place the needle in the joint space at the first attempt, local anaesthetic should be used to anaesthetize the skin and periarticular structures. The needle route should avoid the major tendons anterior to the ankle and the dorsalis pedis artery. If joint fluid is not obtained on the first attempt, then the needle should be slightly repositioned.

The synovial fluid obtained should be examined promptly; including macroscopic appearance, cell count, Gram stain, polarized light microscopic examination for crystals and culture. In Chapter 1 we described the characteristics of synovial fluid in normal and abnormal joints. Here, we will consider only those aspects of synovial fluid analysis that apply to crystal identification. Examination for crystals requires only a tiny amount of synovial fluid (even an apparently 'dry' tap may yield enough) but the examination should be performed immediately. Polarized microscopy allows the identification of urate crystals

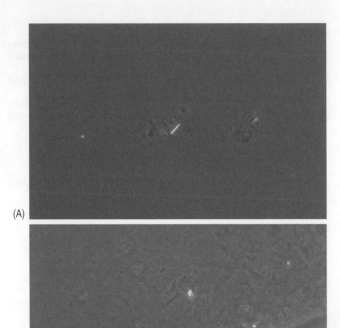

(A)

(B)

Fig. 7.2 Crystals in synovial fluid. (A) Monosodium urate monohydrate; (B) calcium pyrophosphate dihydrate.

(strongly negatively birefringent needle-shaped crystals) and CPPD crystals (weakly positively birefringent rod-shaped or rhomboidal crystals) as shown in Fig. 7.2. The technique is not difficult but the experience of the observer and the adequacy of the microscope (e.g. rotating stage) can make a major difference to accuracy. CPPD crystals are often missed, and thus a repeat examination of a fresh specimen may be appropriate if the diagnosis appears likely, but no crystals are seen initially.

Other investigations

Other investigations can provide useful supplementary information but cannot replace synovial fluid examination. X-rays can detect or help to exclude pre-existing joint or bone disorders, chondrocalcinosis (CPPD deposition in cartilage) and bone trauma. Dual-energy computed tomography (CT) can detect urate crystals with good specificity when examining feet, knees or hands, but only fair sensitivity in early gout where the patient has had only a few attacks. Ultrasound for the detection of intra-articular crystals is dependent on great operator expertise. It is sensible to assess laboratory parameters of inflammation, such as white cell count and ethrocyte sedimentation rate (ESR), for comparison with future results but they assist little in the differentiation of septic from gouty arthritis. The serum uric acid level is of little

Case 7.1 Gout: 2

Investigations

Mr Taufaao's synovial fluid was opaque, creamy-yellow in colour and had reduced viscosity. The cell count was $23.3 \times 10^9/L$, almost all neutrophils. Numerous urate crystals, both extracellular and within neutrophils, were identified using a polarizing microscope. Gram stain and subsequent culture were negative. The diagnosis of acute gout was thus established with certainty. Although, as far as Mr Taufaao was aware, his gout started abruptly, the factors that led to the episode of acute joint inflammation had been operating for years.

help in the setting of possible acute gout. A normal level does not exclude gout and an elevated level does not confirm gout. However, the uric acid level is very important in the long-term management of gout.

Pathophysiology of gouty arthritis

Acute gout is caused by the interaction between the inflammatory system and crystals of monosodium urate monohydrate (urate), with formation of the NLRP3 inflammasome and release and activation of interleukin-1β (IL-1β) being key components. Urate crystals form in and around joints and have a predilection for the cooler areas of peripheral joints (because of the decreased solubility of urate at lower temperatures). Although the inflammatory episode comes on abruptly, the formation of urate crystals probably occurs slowly over weeks to months (there remains some doubt as to the maximum speed of urate crystal formation *in vivo*). Urate crystals can only form in a supersaturated solution of sodium urate, which approximately equates to a uric acid concentration above 0.41 mmol/L (6.8 mg/dL). Thus the attack of acute gout is the culmination of a sequence of events:

1. chronic hyperuricaemia

2. urate crystal formation

3. interaction between the inflammatory system and the urate crystals (Fig. 7.3).
   We will explore these three stages further.

Uric acid metabolism and hyperuricaemia

Persistent hyperuricaemia is necessary for urate crystal formation. Hyperuricaemia, however, is not sufficient in itself to cause urate crystal formation, as reflected by the finding that only about 20% of subjects with uric acid levels in excess of saturation (0.42 mmol/L) ever develop gout. Nevertheless, there is a strong correlation between the degree of hyperuricaemia and the risk of developing gout, and hyperuricaemia is the only proven independ-

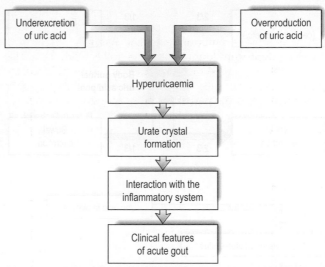

Fig. 7.3 Outline of the pathogenesis of gout.

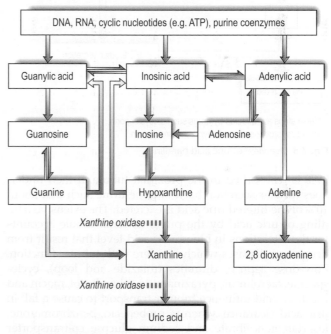

Fig. 7.4 Outline of purine metabolism.

ent risk factor for the development of gout. For patients previously free of gout with a uric acid level of 0.42–0.47 mmol/L, 2% will have experienced an attack of gout after 5 years, compared with 30% of those with a uric acid level of >0.60 mmol/L.

Uric acid is a final breakdown product of purine nucleotide turnover (Fig. 7.4). Of uric acid in the body, approximately two-thirds comes from endogenous sources and approximately one-third from food purines, but there is marked variability between individuals (Fig. 7.5). Excretion of uric acid from the body normally occurs mainly via the kidney (accounting for about two-thirds) with the remainder being excreted by the bowel. Uric acid is almost completely filtered at the glomerulus, and then

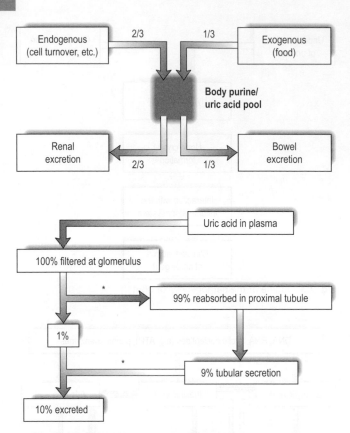

* These steps are affected by drugs such as cyclosporin, diuretics, probenecid, sulfinpyrazone and aspirin.

Fig. 7.5 Overview of uric acid handling.

of nucleic acids, such as myeloproliferative and lymphoproliferative disorders, multiple myeloma, secondary polycythaemia and chronic haemolytic anaemias. Rare enzyme abnormalities (hypoxanthine guanine phosphoribosyl transferase (HGPRT) deficiency, phosphoribosyl pyrophosphate (PRPP) synthetase overactivity, glucose-6-phosphatase deficiency or fructose-1-phosphate aldolase deficiency) can result in marked uric acid overproduction and familial premature gout.

More than 90% of gouty subjects have impaired renal urate clearance, usually in the absence of any other evidence of renal dysfunction.

Urate crystal formation

Although hyperuricaemia is necessary for urate crystal formation to occur, and the likelihood of urate crystal formation increases with increasing uric acid levels, in the majority of hyperuricaemic subjects, urate crystal formation and gout never occur. When urate crystal formation does occur, it preferentially involves peripheral joints, particularly in the lower limbs, subcutaneous tissue, skin, bone and tendon. The process of urate crystal formation is slow (weeks to months) and does not produce symptoms.

Crystal-induced inflammation

Most of the time, the body's inflammatory system largely, although not completely, ignores the urate crystals, but eventually the crystals incite an inflammatory response that results in acute gout. Acute attacks of gout can be precipitated by any cause of a rapid fall in the serum uric acid level, acute illness, trauma, surgery, alcohol and food binges. The mechanism by which these insults precipitate acute gout has not been clarified but alteration of the protein coating of the urate crystals is a plausible explanation. Subsequently, usually after many years, chronic inflammatory responses to the crystals and the physical presence of lumps of crystals (tophi) can lead to joint and bone damage. In male-pattern gout, tophi do not usually develop until many years after the initial attack. In postmenopausal women, however, tophi, particularly in osteoarthritic distal interphalangeal joints, occur early and may be seen at initial presentation. Multiple components of the inflammatory system are involved in the production of acute gouty inflammation. *In vivo*, urate crystals are coated by proteins that markedly influence their ability to induce an inflammatory response. Most crystal surface proteins (especially apolipoprotein B) inhibit the production of inflammation. In contrast, IgG on the crystal surface promotes interaction with the inflammatory system. Urate crystal phagocytosis by monocytes leading to interaction with the NLRP3 inflammasome, activation of caspase-1, in turn, IL-1β and then release of proinflammatory cytokines with resultant neutrophil migration into joints are key components of urate crystal-induced inflammation.

99% is reabsorbed in the proximal tubule. It then undergoes tubular secretion back into the urine such that about 10% of the filtered uric acid is excreted. The extensive handling of uric acid by the proximal renal tubule accounts for the alterations in blood uric acid level that result from drugs and diseases which interfere with tubular function. Low-dose aspirin, diuretics (thiazide and loop), cyclosporine, tacrolimus, pyrazinamide, ethambutol, niacin and nicotinic acid influence tubular transport to cause a fall in uric acid clearance, whereas probenecid, benzbromarone, losartan, fenofibrate and sodium glucose co-transporter 2 (SGLT2) inhibitors all influence tubular transport such that uric acid clearance is increased. Certain racial groups (e.g. Polynesians) have reduced renal clearance of uric acid despite otherwise normal renal function. Oestrogen increases renal uric acid clearance, whereas alcohol, fructose (soft drinks) and obesity decrease it.

Renal insufficiency due to all causes results in reduced uric acid clearance and hence an increased prevalence of hyperuricaemia and gout. Those renal diseases with predominant tubular involvement result in hyperuricaemia disproportionate to the reduction in glomerular filtration rate (e.g. lead poisoning, medullary cystic disease, polycystic disease, cystinuria and analgesic nephropathy).

Less than 10% of gouty subjects demonstrate uric acid overproduction (measured by 24-hour urine collection). In this group are diseases with chronic increased turnover

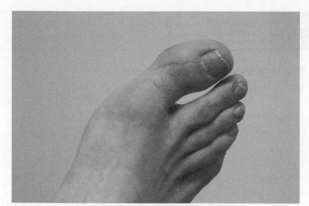

Fig. 7.6 Acute gouty arthritis, here involving the most frequently affected joint – the first metatarsophalangeal joint.

During the inflammatory response, many mediators are released (chemotactic factors, lysosomal enzymes, eicosanoids (e.g. prostaglandins), IL-1β, tumour necrosis factor (TNF), IL-6, IL-8, reactive oxygen species and collagenase) and adhesion molecule expression (E selectin) on synovial endothelial cells is increased. Attacks of gout resolve even without treatment, and resolution appears to be mainly due to the switching off of the inflammatory reaction rather than removal of the urate crystals.

Treatment of acute gout

Acute gout is extremely painful (Fig. 7.6) and demands prompt effective therapy. Minimizing the delay between the onset of the acute attack and the commencement of therapy is more important than which form of therapy is used. For patients who are otherwise well, oral non-steroidal anti-inflammatory (NSAID) medication is usually used. Which NSAID is chosen is not so important and the usual full dose (not higher) should be used. Intra-articular corticosteroid is also very effective and is a particularly good choice in patients with a contraindication to NSAID therapy (such as a history of peptic ulceration, heart failure, renal insufficiency, unstable haemodynamic situation such as following major surgery, anticoagulant therapy, or in situations where interference with platelet function could cause problems, such as in the early postoperative period).

Systemic corticosteroid therapy (synthetic adrenocorticotrophic hormone (ACTH) intramuscularly, triamcinolone intramuscularly, or prednisone orally 20–50 mg daily rapidly reducing to zero over 7–10 days) is also effective and acceptably safe. Colchicine 1.0 mg stat, 0.5 mg after one hour and no further colchicine for 24 hours is as effective and much better tolerated than higher dose regimes which should no longer be used. Low-dose colchicine (0.5 mg twice daily, if renal function is normal) is a useful adjunct to other therapies in acute gout and is effective at preventing recurrence after one-off treatments, such as synthetic ACTH, intramuscular triamcinolone or intra-articular corticosteroid.

If the diagnosis of gout appears likely but synovial fluid cannot be aspirated and thus the diagnosis remains in doubt, the above therapies remain appropriate. It is essential not to use oral antibiotic therapy in this situation because, if the correct diagnosis is septic arthritis, oral antibiotics may suppress the disease and further delay diagnosis. Oral antibiotic therapy is not sufficient treatment for septic arthritis, as discussed in Chapter 11. If what is thought to be acute gout does not respond promptly to the above therapies, then the diagnosis should be reconsidered and further efforts made to obtain synovial fluid from the joint.

Hyperuricaemia can be associated with obesity, hypertension, hyperlipidaemia, insulin resistance, coronary heart disease, excess alcohol ingestion, medication use, renal disease and renal calculi. Many of these conditions warrant intervention in their own right. The risk of gout occurring increases with increasing uric acid levels but is never so high as to warrant drug treatment on that basis prior to an attack of gout. Studies of the effect of hyperuricaemia (in the absence of gout or renal calculi) on renal function and coronary artery disease have not demonstrated benefit from urate-lowering drug therapy (ULT). Hence, asymptomatic hyperuricaemia should not be treated with drug therapy except when there is a possibility of tumour lysis syndrome leading to acute uric acid nephropathy or in the rare patient with a familial cause of uric acid overproduction or familial juvenile hyperuricaemic nephropathy.

Interesting facts

Restriction of dietary purines, within the range that is feasible for a palatable long-term diet, makes relatively little difference to the serum uric acid concentration. Dietary efforts can reduce the occurrence of acute attacks related to excessive dietary intake and should also focus on weight reduction and avoidance of excessive alcohol and/or fructose (soft drinks).

Treatment of chronic gout

The indications for ULT for gout are:

1. features or complications of chronic gout such as tophi, erosions on X-ray, renal calculi, or failure of symptoms to resolve completely between attacks

2. the presence of disorders that make the treatment of acute gout hazardous, such as contraindications to NSAIDs

3. renal insufficiency (because of the increased difficulty of achieving the target serum uric acid level and overall control of gout if the total body load of urate crystals is high)

4. recurrent attacks that have been sufficiently frequent and inconvenient for the patient to prefer to use lifelong daily prophylactic therapy rather than treat the acute attacks as they occur.

Management in relation to risk factors

Although Mr Taufaao was most concerned about his painful ankle, his general practitioner noted that he was Polynesian, overweight, hypertensive, consumed excess alcohol and had a family history of premature vascular disease. This was no coincidence. Hypertension, obesity, insulin resistance, hyperlipidaemia (particularly hypertriglyceridaemia), alcohol excess and Polynesian/Maori race are all associated with hyperuricaemia and gout. Recognition of these other problems in a patient presenting with acute gout can allow intervention to avoid serious consequences in the future.

Primarily to reduce his risk of coronary artery disease and diabetes, Mr Taufaao should modify his diet, reduce alcohol intake and lose weight. Obesity, alcohol and fructose intake are the most important dietary influences on the uric acid level but dietary and lifestyle changes are rarely sufficient to achieve the target serum uric acid level. While it is appropriate to support patients in their efforts to improve lifestyle, to suggest that dietary modification will be sufficient to prevent further gout is wrong and sets the patient up for failure.

Management of chronic gout

Mr Taufaao elected not to use ULT, but he did reduce his alcohol consumption and managed to lose a small amount of weight. His uric acid level fell from an average of about 0.50 mmol/L to about 0.45 mmol/L. Over the subsequent 2 years, he suffered four further attacks of gout with the last two attacks in close succession. He also noted that his most recent two attacks, although less severe at their peak, were slower to resolve and they caused him to lose days from work. After further consultation, Mr Taufaao elected to commence drug therapy with the understanding that he would need to continue the treatment lifelong.

The diagnosis of gout should have been established with near certainty, preferably via the detection of urate crystals in synovial fluid. If crystal confirmation is not possible, an assessment of the degree of certainty of the diagnosis can be obtained using https://goutclassificationcalculator.auckland.ac.nz/. In many patients with probable gout, the diagnosis has not been confirmed. Although it is appropriate to treat probable acute gout without confirmation of the diagnosis, committing a patient to lifelong prophylactic therapy without a high degree of certainty of the diagnosis is inappropriate. Prophylactic therapy for gout is never urgent and, in the long run, it is better to defer until the diagnosis has been established. The most common reason for failure of long-term gout therapy is poor compliance. It is essential that the patient plays an active role in the decision to use ULT and that the patient fully understands the need to continue that therapy lifelong (with rare exceptions). Unless the uric acid level is markedly elevated, it is not usually appropriate to commence long-term ULT after only a single attack of gout.

Urate-lowering drug therapy

In most gouty patients, adequate control of the uric acid level can be achieved with the use of allopurinol or febuxostat, which inhibit xanthine oxidase and hence reduce uric acid production, or with the use of probenecid, which increases uric acid clearance through the kidney. Allopurinol is most commonly chosen because of familiarity, daily dosing, lack of expense and cardiovascular safety. It is suitable for both under-excreters and over-producers. Febuxostat, a non-purine xanthine oxidase inhibitor, is also very effective, does not require dosage modification in mild or moderate renal impairment and has daily dosing. An increase in all-cause and cardiac mortality compared with allopurinol was demonstrated although further studies have not confirmed the increased risk. It is currently not recommended for patients with cardiovascular disease. ULT is best introduced at a low dose so that a gentle fall in the serum uric acid is achieved. The dose is then increased to achieve a uric acid level below 0.36 mmol/L (or for tophaceous gout below 0.30 mmol/L). The approved maximal doses of ULTs vary between countries and should be respected. Reasonable starting and maximal doses are: allopurinol 100 mg daily (start even lower in renal insufficiency), increasing up to 900 mg daily; febuxostat 40 mg daily, increasing up to 80 mg daily (Australia) or 120 mg (New Zealand); probenecid 500 mg daily, increasing up to 1 g twice daily.

Uricosuric therapy is ineffective in patients with moderate to severe chronic kidney disease (stage >3), should not be used in patients with known renal calculi and requires adequate hydration. Aspirin antagonizes the effect of probenecid and, if the two drugs must be used in the same patient, the interval between consumption of the two medications should be at least 6 hours.

Any rapid reduction in the serum uric acid level increases the risk of acute gout, and the introduction of ULT is the commonest example. Patients are unlikely to be impressed by their doctor if they suffer their worst

Interesting facts

Drug therapy options for lowering the serum uric acid level have continued to evolve. Allopurinol remains the most commonly used and the appropriate first choice; febuxostat, a non-purine xanthine oxidase inhibitor, suitable for many patients with allopurinol allergy, carries cardiovascular safety concerns. The uricosuric agents probenecid, benzbromarone, losartan and fenofibrate all continue to provide benefit in selected circumstances.

ever attack of gout soon after commencing medication which has been promised to rid them of gout in the long term. Low-dose colchicine (0.5 mg b.d. if adequate renal function) for 3–6 months is an effective means of preventing acute gout during the introduction of ULT.

The risk of an acute attack should be discussed in advance and the patient should know what action to take should an acute attack occur. Unless there is a contraindication, the advice is usually to continue the ULT and low-dose colchicine, and to introduce an NSAID or corticosteroid promptly. If a patient suffers an attack of gout soon after ceasing colchicine, it should usually be recommenced and continued for a further 3 months.

Provided the target uric acid level (<0.36 mmol/L or <0.30 mmol) has been achieved, there is no reason to alter the dose of ULT just because the patient continues to suffer attacks of gout during the first few months of therapy. The urate crystals that have formed slowly in the body over months and years can continue to cause attacks of gout until they have dissolved, even if the uric acid level has been brought down into the ideal range.

Patients who have a need for NSAID medication for reasons other than to cover the introduction of ULT can usually continue their anti-inflammatory in place of colchicine.

Interesting facts

Uric acid excretion is primarily dependent on renal tubular function. Drugs and diseases that affect tubular function have a greater effect on uric acid levels than those which mainly affect glomerular function.

Patients with renal impairment

The presence of renal impairment reduces uric acid clearance, and uricosuric therapy is less or not effective. The allopurinol hypersensitivity syndrome (skin rash, hepatitis, interstitial nephritis, substantial mortality) occurs with increased frequency in patients with renal impairment and higher starting (but not maintenance) doses of allopurinol. Allopurinol is the preferred ULT, including in moderate to severe chronic kidney disease (stage ≥3). Using a low starting dose (allopurinol dose in mg = 1.5 × eGFR mL/min/1.73 m^2 is a good starting dose) and up-titrating monthly to achieve the target serum uric acid, minimizes safety issues specific to allopurinol hypersensitivity syndrome.

Uncommonly, it is impossible to achieve an ideal uric acid level in the face of renal failure. Although chronic colchicine toxicity is more likely to occur in patients with renal failure than in other situations, low-dose colchicine (0.5 mg daily) is often helpful in minimizing the severity of acute gouty episodes, even although the drug does not reduce uric acid levels nor retard chronic gouty joint and bone damage.

Organ transplant recipients may receive cyclosporin or tacrolimus (which inhibit renal uric acid clearance)

Case 7.2 Chondrocalcinosis: 1

Case history

Mr Steele, a 41-year-old carpenter, sought medical advice because of a gradual onset of discomfort and brief morning stiffness in both hands. On specific questioning, he also admitted to right groin pain at the end of the day's work over the last 6 months. He had noted fatigue for several months but had attributed that symptom to his work.

He had no significant past history and he was not aware of any illness in his family. He did not smoke and he drank only a small amount of alcohol.

On examination he had hard enlargement of the index and middle metacarpophalangeal (MCP) joints of both hands. There was thickening of the skin of both palms in keeping with regular physical work as a carpenter. There was no definite evidence of arthritis of the other small joints of the hands and his other upper limb joints were clinically normal. There was mild restriction of internal rotation of the right hip, but otherwise his lower limb joints were normal.

X-rays demonstrated osteoarthritic change in the index and middle MCP joints of both hands and in the right hip. Chondrocalcinosis was present in the triangular fibrocartilage of both wrists, both hips, the pubic symphysis and the menisci of both knees.

or azathioprine (which can be lethal in combination with allopurinol because allopurinol inhibits the metabolism of the active metabolite of azathioprine, 6-mercaptopurine).

Allopurinol allergy is potentially life threatening. Allopurinol desensitization is now rarely appropriate as other ULTs can usually achieve the target uric acid level. Febuxostat, if necessary in combination with a uricosuric such as probenecid, is usually the best option for allopurinol-allergic patients. Of allopurinol-allergic (skin reaction) patients, 10%–20% are also allergic to febuxostat. Gout therapy can produce several important drug interactions. Azathioprine and allopurinol in combination are potentially lethal. In those rare circumstances when the two drugs need to be used concurrently, the dose of azathioprine needs to be reduced markedly. Probenecid interferes with the excretion of methotrexate and can result in increased toxicity. Concurrent aspirin therapy inhibits the uricosuric effect of probenecid. Allopurinol and ampicillin in combination lead to skin rash in about 20% of cases.

Chondrocalcinosis

Chondrocalcinosis (literally calcification of the cartilage) is a term used to describe the radiological appearance of CPPD crystal deposition within either fibrocartilage (e.g. menisci) or hyaline cartilage. Chondrocalcinosis

Chondrocalcinosis: 2

Investigations and management

The distribution of joint involvement suffered by Mr Steele (index and middle MCP joints, hip joint) is characteristic of the arthropathy of haemochromatosis and that diagnosis was confirmed, initially by the finding of elevated transferrin saturation and elevated ferritin, and subsequently by genetic testing. He was found to have abnormal liver function tests and mild hepatic fibrosis on liver biopsy, and he was referred for endocrinological assessment, which fortunately excluded diabetes, testicular failure and pituitary disease, all of which can occur as a consequence of excessive iron deposition in haemochromatosis. He commenced regular venesection and his liver function tests returned to normal. His arthritis, however, continued to deteriorate and he subsequently required a right hip replacement. The arthropathy of haemochromatosis, once it is established, does not respond to venesection.

becomes increasingly frequent with advancing age such that it can be found in 20% of the population aged in excess of 60 years. At less than 50 years of age, however, it is uncommon and, in this group, the possibility of an underlying cause should be considered. Haemochromatosis, hypomagnesaemia, hypophosphatasia and primary hyper-parathyroidism are all associated with chondrocalcinosis.

Diagnosis

CPPD deposition can be (1) an asymptomatic radiologic finding, (2) associated with osteoarthritis, (3) the cause of acute calcium pyrophosphate crystal arthritis (pseudogout), (4) associated with chronic calcium pyrophosphate crystal inflammatory arthritis and (5) rarely associated with rapidly destructive arthritis resembling neuropathic arthropathy. Knee or wrist involvement in an elderly patient is typical. Although the diagnosis can be suspected by the finding of chondrocalcinosis on X-ray of the involved joint, the definitive diagnostic investigation is synovial fluid examination to confirm the presence of CPPD crystals (weakly positively birefringent rod-shaped or rhomboidal crystals) and to exclude infection. If the clinical features suggest the presence of both osteoarthritis and rheumatoid arthritis, the possibility that all of the manifestations are due to CPPD-associated arthropathy should be considered.

Basic BCP (mainly hydroxyapatite) are found in association with tendon and bursal inflammation (e.g. supraspinatus tendonitis) and the crystals are commonly found in fluid removed from osteoarthritic joints. The role the crystals play in osteoarthritis remains unclear and, at this stage, the finding of BCP crystals in an osteoarthritic joint does not alter clinical management.

Treatment of calcium crystal associated arthritis

Acute joint inflammation in association with CPPD crystals or acute tendon or periarticular inflammation in association with BCP crystals should be treated in a similar manner to acute gout. Prompt treatment with an oral NSAID or intra-articular/intrabursal corticosteroid is most commonly used. The management of CPPD associated with osteoarthritis is the same as for other osteoarthritis. There is no safe and effective means of dissolving or removing calcium crystals from joints or periarticular sites. Magnesium supplementation may retard progression of CPPD deposition in patients with hypomagnesaemia.

Summary

Crystal arthropathies are very common, can mimic joint infection and can be diagnosed with certainty by analysis of synovial fluid aspirated from the involved joint. Successful long-term management of gout is dependent on all involved knowing the target serum urate concentration, safely using ULT to achieve the target and, most difficult of all, ensuring life-long adherence.

Further reading

FitzGerald, J.D., Dalbeth, N., Mikuls, T., et al., 2020. 2020 American College of Rheumatology Guideline for the management of gout. Arthritis & Rheumatology 72 (6), 879–895. https://doi.org/10.1002/art.41247.

Moore, K.L., Dalley, A.F., 2006. Clinically Oriented Anatomy, fifth ed. Williams & Wilkins, Baltimore.

SKELETAL MUSCLE AND ITS DISORDERS

8

Matthew J.S. Parker

Chapter objectives

After studying this chapter, you should be able to:

1. Understand the structure and function of skeletal muscle.

2. Describe the pathological changes that occur in inflammatory myopathies.

3. Appreciate what investigations are appropriate in a patient with primary muscle disease.

4. Understand the common endocrine and metabolic muscle disorders.

5. Describe the use of various drugs in the treatment of muscle disorders.

6. Understand the basic clinical features of the common inherited muscle disorders.

7. Appreciate the clinical features of fibromyalgia.

Introduction

Skeletal muscle is one of the major tissue components of the human body. Its main function is to convert chemical energy into mechanical work. It is usually under the voluntary control of the central nervous system.

Skeletal muscle has other functions; it contains about 80% of the body's content of water and is a reservoir for intracellular ions such as potassium. It also functions as a source of energy-rich compounds and is an important producer of body heat.

A myopathy is a primary disorder of the muscle. The acquired myopathies include IIM, and endocrine and drug-induced myopathies. The inherited myopathies are rare but need to be considered in someone presenting with weakness because they have very different implications for treatment and prognosis.

This chapter will review the relevant anatomy and physiology of skeletal muscle followed by an overview of the primary muscle disorders. It will not discuss muscle disorders secondary to neuromuscular junction disease or diseases of the peripheral and central nervous system.

Anatomy of skeletal muscle

The muscle fibre

Muscles are made up of a collection of individual muscle fibres (Figs 8.1 and 8.2). Each fibre is a multinucleated cell, which can be up to 10 cm in length with a diameter ranging from 10 to 100 μm. Normal muscles have the nuclei arranged around the periphery of the cells. The size of the muscle varies in proportion to the size of the fibres with larger fibres being present in larger muscles. Consistent physical exercise can increase the muscle fibre diameter.

Case 8.1 | **Myopathy: 1**

Case history

Mr Colin Brown is a 47-year-old man who presents to his general practitioner complaining of weakness in both legs when getting out of a chair. He first noticed muscle weakness about 6 months earlier, when he had difficulty walking up and down the stairs at work. He also noticed that his arm and leg muscles were often painful after exercise and occasionally his thigh muscles would be tender. Over the last 2 months, he has noticed increased tiredness.

The history raises the possibility of a disorder of skeletal muscle. It would be important to consider what other clinical information is required and what should be specifically looked for on physical examination.

The muscle cell membrane is called the sarcolemma and the cytoplasm, the sarcoplasm. The sarcolemma has the property of excitability and can conduct the electrical impulses that occur during depolarization. A system of tubules, the transverse tubules or T-tubules, begin at the sarcolemma and extend into the sarcoplasm. They allow rapid distribution of the signal to coordinate contraction throughout the muscle fibre.

The muscle fibre contains numerous myofibrils, which are 1–2 μm in diameter and are arranged longitudinally along the length of the cell, attached to the sarcolemma at each of its ends (Fig. 8.1A). Myofibrils are the structures responsible for muscle contraction. Mitochondria and glycogen granules are situated between the myofibrils.

The myofibrils consist of bundles of filaments, which are made up of the proteins actin and myosin, and are organized in repeating functional units called sarcomeres. Sarcomeres are the smallest functional units of the muscle fibre (Fig. 8.1C). The actin filaments are thin and the myosin filaments are thick. The thick filaments lie at the centre of the sarcomere with the thin filaments at either end. On either side of the centre, there is an area of overlap between the thin and thick filaments in which each myosin filament is surrounded by a hexagonal array of actin filaments. The arrangement of the myosin and actin filaments gives a banded appearance to the muscle and is the reason it is called striated muscle. The sarcomeres are separated by a dense area called the Z line. The M line is at the middle of the sarcomere and consists of proteins that bind the thick myosin filaments. The actin and myosin filaments are joined by molecular cross-bridges and, during contraction, these cross-bridges repeatedly disengage and engage at successive sites, with the result that the actin and myosin filaments slide upon one another and the myofibrils shorten.

The myofibril is surrounded by a sheath of membranes called the sarcoplasmic reticulum. At the zone of overlap between the thick and thin filaments, the tubules of the sarcoplasmic reticulum enlarge and form chambers called terminal cisternae. A T-tubule is situated between two terminal cisternae and the resulting complex is called a triad. The cisternae contain large stores of calcium ions and the release of calcium from these structures, stimulated by electrical signal transmitted by the T-tubules, initiates the muscle contraction.

Skeletal muscle structure

Each fibre is surrounded by a thin layer of collagen, called the endomysium. The fibres are then joined together in bundles to form fascicles, which are surrounded by a further layer of connective tissue called the perimysium (Fig. 8.1A). Groups of fascicles form the whole muscle, which is surrounded by a strong layer of collagen, called the epimysium. The epimysium merges with the peritenon of the tendon and the periosteum.

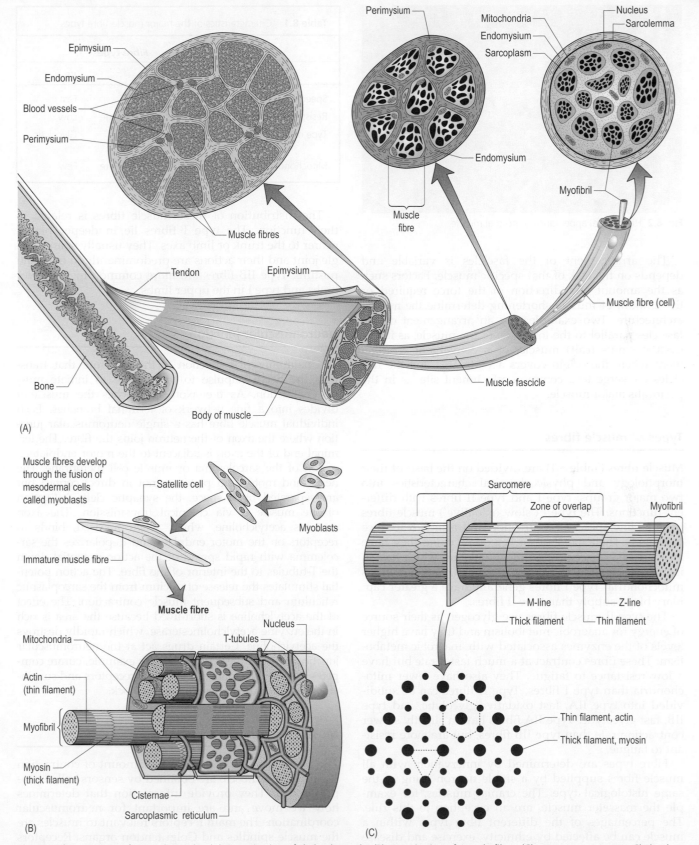

Fig. 8.1 The structure of normal muscle. (A) Organization of skeletal muscle; (B) organization of muscle fibre; (C) sarcomere structure. Skeletal muscle consists of fascicles enclosed by the epimysium. Bundles are separated by the connective tissue fibres of the perimysium and, within each bundle, the muscle fibres are surrounded by the endomysium. Each myofibril consists of a linear series of sarcomeres.

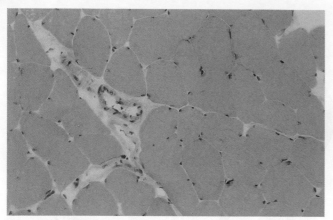

Fig. 8.2 Histological appearance of normal muscle.

Table 8.1 Characteristics of the major muscle fibre types

	Fibre type		
	I	*IIA*	*IIB*
Speed of conduction	Slow	Fast	Fast
Resistance to fatigue	High	Intermediate	Low
Type of metabolism	Oxidative	Oxidative/ glycolytic	Glycolytic
Mitochondria	Many	Intermediate	Few

The arrangement of the fascicles is variable and depends on the task of that specific muscle. Factors such as the amount and direction of the force required or the amount of muscle shortening determine the muscle architecture. Two examples are an arrangement of the fascicles parallel to the long axis of the muscle, as in the gastrocnemius (calf) muscle, or a convergent arrangement where the origin covers a wide area and the fascicles converge to a common attachment site, as in the pectoralis major muscle.

Types of muscle fibres

Muscle fibres (Table 8.1) are divided on the basis of their morphology and physicochemical characteristics into two major groups: type I and type II fibres with different functions. The type I ('slow oxidative') muscle fibres have a slow speed of contraction and a high resistance to fatigue. Their metabolism is oxidative and they have an increased concentration of myoglobin, which has an increased capacity to transport oxygen, and numerous mitochondria. Type I fibres generally have a greater capillary blood supply than type II fibres.

The type II muscle fibres use glycogen as their source of energy for anaerobic metabolism and they have higher levels of the enzymes associated with anaerobic metabolism. These fibres contract at a much faster rate but have a low resistance to fatigue. They also have fewer mitochondria than type I fibres. Type II fibres can be subdivided into type IIA, fast oxidative-glycolytic, and type IIB, fast glycolytic. Type IIA fibres have a slightly slower contraction rate than type IIB fibres, but are more resistant to fatigue.

Fibre types are determined by innervation, with all muscle fibres supplied by a single neuron being of the same histological type. The cranial muscles, for example the masseter muscle, are an exception to this rule. The percentages of the different fibre types within a muscle can be affected by ethnicity, exercise and disease amongst many other factors and, therefore, there is considerable variation between individuals.

The distribution of these muscle fibres is related to their function. The type I fibres lie in deeper planes nearer to the trunk or limb axes. They usually span a single joint and their actions are predominantly to maintain posture. Type IIB fibres are more common in the lower limbs and type I in the upper limbs.

Neuromuscular junction

The neuromuscular junction is the structure that transmits the nerve impulse to the muscle to initiate muscle contraction. As the axon approaches the muscle it divides into a fine network of terminal branches. Each individual muscle fibre has a single neuromuscular junction where the axon of the neuron joins the fibre. The terminal end of the axon is adjacent to the motor endplate, a region of the sarcolemma or muscle cell membrane. The nerve and motor end plate are not in direct contact but are separated by a space, the synaptic cleft. Activation of the muscle is via chemical transmission. The axon contains acetylcholine, which, when released, binds to receptors on the motor endplate and depolarizes the sarcolemma with rapid spread of the action potential down the T-tubules to the interior of the fibre. The action potential stimulates the release of calcium from the sarcoplasmic reticulum and subsequent muscle contraction. The effect of the acetylcholine is short-lived because the area is rich in the enzyme acetylcholinesterase, which rapidly destroys the acetylcholine. Certain drugs act at the neuromuscular junction to affect these processes, for example, curare competes with acetylcholine for endplate receptors and suxamethonium produces a depolarization block.

Muscle and tendon receptors

The position of the joints and the amount of contraction required by a muscle are obtained by sensors called proprioceptors. They provide information that determines how we move and are important for neuromuscular coordination. The main receptors relevant to muscles are the muscle spindles and Golgi tendon organs. Receptors in the ligaments and joint capsule are important for joint position sense.

A muscle spindle is a spindle-shaped stretch receptor found in most muscles but especially concentrated in muscles that exert fine motor control, such as the small muscles of the hand. The muscle spindle is about 100 μm in diameter and up to 10 mm in length. Muscle spindles receive a sensory innervation from groups Ia and II afferent nerve fibres and a motor supply from dynamic γ and static δ motor axons (see Ch. 3 for revision of nerve fibre types).

Another type of stretch receptor is the Golgi tendon organ formed by the terminals of a group Ib afferent nerve fibre. Golgi tendon organs are arranged in series within the tendon adjacent to the musculotendinous junction. They can be activated by either stretch or muscle contraction. Golgi tendon organs signal the force that develops in the tendon on muscle contraction, whereas muscle spindles provide feedback about the amount and rate of muscle stretch.

Interesting facts

The position of the joints and the amount of contraction required by a muscle are obtained by sensors called proprioceptors. They provide information that determines how we move. The main proprioceptors that affect muscles are the muscle spindles and Golgi tendon organs. Proprioceptors in the ligaments and joint capsule are important for joint position sense.

Muscle metabolism

Muscle requires a large amount of energy to function adequately. Muscle contains large energy reserves, these being adenosine triphosphate (ATP) and other high-energy compounds, especially creatine phosphate and glycogen.

Resting muscle generates ATP, which is stored among the myofilaments. The cell produces more ATP than can be stored, and excess is used to generate creatine phosphate. The enzyme creatine kinase (CK) (see Investigations) catalyses the conversion of creatine to creatine phosphate using the excess ATP. At rest, the muscle contains six times as much creatine phosphate as ATP. When energy is required, the reverse reaction occurs, producing ATP (and creatine).

When the ATP and creatine phosphate supplies are exhausted, glycogen becomes the energy source. Glycogen is broken down into glucose, which is ultimately metabolized to ATP. This can be done by aerobic or anaerobic respiration depending on the supply of oxygen. Mitochondria produce ATP from glucose by aerobic respiration.

At low levels of muscle activity, aerobic respiration is sufficient to provide energy for the muscle. At maximum muscle activity, mitochondria produce about one-third of the required ATP, and the rest is produced by anaerobic glycolysis. Anaerobic glycolysis as a method of energy production has some disadvantages. It is relatively inefficient, requiring 18 molecules of glucose to provide the same amount of energy as from one glucose molecule by aerobic metabolism. It also results in the production of lactate which has important (generally negative) metabolic consequences.

Muscle contraction

Muscle contraction occurs as a result of the actin and myosin filaments sliding alongside each other – the molecular mechanism for muscle contraction is known as the cross-bridge cycle or sliding filament theory. At rest, the interaction between actin and myosin is prevented by the proteins tropomyosin and troponin. As sarcoplasmic calcium levels rise rapidly after sarcolemmal depolarization, conformational changes in troponin and tropomyosin remove this inhibition and allow the myofibrils to shorten in the presence of sufficient ATP. Contraction stops as a result of active removal of the calcium from the cell.

There are two main types of muscle contraction, isotonic and isometric. Isotonic contractions result in a change in length of the muscle and can be either concentric (shortening) or eccentric (lengthening). Isometric contractions do not result in a change in length but result in increased tension, for example when maintaining posture. A muscle will contract most efficiently until it has shortened by about 30%. If the muscle is significantly contracted (or overstretched) it becomes less efficient.

Muscles work in groups and, on the basis of their actions, can be described as agonists, synergists or antagonists. Agonists are the muscles primarily responsible for producing the desired movement, synergists assist the prime mover or stabilize the joint and antagonists oppose the desired movement to provide more control. Using shoulder abduction as an example, the deltoid muscle would be the agonist, the supraspinatus muscle would be a synergist (in early abduction) and the pectoralis major and latissimus dorsi muscles act as antagonists.

Control of muscle function

A motor unit comprises a single motor neuron and all of the muscle fibres it innervates. These fibres are scattered throughout the muscle and contract together under the influence of the motor neuron. All muscle fibres of an individual motor unit will be of the same type (either type I or type II). The number of fibres per motor unit varies widely depending on the function of the muscle. It may comprise 2000 fibres in a muscle such as the gastrocnemius that is used for rapid and powerful contractions as when sprinting, but only three in the extraocular muscles that require rapid, precise movement with little power.

The nervous system controls the force of the contracting muscle by varying the number of motor neurons activated at any one time. For each movement, there is a progressive increase in the number of motor units contracting to provide an even increase in tension. Maximum tension in a muscle occurs when all the motor units are contracting.

Muscle tone refers to the resting tension in a skeletal muscle and is important for maintaining normal posture, providing support for the joints to stabilize their position and to help prevent sudden changes in position. Muscle tone is maintained by a reflex arc, whereby a signal is sent from the muscle spindles to a lower motor neuron in the posterior root ganglion which then sends a signal to the appropriate muscles to adjust the extent of their contraction to maintain constant tension. This reflex arc is also under the influence of the central nervous system.

Interesting facts

Myotonia is delayed relaxation of the muscle after contraction. It is an important feature of dystrophia myotonica but can be due to other causes, where it is less severe, which include hypothyroidism, prolonged cold exposure, extreme physical exercise and medication, e.g. propranolol.

Muscle fatigue and pain

Muscle fatigue is a transient and recoverable reduction in the force of muscle contraction which occurs during exercise. There are numerous causes for fatigue and their role and interactions are not clearly understood. Fatigue can be influenced by local muscle factors, the central nervous system and general fitness. The type of exercise also influences fatigue, with the factors that cause fatigue during high-intensity exercise, for example sprinting, being different to those during low-intensity endurance exercise, for example long-distance running. Muscle fatigue can occur earlier than expected depending on various factors that include reduced blood flow or low energy reserves because of poor diet, illness or metabolic disorders. The recovery period after exercise can take from several hours to about a week, depending on the exercise.

Cramp is a prolonged, painful muscle contraction, which can occur following intense exercise. During cramp, the muscle fibre membrane conducts action potentials at abnormally high frequencies in the absence of nerve stimulation. This is due to changes in membrane permeability brought about by changes in ion concentration in the tissue fluids secondary to dehydration and loss of electrolytes.

Muscles contain sensory free nerve endings which act as nociceptors primarily sensing the presence of extracellular ATP (as occurs in tissue damage) or H+ (which increases in concentration in the setting of tissue ischaemia and/or anaerobic respiration). The relationship between the triggering of nociceptors and the subjective experience of pain is complex, multifactorial and far from understood.

Ageing and the muscular system

There are several changes in muscle with ageing that result in a reduction of anaerobic and aerobic performance by 30%–50% at the age of 65 years. These include selective type II fibre atrophy, a reduction in the number of myofibrils and reduced mitochondria and glycogen reserves. There is also an increase in fibrous tissue throughout the muscle, which reduces its flexibility. The number of motor units also falls with age due to a sporadic death of motor units, which cannot regenerate. There is a sprouting from the surviving axons to reinnervate the denervated muscle which increases the size of the surviving motor units but this process is limited. Conduction velocities along motor nerves slow with ageing. With these factors combined, there is a general decline in both strength and fine motor control with ageing. Ongoing exercise is a powerful mitigating factor in this decline and there is evidence for its use at any stage of the life course.

Investigations

In patients presenting with potential 'muscle' disease there is a very broad differential and investigations will be targeted on the basis of a thorough history and examination. In general, it is important to exclude easily detectable and treatable causes such as electrolyte disturbance and endocrinopathies early with some simple blood tests. There are a few investigations commonly done specifically relating to skeletal muscle itself worthy of particular mention.

Muscle enzymes

Various muscle enzymes appear in blood when muscle damage occurs, making them useful serum markers of muscle pathology. CK is the most clinically useful enzyme and is elevated sometimes many hundred-fold above reference ranges in severe muscle injury. It is important to remember that CK is also present in cardiac muscle and brain tissue where it exists in different isoforms – these can be measured individually to help identify the site of damage if this is unclear. There is substantial interindividual variation in baseline CK levels so mild elevations should not be overinterpreted unless there are associated symptoms or signs of pathology. Other enzymes that increase in serum as a result of muscle pathology include alanine aminotransferase (ALT) and aspartate aminotransferase (AST), traditionally considered 'liver tests', lactate dehydrogenase (LDH), aldolase and Troponin T.

Electromyography

Neurophysiological testing (electromyography – EMG) can be very useful in differentiating which element of the motor unit is dysfunctional – the motor neuron, the neu-

Case 8.1 Myopathy: 2

Case note: Clinical examination

We can now answer the question of what other clinical information is required in Mr Brown's case. Muscle disorders usually present with a limited number of symptoms. Pain and weakness are the most common presenting symptoms. Tenderness, twitching and cramps are less common. Muscle wasting and contractures usually occur late in the illness. However, the clinical history is still important, as it is essential to try to determine the cause of the muscle symptoms as well as the appropriate investigations required to make the diagnosis.

It is important to determine whether there are any other neurological symptoms, e.g. numbness, 'pins and needles', dysaesthesia or cranial nerve symptoms, to help determine whether it is a primary muscle disorder or secondary to peripheral nervous system involvement. Enquire about symptoms of connective tissue disease, e.g. photosensitivity, skin rash, Raynaud's phenomenon, arthritis, pleurisy or pericarditis. Family history is important to exclude a congenital problem, e.g. muscular dystrophy. Congenital conditions, however, are usually manifest in childhood or the early 20s. It is also important to take a history of current drug exposure, as a variety of drugs have been associated with muscle disease, as discussed below. Tiredness and fatigue are features of many diseases but can occur in some endocrine disorders, so it is important to determine whether there are other symptoms relevant to an endocrine disorder such as hyper/hypothyroidism.

With regard to the physical examination, it is important to try to determine whether the muscle pain and weakness are due to a primary muscle disorder or secondary to involvement of the nervous system. Neurological abnormalities, in particular lesions of the spinal cord or peripheral nerves, may have associated sensory symptoms and signs. This indicates that the problem is not a primary muscle disorder.

The clinical examination should carefully evaluate all muscle groups both proximally and distally, including the trunk and cervical muscles. This will give you information about the muscle groups involved; whether they are proximal or distal, symmetrical or unilateral, diffuse or related to a particular nerve root distribution. A full neurological examination should be performed to determine whether there is any other neurological abnormality.

The examination of muscle strength involves general functions as well as testing of specific muscles or muscle groups. The patient should be observed walking, getting out of a chair, using a step(s), sitting up from a supine position and holding arms above the head.

Specific muscle testing involves isometric contraction against resistance. The grading system for power is that described in the Medical Research Council Memorandum of 1943 (*Aids to the investigation of peripheral nerve injuries,* War Memorandum No. 7), which is as follows:

Grade 0, no contraction
Grade 1, flicker or trace of contraction
Grade 2, active movement with gravity eliminated
Grade 3, active movement against gravity
Grade 4, active movement against gravity and resistance – this can be subdivided into 4– , 4 and 4+ to indicate slight, moderate and strong resistance
Grade 5, normal power.

This is a subjective scale but is the most appropriate for routine clinical use. There are numerous devices for accurately measuring muscle power, but size or cost precludes their use in the clinical setting.

A general physical examination is also required. Sometimes muscle disorders can be part of a more diffuse disorder, e.g. systemic lupus erythematosus, and there may be other clinical signs, such as a skin rash or arthritis (see Ch. 9). Hyperthyroidism and hypothyroidism can also be associated with muscle disorders and once again, examination should be able to determine whether the patient is clinically euthyroid.

---

romuscular junction or the myocyte. It is a specialized test but when performed by an experienced clinician can be invaluable. Findings can occasionally be almost pathognomic for specific diagnoses such as in myasthenia gravis or certain channelopathies

Muscle imaging

Magnetic resonance imaging (MRI) is becoming increasingly useful in the investigation of muscle disease. It can reliably identify muscle oedema ('myoedema'; synonymous with muscle inflammation) and/or fatty infiltration of muscle which can happen as a result of chronic myopathies. The pattern of muscle involvement is helpful in characterising the underlying pathology and the

MRI result can help target an appropriate site for biopsy. Other forms of imaging (e.g. ultrasound, positron emission tomography) are less useful currently but areas of ongoing research.

Muscle biopsy

When the diagnosis is uncertain, a muscle biopsy is usually very helpful. Muscle biopsies are most commonly taken from a thigh muscle or the deltoid. Interpretation of muscle biopsies is a highly specialized field and it is important that full clinical details are available to the neuropathologist to help properly interrogate the results. There are many different potential findings but in brief they will look at the overall architecture and appearance of the sample (e.g. is there muscle fibre atrophy or hypertrophy), look for evidence of inflammation and look for other features to suggest the underlying pathology (e.g. angular fibres with fibre type grouping in nerve pathology, perifascular atrophy with perimysial inflammation in dermatomyositis). There are a series of stains performed to investigate for specific myopathies (e.g. dystrophin to investigate for muscular dystrophies) depending on the clinical context.

Genetic studies

There are an ever-increasing number of genetic myopathies described and technology to investigate for these is improving at an exciting rate. It is still common practice to use the investigations described above to help focus any genetic investigation rather than perform genetic tests 'blind'. Any genetic investigation has potentially far-reaching consequences for the individual and their family and should be appropriately considered and counselled.

Specific muscle diseases

Muscle disease can be divided into two broad groups, acquired and inherited.

Acquired muscle diseases

Idiopathic inflammatory myopathies

This group of muscle disorders are primarily autoimmune in aetiology and are often referred to by clinicians collectively using the term 'myositis'. Given that myositis simply means muscle inflammation and many different muscle pathologies result in muscle inflammation, this term is not ideal. A potentially confusing feature of these conditions is that they commonly result in other (extramuscular) disease manifestations such as arthritis, gastrointestinal, pulmonary and cutaneous involvement. Occasionally these extramuscular manifestations will predominate and the muscle involvement is relatively minor or even absent ('clinically amyopathic'). These conditions are being intensively researched and the nomenclature of various subtypes as well as the assorted diagnostic tests is constantly evolving.

Epidemiology

IIM are rare with an incidence of around 20 per 100 000 person years. They can present at any age but have a bimodal distribution with a peak in childhood and again in middle age. They are globally distributed although there is some regional variation when considering certain subtypes. There is a female preponderance for most subtypes.

Classification

There has been an increasing recognition that there are a number of distinct clinical syndromes within the IIM. Currently, the following disease subtypes are widely accepted: dermatomyositis, antisynthetase syndrome, immune-mediated necrotising myopathy (IMNM, also known as necrotising autoimmune myopathy by some clinicians), inclusion body myositis (IBM), polymyositis and 'overlap myositis' (where patients have autoimmune myositis in conjunction with another connective tissue disease such as systemic sclerosis or mixed connective tissue disease). It is beyond the scope of this chapter to discuss these in turn but some will be discussed below.

Clinical features

The cardinal presenting feature of IIM is weakness which is typically progressive, proximal and painless. Patients may not describe weakness *per se* but instead describe the functional consequences of proximal weakness such as difficulty climbing stairs, rising from a low chair or reaching above their head. Symptoms are usually symmetric and involve both upper and lower limbs. Pain is not usually present and almost never a more significant symptom than weakness – if it is volunteered it should prompt careful consideration of other diagnoses. Without treatment, patients can quickly become significantly impaired and wheelchair or bed bound and therefore this presentation should result in prompt specialist attention. In addition to proximal limb girdle weakness, some patients also develop oropharyngeal dysphagia (the proximal third of the oesophagus is striated rather than smooth muscle) which can be very troublesome and refractory to treatment. Finally, it is important to be alert to respiratory muscle weakness as a life-threatening complication of IIM; this would normally be associated with axial weakness (e.g. unable to sit forward from lying position, neck flexor weakness) and can result in symptoms of orthopnoea and hypercapnic (type II) respiratory failure.

Extramuscular features

Given the IIM are systemic autoimmune processes, it is not surprising that there are a wide range of associated organ manifestations. These include certain skin signs such as those that define the dermatomyositis subtype (Gottron's papules and the heliotrope rash as examples) or the 'mechanic's hands' of antisynthetase syndrome. Arthritis is a relatively common symptom in patients with antisynthetase syndrome and overlap myositis and is usually a small joint non-erosive polyarthritis. The IIM can involve the gastrointestinal tract and any level but by far the most common manifestation is dysphagia, discussed above, which can happen with any IIM subtype but especially in IBM and immune-mediated necrotising myopathy. Raynaud's phenomenon and occasionally associated digital ischaemia can occur in antisynthetase syndrome or overlap myositis. The biggest contributor to mortality in IIM is the development of interstitial lung disease (ILD) which is common in antisynthetase syndrome in particular as well as some dermatomyositis subtypes. Patients can develop rapidly progressive lung fibrosis with a high mortality even despite aggressive treatment. Cardiac involvement is also well described and likely under-appreciated due to the difficulties in diagnosing this when mild.

Investigations

A broad range of investigation is appropriate when considering a diagnosis of IIM as mentioned above. In addition to the tests already mentioned there are an ever-increasing number of autoantibodies described, known as myositis specific autoantibodies (MSA). The MSA are usually mutually exclusive and tightly associate with one of the clinical subtypes described above. These are briefly listed in **Table 8.2**. At least two-thirds of patients with IIM will have a positive autoantibody detected with the remainder being 'seronegative'.

Cancer-associated 'myositis'

Worthy of particular mention is the association of certain subtypes of IIM with malignancy. Overall, around 10% of patients with a newly diagnosed IIM will be found to have an underlying malignancy. This risk is highest in older men with dermatomyositis (especially those with a specific MSA known as anti-TIF1g). It is important to consider investigations for occult malignancy in any patient with new IIM.

Table 8.2	Myositis specific antibodies
Antibody	**Clinical associations**
Antisynthetase antibodies: Anti-Jo1 Anti-PL7 Anti-PL12 Anti-EJ Anti-OJ Anti-KS	Antisynthetase syndrome with myositis, interstitial lung disease, Raynaud's phenomenon and mechanic's hands
Anti-TIF1-γ Anti-NXP2	Malignancy and dermatomyositis
Anti-SRP	Severe necrotizing myopathy, treatment resistant
Anti-MDA5	Severe and rapidly progressive interstitial lung disease
Anti-HMGCR	Statin induced necrotizing myopathy
Anti-Mi2 Anti-SAE	Dermatomyositis

Treatment

Treatment of IIM is complex and will be tailored to the individual patient, influenced by the clinician's own experience and the constantly evolving evidence base. A few general principles apply. Initial treatment can be considered 'induction' treatment; highly potent immunotherapy intended to achieve rapid disease control. Subsequent treatment can be considered 'maintenance' treatment where medications are used to maintain disease remission and is usually substantially less potent than induction treatment and influenced by concerns about long-term cumulative treatment toxicity from

> ### Case 8.1 Myopathy: 3
>
> #### Case note: Diagnosis
>
> Further history taking revealed that Mr Brown had had asthma for 6 years, requiring oral corticosteroids for the past 3 years. There was no other significant past history or symptoms. His family history does not include muscle disorders. Physical examination showed symmetrical proximal muscle weakness, more marked in the legs than the arms. The remainder of the neurological examination was normal; in particular there was no evidence of sensory impairment. He did not have any rash. The remainder of the physical examination was normal.
>
> The most likely diagnosis is polymyositis or its variants, for example, inclusion body myositis. Steroid myopathy should be considered. The absence of other features made an associated connective tissue disorder or endocrine disorder unlikely. Specific tests include measurement of serum creatine kinase, which was elevated at 2500 IU/L (normal 40–300 IU/L).
>
> Mr Brown was subsequently referred to a rheumatologist for further investigation. Chest X-ray was normal and respiratory function tests showed a mild impairment of diffusing capacity but were otherwise normal. There was an antibody to Jo-1. A muscle biopsy showed irregularity in the size and shape of muscle fibres, including necrotic fibres, regenerative fibres and a variable inflammatory infiltrate. These changes were consistent with polymyositis (Fig. 8.3).
>
>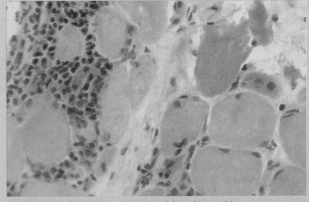
>
> **Fig. 8.3** Histological appearance with polymyositis.

certain medications such as glucocorticoids. The backbone of most induction regimens is high-dose glucocorticoids such as prednisolone 0.5–1 mg/kg tapered to more moderate doses over a few months once patients have improved. Only a minority of patients will achieve complete remission on even high dose glucocorticoid monotherapy and therefore a 'second agent' is typically used at induction with the most commonly chosen including cyclophosphamide, methotrexate, intravenous immunoglobulin (IVIG) and rituximab. Once patients have improved significantly or are ideally in remission, medications used for maintenance include methotrexate, mycophenolate, azathioprine or tacrolimus and these can be combined especially if there are difficulties maintaining remission whilst the dose of glucocorticoid is tapered. Despite conventional treatment some patients with IIM do not respond or do so only partially and there remains substantial morbidity and mortality. It is likely that new and more effective treatments will be available for certain subtypes in the near future.

Inclusion body myositis

Although IBM is currently classified as an IIM, it has features that are somewhat at odds with the other subtypes. In particular, there is very little evidence that current immunosuppression works and therefore it is an important condition to recognize to avoid iatrogenic harm. Patients with IBM are older (very unusual for symptoms to begin prior to the age of 50), typically male (3:1) and have a characteristic pattern of weakness (distal upper limb and proximal lower limb). Symptoms related to weakness present insidiously, worsening over years compared to the much more sudden presentation in most other IIM. Because of the pattern of weakness these patients often experience difficulty with grip strength (finger flexor involvement) and early falls, often when going down stairs or hills (quadriceps weakness). There are specific features on muscle biopsy ('rimmed vacuoles') and some patients have a specific autoantibody (anti-CN1a) but it can still be difficult for this condition to be differentiated from other IIM and causes of myopathy early in the disease.

Selected other acquired muscle diseases

Endocrine myopathies

Muscle weakness occurs with several endocrine disorders, where it can occasionally be the presenting symptom. If any of these endocrine disorders is suspected, then the appropriate additional endocrine investigations are also required. With all these endocrine disorders, correction of the endocrine abnormality results in the return of muscle function to normal.

Thyroid disease

Both hyper- and hypothyroidism can present with significant weakness and it is an important differential to consider as these are readily diagnosed and treated. Hyperthyroidism produces generalized weakness and occasionally there may be associated paralysis of the extraocular muscles. Proximal muscle weakness is usually the presenting symptom, although there is usually less obvious distal muscle weakness. The CK level is normal or only slightly elevated. There are usually other clinical signs of hyperthyroidism such as tremor or hyperreflexia. Hypothyroidism can result in significant proximal muscle weakness and patients are more likely to have myalgia or early muscle fatigue. There is often slowness of contraction, delayed relaxation after contraction (pseudomyotonia) and delayed relaxation of the deep tendon reflexes ('Woltman's sign'). Occasionally patients can present with even more marked myopathy, muscle stiffness and pseudohypertrophy (Hoffman's syndrome) which can mimic the appearance of muscular dystrophy. In contrast to hyperthyroidism, the CK level is often elevated, sometimes markedly. The weakness and CK level can take months to improve even after thyroxine is replaced. The muscle biopsy is not usually helpful in making these diagnoses as there are no specific features of thyroid disease.

Cushing's syndrome

Cushing's syndrome is a result of increased glucocorticoid exposure (either endogenous or exogenous) and is associated with proximal muscle weakness due to the effect of cortisol on muscle cell metabolism. The CK level will be normal and, if a biopsy is performed, there is usually evidence of selective type II fibre atrophy (this is not a specific finding).

Acromegaly

Acromegaly (excess production of growth hormone) is commonly associated with mild proximal weakness even though skeletal muscle mass is increased. The CK level can be elevated. The muscle histology shows type I fibre hypertrophy and type II fibre atrophy.

Disorders of calcium metabolism

As would be anticipated from the critical role of calcium in muscle physiology, both hyper- and hypocalcaemia from any cause can be associated with muscle weakness. CK level is usually normal and the histological changes if present include type II fibre atrophy.

Infections and muscles

Myalgia is the commonest muscle symptom associated with infections, and occurs with most viral infections. It resolves with the illness, there is no weakness and the CK is normal.

True myositis ranging in severity up to rhabdomyolysis has been described with numerous viruses, particularly influenza and Coxsackie viruses. Patients may present any or all symptoms of rhabdomyolysis; muscle pain and swelling, fever, myoglobinuria (dark coloured urine) and associated acute renal failure. The CK can be extremely elevated but will rapidly improve if supportive care is successful. Human immunodeficiency virus (HIV) has been associated with a chronic myopathy which can mimic either polymyositis or IBM. Pyomyositis is a bacterial infection of muscle which is usually localized and therefore easy to distinguish from more widespread myopathies and relatively rare. Parasitic infections can cause myositis and include toxoplasmosis and trichinosis. They usually result in diffuse muscle pain.

Drug- and toxin-induced muscle disease

A wide range of drugs can affect muscle function because of a direct effect on the muscle. It is important to remember that drugs can also affect the nerves or neuromuscular junction, and this will have a secondary effect on muscle function. The true frequency of drug-induced muscle involvement is not known. The clinical features are usually muscle pain, tenderness and weakness. The weakness is usually proximal and the CK level may be elevated.

Because a wide range of drugs have been described as causing muscle disease, any history of a patient with muscle disease should include a detailed history of medications. A temporal association between first taking the drug and the onset of muscle symptoms is important. Sometimes the only way to determine if the drug is the cause is to stop it. The drugs more commonly associated with muscle disease are shown in Box 8.1.

Probably the commonest cause of drug-induced myopathy is statins. Around 1 in 5 patients taking statins will describe a perceived muscle side effect although there is a well-established powerful 'nocebo' effect at play; when comparing incidence of muscle side effects in patients on statins versus matched controls on placebo there is an absolute rate increase of around 1 in 100 patients. Statin-induced myopathy can range from mild myalgia to severe rhabdomyoly-

Box 8.1 Drugs commonly associated with muscle disease

Cholesterol-lowering drugs:
 Clofibrate
 HMG-CoA enzyme inhibitors
Alcohol
 Hydroxychloroquine
 Colchicine
Zidovudine
Vincristine
Lithium
Cimetidine
Phenothiazines and other antipsychotics

sis. It is more common in the first few months after starting the statin but can occur at any time. Stopping the statin should result in rapid resolution of the muscle disorder. A very rare complication of statin therapy has only been established in the last decade and is called statin-associated immune-mediated necrotising myopathy. It is thought that statin therapy in genetically predisposed patients triggers an autoimmune myositis that can be severe and will persist even if the statin therapy has been ceased. Patients who have severe weakness and/or who do not improve rapidly with statin cessation should be discussed with a specialist.

Corticosteroids are another very common cause of myopathy with clinical features consistent with Cushing's syndrome (see above). The effect of the corticosteroid on the muscle is dose dependent but there is substantial interindividual variation in the doses required to cause myotoxicity. Myopathy is more common with fluorinated steroids, particularly triamcinolone and betamethasone. Alcohol can result in two major types of myopathy. Individuals with chronic alcoholism may develop slowly progressive proximal muscle weakness. There may be a neuropathic component to the weakness. Acute alcoholic myopathy can occur after an episode of heavy drinking. There is pain, cramps and muscle swelling that can lead to rhabdomyolysis with very high serum CK levels. The alcoholic myopathies improve when alcohol consumption is stopped.

Interesting facts

The nocebo effect is the opposite of the placebo effect, where a side effect may occur due to the belief that a medication will cause the side effect. Statin medications are well known to cause myalgia and less commonly myopathy and even rhabdomyolysis. Placebo studies suggest that the nocebo effect is the major cause of myalgia in most (but not all) people taking statins.

Inherited muscle disorders

Although individually rare, when taken collectively the incidence of genetic myopathies is very similar to the incidence of IIM and many genetic myopathies can closely mimic inflammatory myopathy. Some clinical clues that should prompt particular consideration of a genetic myopathy include a long history of slowly progressive symptoms, selective muscle group involvement (e.g. marked deltoid wasting but normal trapezius bulk in patients with fascioscapulohumeral dystrophy, see below), pathological muscle hypertrophy (technically pseudohypertrophy classically described in Duchenne's and Becker's muscular dystrophy), prominent muscle pain rather than weakness, other suggestive clinical features (e.g. bilateral ptosis, cardiomyopathy, respiratory muscle weakness in myotonic dystrophy, see below), a family history of neuromuscular symptoms or in any patient refractory to immunotherapy. It is far beyond the scope of this chapter to discuss genetic myopathies in any detail but a few are discussed here to represent the breadth of presentations and clinical features.

Muscular dystrophies

These represent a group of heterogeneous disorders with over 30 subtypes recognized and many more likely to emerge with advances in genetic diagnoses. In addition to skeletal muscle involvement, some subtypes of muscular dystrophy result in other organ involvement such as cardiac and respiratory systems. All modes of inheritance have been observed. An X-linked inheritance pattern is seen for Duchenne and Becker muscular dystrophy, both caused by mutations in the dystrophin-encoding *DMD* gene (on the X chromosome). These are the most common dystrophies seen in children and adolescents and can severely limit mobility and life expectancy (patients with Duchenne muscular dystrophy are wheelchair dependent by their adolescence and may not live past their early 20s). Myotonic dystrophies (type I and II; DM1 and DM2) are the most common dystrophies seen in adult patients. Inheritance is autosomal dominant and, as they are tri- and tetra-nucleotide repeat disorders respectively, can show generational anticipation. The characteristic finding of myotonia can be subtle, especially in DM2, but other clinical features include early cataract formation, bilateral ptosis and cardiac arrhythmia. Other more common subtypes of muscular dystrophy are the limb girdle muscular dystrophies (LGMD; characterized by proximal upper and lower limb muscle weakness) and facioscapulohumeral dystrophy (FSHD; characterized by weakness of the facial and proximal upper limb muscles). There are additional muscular dystrophies, especially those that present in infancy or very early childhood, which are beyond the scope of this review.

Metabolic myopathies

These result from genetic defects in enzymes necessary for the metabolism of carbohydrate or lipid. Symptoms occur as muscle is unable to produce sufficient energy. For this reason many patients will experience exercise-induced myalgia, cramping, lactic acidosis and recurrent episodes of rhabdomyolysis. The circumstances of symptoms can serve as a clue to the metabolic pathway affected – for example the early onset myalgia with 'second-wind phenomenon' seen in McArdle's disease, a disorder of carbohydrate metabolism, compared to episodes of rhabdomy-

olysis after prolonged endurance exercise especially after fasting in fatty acid oxidation defects. Metabolic myopathies include the subtypes of glycogen storage disease (most relevant being Pompe disease and McArdle's disease) and lipid storage diseases. In addition to the history, muscle biopsy can be very helpful in identifying these conditions.

Mitochondrial myopathies

As discussed previously, muscle has a very high concentration of mitochondria to perform oxidative phosphorylation (aerobic respiration) and supply ATP for muscle activity. The symptoms of a mitochondrial myopathy can overlap somewhat with metabolic myopathies and include early muscle fatigue and myalgia, proximal weakness and lactic acidosis. Mutations can be present in either the mitochondrial DNA (in which case there is a maternal mode of inheritance) or nuclear DNA (when all other forms of inheritance can be seen). Many genetic mitochondrial disorders have been described and, as well as skeletal muscle involvement, other clinical features include ptosis and chronic progressive external ophthalmoplegia and central nervous system involvement (especially episodes of encephalopathy). Muscle biopsy can appear normal but often has specific features suggestive of mitochondrial pathology.

Congenital myopathies

These disorders usually present at birth or in early life with generalized weakness, poor muscle bulk and, often, respiratory muscle weakness. Unlike the dystrophies, they usually have normal or only mildly elevated CK levels. Causes include the nemaline myopathies (with their characteristic rod-like inclusions seen on muscle biopsy), core myopathies (including the myopathy caused by mutations in the *RYR1* gene that also results in susceptibility to malignant hyperthermia on exposure to certain anaesthetic agents) and centronuclear myopathy (again with characteristic muscle biopsy features).

'Channelopathies'

These conditions result from mutations in various ion channels that consequently interfere with appropriate muscle contraction and relaxation. Causes include myotonia congenita and paramyotonia congenita as well as the hereditary periodic paralyses. Symptoms from these conditions are usually intermittent and transient and triggered by certain reproducible stimuli (such as temperature, electrolyte disturbance). Neurophysiology can be particularly important in making a diagnosis.

Disorders in which muscle pain is the main feature

Myofascial pain syndromes

Myofascial pain refers to a localized area of pain within a muscle. It is usually caused by acute overload of a muscle, fatigue due to chronic overuse or direct trauma. Any muscle group can be involved and there is a characteristic pain pattern for each muscle. The pain is usually over the involved muscle but there is also a referred pain pattern that is specific for each muscle.

The other feature of myofascial pain is a localized tender area, often called the 'trigger point', within the involved muscle. Sometimes bands of tight muscle fibres can be palpated within the muscle.

There is restriction of movement on stretching the involved muscle group and there may be weakness on isometric contraction. Myofascial pain is distinguished from other causes of muscle pain and weakness because it is usually restricted to one or two muscle groups. A careful clinical examination is required to identify the involved muscle. A correct diagnosis is important, because therapy has to be directed at the involved muscle.

Levator scapulae myofascial pain

The levator scapulae muscle is one of the more common muscles that have myofascial pain symptoms. The muscle extends from the upper medial border of the scapula to the transverse processes of the first four cervical vertebrae. The levator scapulae muscle, in conjunction with the other shoulder muscles, has an important action in stabilizing and moving the scapula and is associated with movement of the shoulder.

Levator scapulae pain is experienced at the angle of the neck and may radiate down the medial border of the scapula or out to the posterior aspect of the shoulder joint. Associated with this will be some restriction of neck movements and pain on stretching the levator scapulae muscle. Tenderness is maximal over the angle of the neck along the line of the muscle. Levator scapulae myofascial pain is often precipitated by using a keyboard in an abnormal position with the neck rotated but can occur in sports, for example, swimming, where frequent neck rotation is required. Treatment consists of stretching and strengthening exercises for the individual muscle and correction of the precipitating cause.

Fibromyalgia

Fibromyalgia is a condition characterized by widespread muscle pain in combination with widespread tenderness. It occurs most frequently in the 30–60 year age group, and 80%–90% of patients are female, though the syndrome may be underrecognized in men. Fibromyalgia may occur on its own or be associated with rheumatic

Case 8.1 Myopathy: 4

Case note: Treatment

You will recall that investigations in Mr Brown were consistent with a diagnosis of idiopathic polymyositis. Steroid myopathy was unlikely because of the high creatine kinase (CK) level and the absence of type II fibre atrophy on muscle biopsy. However, Mr Brown may develop type II fibre atrophy secondary to the increased prednisone required for the polymyositis.

Mr Brown was instructed by his rheumatologist to increase his prednisone to 50 mg/day and start taking azathioprine at 100 mg/day. After 6 weeks, his muscle power had returned to normal and his CK was 145 IU/mL. The prednisone was reduced over the next month to 10 mg/day and the over the next 3 months to 5 mg/day. Mr Brown's muscle power and CK level remain normal. Lung function tests remain unchanged.

disorders. Fibromyalgia that is associated with other rheumatic disorders, for example, rheumatoid arthritis and systemic lupus erythematosus (SLE), is clinically identical to fibromyalgia occurring on its own. It is increasingly thought of as a nociplastic pain disorder, characterized by central sensitization to pain, often in association with depression and sleep disturbance.

Clinical features

The pain most commonly involves muscles of the axial skeleton, including the shoulder and pelvic girdles. There is no diurnal variation in symptoms.

The pain is poorly localized but there are specific areas of tenderness, tender or trigger points.

Associated features of fibromyalgia are common and include sleep disturbance, irritable bowel syndrome, headaches, paraesthesia, urinary urgency and anxiety.

The disturbed sleep pattern is an important feature of fibromyalgia. The electroencephalographic changes during sleep in patients with fibromyalgia have shown a disturbance of Stage IV, non-rapid eye movement sleep. It is associated with non-restorative sleep and waking unrefreshed in the morning. Induction of this type of sleep pattern has been shown to produce symptoms and signs of fibromyalgia in otherwise healthy volunteers.

All investigations are normal, including erythrocyte sedimentation rate, C-reactive protein (CRP) and CK levels. If any of the laboratory tests are abnormal, then causes other than fibromyalgia need to be considered for the myalgia.

Management

It is important to make a positive diagnosis of fibromyalgia to distinguish it from other conditions that have overlapping symptomatology but different management. In particular, immunosuppression is not effective in fibromyalgia and should be avoided to prevent potential harm. Physical activity and ideally a graduated objectively measured or supervised exercise program is the most important and useful therapeutic intervention. Improvement is often relatively slow with function improving (i.e. able to do more despite ongoing pain) before pain reduces in intensity. It is difficult for patients with fibromyalgia to engage in regular activity and they should be set shared achievable goals, especially early on, to prove the benefit of physical therapy. Pharmacotherapy has a limited role in fibromyalgia. Some patients may derive some benefit from analgesics but this has to be weighed against the potential for harm. In particular, opiates should be avoided as is the case in chronic pain more generally. There is some evidence for antidepressants, especially in patients who have substantial relevant psychiatric co-morbidity or substantial sleep disturbance. Psychological interventions can be useful in subsets of patients.

Prognosis

The condition is chronic and is often difficult to treat. It tends to remain stable without any significant deterioration and about 60% of patients still have moderate symptoms 3 years after diagnosis. An understanding of the illness helps the patients' anxiety and improves their ability to cope with the disease.

Further reading

Firestein, G.S., Budd, R.C., Gabriel, S.E., et al., 2020. Firestein and Kelley's Textbook of Rheumatology, eleventh ed. Elsevier Saunders, Philadelphia.

Standring, S., 2021. Gray's Anatomy, forty-second ed. Philadelphia, Elsevier Limited.

West, S.G., 2020. Kolfenbach J: Rheumatology Secrets, fourth ed. Elsevier Saunders, Philadelphia.

AUTOIMMUNITY AND THE MUSCULOSKELETAL SYSTEM

9

Sean O'Neill

Chapter objectives

After studying this chapter, you should be able to:

1. Understand the features of autoimmune disease in the musculoskeletal system.

2. Understand the basis of immune complex disease pathogenesis.

3. Understand the use and interpretation of autoantibodies in diagnosis.

4. Understand the clinical features of systemic lupus erythematosus (SLE).

5. Understand the clinicopathological correlation of symptoms and signs in SLE.

6. Understand the treatment of SLE.

Introduction

Systemic lupus erythematosus (SLE) is the prototypic autoimmune disease, characterized by excessive autoantibody production, immune complex formation and immunologically-mediated tissue injury at multiple sites. It is a clinically heterogeneous disorder with a broad spectrum of presentations. Although the immune mechanism/s responsible for the breakdown of tolerance against self-antigens is unknown, a genetic influence in disease predisposition has been clearly demonstrated. Like most other connective tissue disorders, autoantibody testing can be of value in making the diagnosis. These results must always be correlated with the patient's symptoms and signs for correct interpretation. Treatment is symptomatic and aimed at suppressing an altered immune system that causes end-organ damage. In Chapter 1 we dealt with another autoimmune disease – rheumatoid arthritis (RA). This chapter will be illustrated by a case of SLE that tracks its course over several years to illustrate its clinical and immunological features.

Interesting facts

Lupus with its characteristic butterfly rash was long considered a skin disease. Kaposi in 1870 recognized that lupus had other extracutaneous manifestations such as arthritis and at the turn of the century, Osler recognized the systemic nature of the disease. In the 1920s Libman and Sacks differentiated the effects of lupus on the heart from that of rheumatic fever and, in 1938, Hargraves noted the Lupus Erythematosus-cell phenomenon, which later became the test for lupus. Steroids revolutionized the treatment of lupus in the 1950s; antinuclear antibodies were introduced for the identification and diagnosis of lupus in the 1960s. The survival of lupus patients has dramatically increased over the last 50 years. In 1953, 4 years after diagnosis 50% of patients had died. Nowadays, although the great majority of patients survive well beyond 4 years, the profound morbidity of the disease and its treatment remain challenging.

Immunology

Autoimmunity

Despite the heterogeneity of clinical features of SLE discussed later in this chapter, one characteristic laboratory finding is the presence of antibodies generated by the person's own immune system against a wide range of 'self' antigens, such as deoxyribonucleic acids (DNA) and ribonucleoproteins (RNPs). Since these antibodies are directed against 'self' antigens they are called 'autoantibodies'. A schematic representation of an anti-

Case 9.1 SLE: 1

Case history

Melanie, an 18-year-old woman, initially presented to her general practitioner (GP) complaining of joint pain in both hands. On specific questioning it was noted that she had felt unwell over the preceding several months and was experiencing increasing lethargy which was disproportionate to her daily activities. Other features noted in her history were the presence of facial rash, alopecia (hair loss) and mouth ulcers. There was no history of drug ingestion, overseas travel, diarrhoea, urinary tract symptoms or recent upper respiratory infection. The patient had a twin sister and two other siblings who were well. There was no family history of arthritis.

Physical examination revealed an ill-looking woman with a malar rash in a butterfly distribution over the face. The hair was sparse and there were mouth ulcers in the buccal cavity. Examination of the musculoskeletal system revealed tenderness in the proximal interphalangeal and metacarpophalangeal joints of both hands consistent with a symmetrical polyarthritis. There were small effusions present in both knees. There were no nodules or psoriatic skin changes. Heart sounds were dual with no murmurs and breath sounds were normal.

A presumptive diagnosis of systemic lupus erythematosus (SLE) was made. To confirm the clinical suspicion and to assess the extent of disease activity, she underwent a variety of serum and urine tests including testing for various autoantibodies. The serum tests showed a mild anaemia, elevated erythrocyte sedimentation rate (ESR), a positive antinuclear antibody (ANA) at a titre of 1:640 with a homogeneous pattern and positive antibody to the Sm antigen. Biochemistry and urinalysis were normal. The patient was started on hydroxychloroquine and low-dose prednisone that was tapered and ceased over several months.

gen–antibody (immune) complex is shown in Figure 9.1. The exact reason for this breakdown of immune tolerance is still unclear. There is evidence for abnormal function in most key facets of the immune system in SLE, beginning with failure of apoptosis leading to increased dendritic cell interaction with modified self antigens. Excessive activity of these antigen-presenting dendritic cells leads to activation of the interferon alpha pathway and increased antigen presentation to T cells. Reduced number and function of T regulatory cells has been observed, along with increased activity of antibody producing B cells. The consequence of this activity is autoantibody–antigen immune complex deposition in many vascular beds throughout the body results in a wide variety of clinical presentations. These manifestations are dictated by the site and extent of the inflammatory process, triggered by the antibody–antigen complex.

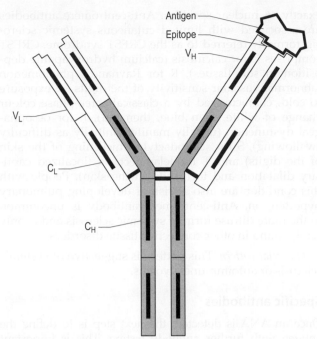

Fig. 9.1 Interaction of an antibody with antigen. Key for abbreviations: V_L = variable region of the light chain, V_H = variable region of the heavy chain, C_L = constant region of the light chain and C_H = constant region of the heavy chain. The epitope refers to the component of the antigen that binds to the antibody.

Immunopathology

An autoimmune disease like SLE is characterized by the production of many autoantibodies. Their exact role in disease aetiopathogenesis remains unclear. Some autoantibodies have been shown to contribute directly to the clinical picture by causing cell death. For example, anti-erythrocyte antibodies result in haemolysis (red cell lysis) and lymphocytotoxic antibodies are responsible for the reduced lymphocyte count (lymphopenia) that occurs in active lupus. An alternative mechanism of tissue injury is deposition of antigen–antibody complexes with subsequent complement activation. This is seen particularly in the kidney and skin. Complement and pro-inflammatory cytokine production result in polymorph trafficking into the area in question. Further release of pro-inflammatory mediators from mast cells, basophils and polymorphs perpetuate the inflammatory cascade. Platelet aggregation and clot formation result in microthrombi formation and tissue ischaemia. This is compounded by the release of proteases, hydrolytic enzymes and free radicals. Complement activation may also lead both directly (via complement components C5–9) and indirectly to cell lysis. Resultant end-organ damage in various tissues such as the kidney, skin and brain are responsible for the clinical manifestations of the disease. Under normal circumstances, antigen–antibody complexes are rapidly and efficiently cleared by phagocytes. However, defective mechanisms of immune complex clearance may perpetuate the inflammatory response.

Complement receptors (CR) bind different complement fragments produced during complement activation. They are found on erythrocytes (CR1), B cells (CR2) and macrophages and polymorphonuclear cells (CR3, CR4). Deficiency in these receptors may lead to continued inflammation and immune complex deposition. Immune complexes may also be cleared via the immunoglobulin portion of Fc receptors expressed on monocytes, polymorphonuclear cells and other immune cells. The Fc receptors are encoded by genes on chromosome 1 and have different forms (alleles) that may influence immune complex handling.

Cutaneous immunopathology

In skin, the three key features are immune complex deposition, vascular inflammation and mononuclear cell infiltration. Immunoglobulin and complement deposition occurs at the dermo–epidermal junction, presumably because this is highly vascular. This can be detected in a skin biopsy by immunofluorescence and is called the 'lupus band test'. Immunofluorescence involves staining with specific antibody preparations labelled with fluorescent compounds and examining for fluorescence by microscopy. It is not completely specific for SLE, being seen in other autoimmune conditions such as RA.

Renal immunopathology

Immune complex deposition in the glomeruli is the main immunopathogenic mechanism that results in tissue injury. Immunofluorescence often reveals the deposition of IgG, IgM, IgA, C3, C4 and C1q. These deposits are of variable clinical significance and may lead to a range of clinical consequences from very mild to rapidly progressive severe renal disease. This will be discussed again later.

Central nervous system immunopathology

The pathogenesis of central nervous system (CNS) lupus is uncertain, but immune deposition and activation in the cerebral vasculature may result in microvascular and macrovascular thromboses (clots) with resultant cerebral oedema and ischaemia. Other possible mechanisms include a direct effect of autoantibodies on neuronal tissue with resultant dysfunction. Anti-ribosomal P antibodies have been associated with psychosis in SLE. It is important to exclude other diagnoses such as infection, renal failure, malignant hypertension and drug-related effects in an often immunosuppressed patient.

Serological manifestations of autoimmunity

Complement

In autoimmune disease, activation and deposition of complement components induced by antigen–antibody complexes cause tissue damage such as glomerulonephritis (glomerular inflammation) in the kidney. Low serum levels of complement (C3, C4) reflect consumption and are useful in assessing disease activity. Contrary to what may be expected, complement factor deficiency is associated with a predisposition to SLE, possibly due to a decrease in the ability to solubilize immune complexes leading to tissue deposition and inflammation. C1q/r/s and C4 deficiencies show the strongest association with SLE, whereas C2 deficiency may manifest a lupus-like disease with cutaneous manifestations. C3 deficiency is rare.

Antinuclear antibodies

The most typical serologic abnormality in SLE is the presence of antinuclear antibodies (ANA). These antibodies are usually directed against intranuclear proteins involved in DNA packaging, RNA splicing or RNA translation. The two important features of an ANA are: (1) the titre (extent of serum dilution that still gives a detectable pattern) and (2) the pattern of immunofluorescence.

Titre

The titre does not always correlate with clinical activity, since it is the avidity of antibody binding that is important and not the amount. More than 95% of patients with SLE have a positive ANA. ANA-negative SLE is very uncommon and may be due to the presence of anti-cytoplasmic antibodies, the commonest being SS-A (also known as Ro). Our patient had a moderately positive ANA at a titre of 1/640. It is important to remember that a positive ANA is not diagnostic of SLE and can occur with other illnesses, for example bacterial and viral infection, drug therapy and other inflammatory disorders. About 5% of the normal population have a positive ANA at a titre of 1:160 or below.

Staining patterns

Different staining patterns (Fig. 9.2) reflect the nature of the antigen and its distribution. Their disease associations are summarized in Table 9.1. Different patterns include:

Homogenous pattern This pattern is most common in SLE and drug-induced lupus erythematosus. The antigen is usually DNA, histones or deoxyribonucleoprotein.

Rim pattern This pattern is also associated predominantly with SLE. It is thought that rim and homogenous are essentially the same pattern, but appear slightly differently due to sectioning of cells.

Speckled pattern This is the most frequent staining pattern and may occur in people with SLE, but is also commonly occurs in other illnesses and normal people with low titres of ANA.

Anti-centromere pattern This specific speckled pattern is due to antibodies to the centromere and results in

exactly 46 nuclear speckles. Anti-centromere antibodies are associated with limited cutaneous systemic sclerosis, formerly referred to as the CREST syndrome. CREST comprises C for calcinosis (calcium hydroxyapatite deposition in soft tissues), R for Raynaud's phenomenon (abnormal vascular sensitivity of the digits on exposure to cold, characterized by a classical three-phase colour change of white, then blue, then red), E for oesophageal dysfunction (usually manifest initially as difficulty swallowing), S for sclerodactyly (thickening of the skin of the digits) and T for telangiectasia (localized capillary dilatation and tortuosity in the skin). People with this condition are also at risk of developing pulmonary hypertension. Anti-centromere antibody is uncommon in the more diffuse form of systemic sclerosis and is only rarely found in other connective tissue disorders.

Nucleolar pattern This pattern is suggestive of systemic sclerosis or autoimmune myositis.

Specific antibodies

Once an ANA is detected, the next step is to define the antigen with further antibody testing. This is important because specific autoantibodies are associated with particular clinical features and particular autoimmune diseases.

Antibodies to dsDNA

Antibodies to double-stranded DNA (dsDNA) are specific for SLE, but are only present in 40% of patients. Elevated levels are usually associated with active disease, but patients can have elevated DNA antibodies and be clinically quiescent. Rapid rises or falls in DNA antibody levels may precede flares in the disease. Levels may fall with successful treatment. The presence of dsDNA correlates well with the probability of development of lupus nephritis (kidney disease). They have a pathogenic role by complexing with DNA trapped in glomeruli or by direct attachment to glomerular structures. Their complement-fixing ability then results in tissue damage.

Serum complement levels of C3 and C4 are useful in monitoring disease activity in conjunction with dsDNA levels. A rapid rise or fall of dsDNA levels in association with a fall in complement C3 and/or C4, is more likely to be significant than when the complement levels remain normal.

Antibodies to extractable nuclear antigens

The extractable nuclear antigens (ENA) consist of a number of antigens which include RNP, Smith antigen (Sm), SS-A/Ro, SS-B/La, Jo-1, ribosomal-p and Scl-70. Their disease associations are summarized in Table 9.2. Autoantibodies can also be useful in helping with the diagnosis of connective tissue disorders (see Table 9.2). The clinical findings are the most important factor in determining which autoantibody to measure.

Anti-RNP

Antibodies to RNP are present in about one-third of patients with SLE and are the only autoantibodies present in patients with so-called 'mixed connective tissue disease'.

Anti-Sm

Anti-Sm antibody is highly specific for SLE but is present in only about 20% of patients. Therefore, although it is very specific, it is not particularly sensitive. Our patient had a positive anti-Sm antibody.

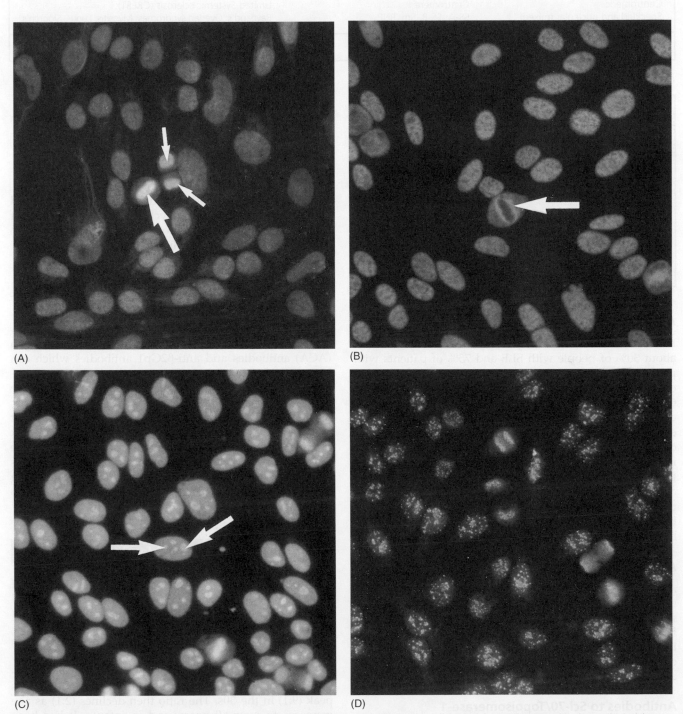

Fig. 9.2 Fluorescence micrographs of ANA staining patterns. (A) Homogeneous: the arrows indicate staining of DNA inside the nucleus. (B) Speckled: the arrow indicates staining of non-DNA fragments. Compare it with (A), where there is clearly staining of DNA. (C) Nucleolar: this indicates staining of the nucleolus (arrows). (D) Centromere: as the antigen is the centromere, there are exactly 46 nuclear speckles. (Courtesy the Immunology Laboratory, Institute of Clinical Pathology and Medical Research, Westmead Hospital.)

Table 9.1 ANA patterns and disease associations

Pattern	Antigen	Association
Homogeneous	Deoxyribonucleic acid, histones	SLE; Drug-induced lupus
Speckled	SS-A, SS-B, Sm, RNP	SLE; Sjögren's syndrome; MCTD
Nucleolar	–	Systemic sclerosis; Polymyositis
Centromeric	Centromere	Limited Systemic sclerosis (CREST)
Speckled and nucleolar (mixed)	SS-A, SS-B, Sm, RNP	Raynaud's; Overlap syndromes; Myositis; Lupus; Sjögren's

ANA, antinuclear antibody; MCTD, mixed connective tissue disease.

Table 9.2 Specific autoantibodies and their disease association

Antibody	Disease association
dsDNA	SLE
Sm	SLE
SS-A/Ro with SS-B/La	Primary Sjögren's syndrome
SS-A/Ro without SS-B/La	SLE, Sjögren's syndrome
Jo-1	Polymyositis/dermatomyositis
RNP	Mixed connective tissue disease
Scl-70	Diffuse systemic sclerosis
Anti-centromere	Limited systemic sclerosis (CREST)

Anti-SS-A/Ro

Anti-SS-A/Ro is a relatively common antibody found in about 30% of people with SLE and 75% of patients with primary Sjögren's syndrome (indeed SS is an abbreviation of Sjögren's syndrome). Some laboratories report anti-Ro 60 and anti-Ro 52 separately as the antibodies bind two different antigens. Sjögren's syndrome is characterized by chronic inflammation of the lacrimal and salivary glands, causing dryness of the eyes and mouth respectively, and is associated with other autoimmune diseases such as RA. People with SLE who have anti-Ro are more likely to have cutaneous involvement. Women with this antibody, when pregnant, are more likely to have children with congenital heart block. This applies particularly if they also have antibodies to SS-B/La.

Anti-SS-B/La

Antibodies to SS-B/La are less common and usually occur in conjunction with anti-SS-A/Ro. They are present in only about 10% of people with SLE and in about 50% of primary Sjögren's syndrome. Their presence may indicate a milder course of disease in SLE. The presence of both SS-A/Ro and SS-B/La is more commonly associated with primary Sjögren's syndrome.

Antibodies to Scl-70/Topoisomerase-1

Antibodies to Scl-70 are highly specific for diffuse systemic sclerosis. They occur in about 50% of patients with diffuse skin involvement.

Antibodies to Jo-1

Antibodies to Jo-1 are present in 30% of people with polymyositis, particularly in those who also have pulmonary fibrosis as discussed in Chapter 8.

Antibodies to ribosomal-p

These antibodies are present in about 15% of SLE, and may be associated with psychiatric manifestations of SLE. However, the association is not strong enough to make them of diagnostic value.

Anti-phospholipid/anti-cardiolipin antibodies

These consist of a number of antibodies that bind to different negatively charged phospholipids of the cell membrane. They include lupus anticoagulant, anti-cardiolipin (ACA) antibodies and anti-β2Gp1 antibodies which can be independently positive. Lupus anticoagulant may prolong the clotting time of various bleeding tests such as the activated partial thromboplastin time (APTT). However, despite the prolonged APTT, the patient is actually at increased risk of thrombosis, as well as increased risk of pregnancy morbidity. How these antibodies induce thrombosis is incompletely understood, though there is evidence for numerous possible mechanisms including binding to specific domains β2Gp1, as well as binding to platelets, macrophages and endothelial cells.

Clinical features and epidemiology

SLE is traditionally considered to present in women of child-bearing age, with a peak incidence between 15 and 40 years of age. However, the onset can range outside of these age groups to involve infants and the elderly.

Some 90% of patients with SLE are female. This strong correlation suggests that hormonal factors may be involved in disease development. The female-to-male ratio of incidence ranges from 5:1 at teenage to its peak (9:1) in the 30s. The ratio then declines (2:1) as age increases to over 60 years, and in infants. It has been postulated that sex hormones play an important role in disease predisposition and may modulate the immune system, either by oestrogens inhibiting and androgens accelerating clearance of circulating immune complexes; oestrogens stimulating antibody production by B cells; and/or androgens stimulating T suppressor/cytotoxic cell activity. Females may develop full-blown SLE after receiving high-dose oestrogens for oral contraception and pregnancy can lead to flares of the disease.

SLE has no geographic limitation and a worldwide prevalence that varies from 15–207/100 000 per head of population. The incidence (number of new cases per head of population per year) rates also vary between studies and range from 1.8–7.6/100 000 per year. In general the prevalence is approximately 1 in 2000, although this may vary depending on geographical (racial) differences, ethnicity and socioeconomic status.

SLE is commoner in Afro-Caribbeans (prevalence rate of 207/100,000) and Asians (49/100,000) compared with Caucasians (20/100,000). Interestingly, despite the high incidence and prevalence of SLE in Blacks in the UK and USA, lupus is thought to be almost non-existent in West and Central Africa. Further epidemiological studies are needed to understand this difference, though the results suggest that there may be more than genetic influences determining susceptibility and that environmental factors are likely to be important.

Pathology

The pathologic findings of SLE are widely distributed throughout the body and reflect tissue damage due to immune complex deposition and primary or secondary infiltration of tissue with mononuclear cells. The pathology is characterized by inflammation, blood vessel abnormalities secondary to immune complex deposition and/or cellular infiltrate. Pathological findings in the kidney are described below.

The kidney in SLE

The WHO classification of lupus nephritis is shown in Table 9.3. Light microscopic examination of the kidney reveals increases in mesangial cells and matrix, an inflammatory cellular infiltrate and basement membrane damage. Mesangial proliferative nephritis has the best prognosis and is characterized by immune complex and complement deposition predominantly in the mesangium with an increase in mesangial cellularity and matrix. Focal and segmental proliferative nephritis has involvement of some parts (segmental) of some glomeruli (focal) only (Class III). This is manifested by an increase in the resident glomerular endothelial and mesangial cells as well as infiltrating inflammatory cells. This form of nephritis is concerning and has a variable prognosis. Diffuse proliferative nephritis is the most serious form of lupus nephritis (Class IV). There are usually significant increases in glomerular cellularity, fibrin deposition and necrosis resulting in crescent formation. On electron microscopic examination, the immune deposits reside in the mesangium and on the subepithelial and subendothelial sides of the glomerular basement membrane. Another form of nephritis is membranous nephritis. This has diffusely thickened capillary loops with marked proteinuria. Advanced sclerosing nephritis is characterized by glomerular fibrosis and sclerosis.

Other clinicopathological correlations

Constitutional symptoms of lethargy, malaise and feeling unwell are common features of active SLE and may herald the onset of a flare. Cytokines produced as a result of inflammation are believed to be responsible for the lethargy and fatigue. Serum levels of tumour necrosis factor alpha (TNF-α), IFN-α, IFN-γ and IL-6 are elevated in SLE while TNF-α levels have been shown to correlate with disease activity in SLE. These symptoms are non-specific and one should be cautious of underlying infection. Fatigue and widespread pain are common symptoms in SLE and it is important to differentiate disease flares from other factors that contribute to fatigue such as depression, thyroid dysfunction, anaemia and sleep disturbance. The major clinical features to examine for are depicted pictorially in Figure 9.4. The common clinicopathological features are discussed below.

Skin

Skin lesions in SLE patients are classified as either acute (butterfly rash, photosensitivity), sub-acute (sub-acute cutaneous lupus erythematosus or SCLE) or chronic (discoid). The characteristic acute malar butterfly rash seen in acute flares presents as an erythematous, elevated and painful photosensitive lesion (Fig. 9.5) that spares the nasolabial fold. The malar rash is the commonest recognized skin manifestation of SLE. Conditions such as cellulitis of the face or rosacea do not spare the nasolabial fold. Other acute lesions include erythema in sun-exposed areas (photosensitivity) or blistering lesions in dark-skinned individuals. It has been found that lymphocytes from SLE patients are activated by light in the near ultraviolet (360–400 nm) wavelength. This heightened activity, along with ultraviolet light induced keratinocyte death and oxidation of self-nuclear antigens may result in tissue damage and exposure of more autoantigen which further stimulates the immune-mediated process occurring in skin. Localized fixed lesions may also be seen and are termed discoid lupus. These are erythematous plaques or papules with a hypopigmented central area that may occur in the presence or absence of systemic manifestations of SLE.

Other non-specific dermatological manifestations of SLE are protean and may include panniculitis, urticaria and vasculitic lesions such as palpable purpura. Histologic examination of the skin reveals non-specific inflammation with abundant immune deposits on immunofluorescence at the dermo–epidermal junction.

Case 9.1 — **SLE: 2**

Case progress

Melanie remained stable for 2 years. At the end of this period, she again became unwell and developed a malar rash, polyarthritis, chest pain, shortness of breath and vasculitic lesions on her hands. An abnormal urinary sediment with haematuria and proteinuria was noted on urinalysis. Proteinuria usually indicates excessive leakiness of the glomerular basement membrane which, in combination with haematuria, almost certainly indicates glomerular inflam-

mation. Accordingly, a renal biopsy was performed and confirmed acute glomerulonephritis (Fig. 9.3). The results of laboratory tests revealed she was anaemic, had an elevated ESR and C-reactive protein (CRP), normal creatinine, low C3 and C4 and her dsDNA was markedly elevated. The patient was commenced on high-dose prednisone and mycophenolate in addition to her hydroxychloroquine. Her clinical picture stabilized with the institution of the above therapy.

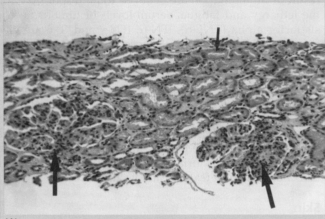

(A)

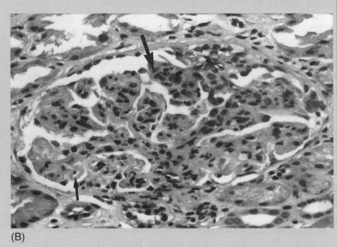

(B)

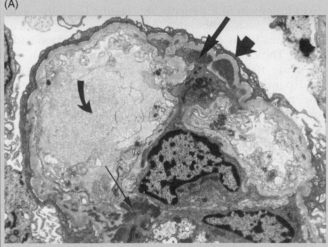

(C)

Fig. 9.3 (A) Low power photomicrograph of a renal biopsy showing two glomeruli *(large arrows)* and normal tubules *(small arrow)*. (B) High power photomicrograph of a glomerulus showing features of a diffuse proliferative glomerulonephritis. There is an increase in mesangial cellularity *(large arrow)* and lobulation as well as thickened capillary loops *(small arrow)*. (C) Electron micrograph of a capillary loop showing fusion of foot processes *(short wide arrow)* in diffuse proliferative glomerulonephritis (Class IV). Other notable features are subendothelial electron-dense deposits *(straight large arrow)* and focal mesangial deposits *(straight thin arrow)*. The curved arrow indicates the capillary lumen (Courtesy Dr Thomas Ng, Institute of Clinical Pathology and Medical Research, Westmead Hospital.)

Musculoskeletal

Arthralgia and/or arthritis are the commonest clinical manifestations of SLE. Synovitis is due to inflammation induced by deposition of antigen–antibody immune complexes with complement activation and release of numerous different inflammatory cytokines reflecting widespread immune activation. The arthritis seen in SLE usually affects the small joints of the hand, wrists and knees. Although most cases of SLE arthritis are symmetric, asymmetric presentations can occur. It

may be distinguished from RA because it is non-erosive. Although nodules are more common in RA, they may also occur in SLE. Tenosynovitis is frequently seen in SLE. Significant joint deformity may occur in SLE. This pattern of non-erosive but deforming disease is termed 'Jaccoud's arthritis' and may be confused with RA. In these patients, the hand deformities include subluxation with ulnar deviation at the metacarpophalangeal joints (Fig. 9.6). This is a non-erosive arthritis and the deformities are reducible – unlike the fixed deformities seen in

Table 9.3 World Health Organization classification of lupus nephritis

Type		Approximate prevalence (%)
I	Normal glomeruli	≤10
II	Mesangial proliferative	10
III	Focal and segmental proliferative	15
IV	Diffuse proliferative	50
V	Membranous	15
VI	Advanced sclerosing	≤10

Adapted from Becker, G.J., Whitworth, J.A., Kincaid-Smith, P., 1992. Clinical nephrology in medical practice. Blackwell, Victoria.

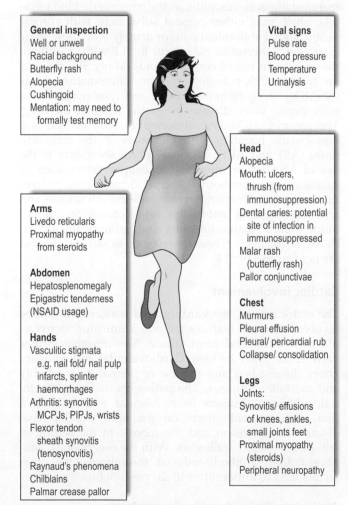

General inspection
Well or unwell
Racial background
Butterfly rash
Alopecia
Cushingoid
Mentation: may need to
   formally test memory

Vital signs
Pulse rate
Blood pressure
Temperature
Urinalysis

Head
Alopecia
Mouth: ulcers,
   thrush (from
   immunosuppression)
Dental caries: potential
   site of infection in
   immunosuppressed
Malar rash
   (butterfly rash)
Pallor conjunctivae

Arms
Livedo reticularis
Proximal myopathy
   from steroids

Abdomen
Hepatosplenomegaly
Epigastric tenderness
(NSAID usage)

Chest
Murmurs
Pleural effusion
Pleural/ pericardial rub
Collapse/ consolidation

Hands
Vasculitic stigmata
   e.g. nail fold/ nail pulp
   infarcts, splinter
   haemorrhages
Arthritis: synovitis
   MCPJs, PIPJs, wrists
Flexor tendon
   sheath synovitis
   (tenosynovitis)
Raynaud's phenomena
Chilblains
Palmar crease pallor

Legs
Joints:
Synovitis/ effusions
   of knees, ankles,
   small joints feet
Proximal myopathy
   (steroids)
Peripheral neuropathy

Fig. 9.4 Clinical manifestations of SLE. This is a multi-system disease.

RA. Radiological examination of the hands reveals only periarticular osteoporosis due to disuse and soft tissue swelling, but no erosions or joint destruction. This is often surprising given that significant deformity may be present clinically.

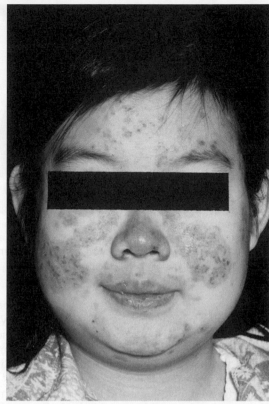

Fig. 9.5 The malar (butterfly) rash of SLE. (Courtesy Professor Les Schrieber, Department of Rheumatology, Royal North Shore Hospital.)

Avascular necrosis of bone may be seen in SLE, particularly in the presence of a positive ACA antibody. It is more commonly seen in the context of corticosteroid usage, however, this diagnosis should always be considered in a patient with SLE who presents with acute onset severe bony pain, regardless of whether or not they are being treated with corticosteroids. The underlying mechanism is presumed to be thrombotic in aetiology.

> **Interesting facts**
>
> Osteoporosis is very common in lupus. It can be a manifestation of the disease or secondary to medications and should be monitored regularly and treated appropriately.

Renal

This is one of the major determinants of morbidity and mortality in lupus. Patients do not usually volunteer symptoms pertaining to this system until late in the course of renal failure. Symptoms may include shortness of breath, headache, oliguria (reduced urine output) and ankle oedema. Lupus nephritis may often be clinically silent. It is worth remembering that urinalysis should be considered as part of the physical examination. It provides an immense amount of clinical information. In this case, it identified the onset of lupus nephritis. Although renal involvement is suggested by an elevated creatinine, proteinuria, haematuria and

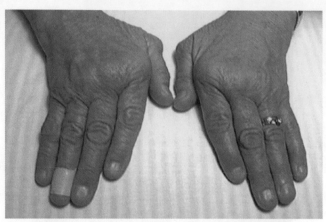

Fig. 9.6 A patient with lupus and Jaccoud's arthritis. The features include a symmetric deforming hand arthritis with ulnar deviation at the metacarpophalangeal joints. Unlike rheumatoid arthritis, the deformities are reducible and there are no signs of joint erosion on X-ray.

presence of casts, the only way to accurately determine the type and extent of renal involvement is by renal biopsy and histologic examination. However, given that a renal biopsy may be complicated by significant morbidity, for example bleeding, it is usually only indicated if an abnormality is detected in one or more of the above parameters.

Once performed, histologic and immunologic examination of the tissue obtained is useful in both diagnosis and prognosis. The presence of acute inflammatory changes such as cellular proliferation, cellular crescents and leukocyte infiltration, necessitates the institution of potent immunosuppressive therapy in an attempt to reverse the inflammatory changes and prevent further renal damage. On the other hand, while the presence of chronic changes such as sclerotic glomeruli and fibrosis may augur poorly for the patient's renal function, it does not require the commencement of immunosuppressive therapy.

Neuropsychiatric

SLE may affect the central and peripheral nervous systems and cause abnormal (psychiatric) behaviour. CNS involvement may be subdivided into: (a) organic brain syndrome, manifested by focal signs, seizures, strokes or chorea; or (b) psychosis, often with depression, dementia, hallucinations and delusions. The diagnosis of neuropsychiatric lupus is difficult and a large number of imaging techniques (e.g. MRI, CT scan, PET) are not specific in making the diagnosis. However, the presence of multiple high-signal lesions on MRI in a young person with appropriate autoimmune serology is highly suggestive of cerebral lupus. These imaging modalities are useful in excluding other causes of CNS dysfunction such as infection in SLE patients. The diagnosis of neuropsychiatric lupus is predominantly a clinical one.

Pulmonary

Lung involvement in SLE may include pleurisy, pneumonitis, pulmonary haemorrhage, pulmonary hypertension and pulmonary embolism. Pneumonitis may simulate pneumonia with clinical features of fever, cough and haemoptysis. Serositis is a generic term for inflammation of serosal membranes lining visceral and thoracic organs. Pleurisy and pericarditis are two examples and may manifest as inflammation or effusions. Pulmonary vasculitis is uncommon but may present precipitously with haemoptysis. The other cause of haemoptysis that requires exclusion is pulmonary emboli, particularly in the setting of the anti-phospholipid antibody syndrome (APAS). Pulmonary hypertension, usually presenting in patients as dyspnoea, may be the result of recurrent pulmonary emboli or pulmonary vasculitis.

Gastroenterology

Abdominal serositis (peritonitis) may manifest as abdominal pain. One of the most feared gastrointestinal manifestations is vasculitis of the mesenteric blood vessels which may either present subacutely with chronic post-prandial abdominal pain or acutely with mesenteric infarction. Pancreatitis may occur in SLE with or without the co-existent use of corticosteroids. Many SLE patients are treated with non-steroidal anti-inflammatory drugs (NSAIDs) for symptomatic relief and thus may present with peptic ulcer disease or gastrointestinal bleeding. The commonest hepatic abnormality seen in SLE is a non-specific hepatitis with elevation of the transaminases (AST and ALT). This may occur secondary to the use of NSAIDs or other immunosuppressives such as azathioprine or methotrexate. Specific autoimmune liver involvement with characteristic anti-smooth muscle and anti-mitochondrial antibodies are features of autoimmune chronic active hepatitis and primary biliary cirrhosis, respectively. These diseases are organ-specific and are not features of SLE.

Cardiac involvement

The endocardium, myocardium and pericardium can be involved. Clinical features include a murmur, tachycardia, arrhythmia and heart failure. Non-infective cardiac valve lesions may be seen. Cardiovascular and coronary artery disease is a major cause of premature morbidity and mortality in lupus. The pathogenesis is multifactorial, with contributions from vascular wall inflammation, corticosteroid effects on the lipid profile, renal disease, hypertension and thrombosis in the setting of anti-phospholipid antibodies. With the exception of anti-phospholipid antibody-induced thromboses, the other factors tend to impact after 10–20 years of lupus activity.

Anti-phospholipid antibody syndrome

These are autoantibodies directed against components of the cellular membrane. The APAS or ACA antibody syndrome has three components: (a) arterial and/or venous thrombosis; (b) thrombocytopenia or a reduced platelet count; and (c) spontaneous abortions associated with persistently positive ACA antibodies, anti-β2Gp1 antibodies or lupus anticoagulant. It may occur as a primary syndrome with no apparent cause or in association with an underlying connective tissue disease such as SLE (secondary). About half of all patients with the APAS have the primary form of the disease. Antiphospholipid antibodies are found in approximately one-third of all patients with SLE, though only one-third of them develop the clinical syndrome. The antibodies are found in up to 2% of normal controls. Both primary and secondary APAS have similar manifestations and the activity of APAS in SLE is independent of the clinical activity of the lupus. Long-term anticoagulation is generally indicated.

Aetiology

Environmental factors

The aetiology of SLE is unclear but probably results from an interplay between susceptibility genes and environmental stimuli. Potential environmental stimuli that could trigger the process include stress, sunlight, drugs/chemicals (TNF inhibitors, procainamide, hydralazine, sulphonamides), pollutants/toxins, hairsprays, diet (alfalfa sprouts) and infections (viruses, bacterial superantigens). As yet, there is no definitive evidence for involvement of a specific infective agent in the aetiology of SLE. Viral agents possibly implicated in SLE are cytomegalovirus (CMV), Epstein–Barr virus (EBV) and retroviruses.

It has been postulated that an environmental agent, such as a microbe, may produce autoimmune disease in a genetically susceptible host by 'molecular mimicry'. That is, the antigen incites antibodies that cross-react with the host's proteins. Alternatively, the inciting agent may alter the structure of proteins in the host, thus resulting in a breakdown of immune tolerance in the host.

Superantigens are antigens that interact with major histocompatibility complex (MHC) class II molecules on the surface of antigen-presenting cells and with specific elements of the T cell receptor (TCR). This mode of immune activation can trigger T cell proliferation and the release of large concentrations of cytokines leading to fever, malaise and, at times, shock. In addition, superantigens may bridge T cells and B cells, allowing rapid polyclonal B cell activation with autoantibody secretion. Superantigens may originate from bacteria and thus may provide the link between infection and triggering of autoimmunity. As yet there is no clear evidence indicating that superantigens may directly trigger SLE in human beings.

Genetics

Persuasive evidence for a genetic influence on SLE predisposition has arisen from twin studies, familial aggregation, studies of ethnicity and experimental animal

---

Case 9.1 SLE: 3

Clinical case

Recall that Melanie was anaemic when she flared. In SLE this can be due to a number of factors, including the anaemia of chronic disease, renal failure, autoimmune haemolysis and iron deficiency due to poor dietary intake or blood loss induced by NSAIDs. In our patient, the two main factors were an anaemia of chronic disease compounded by poor dietary intake. There was no evidence of autoimmune haemolysis on the blood film, her serum creatinine level was in the normal range and she was not on any NSAIDs. Her ESR was markedly elevated at 112 mm/h and her CRP was also elevated. The ESR and CRP are objective markers of inflammation, though the CRP may frequently be normal or only modestly elevated in active SLE – high levels of CRP should raise suspicion for bacterial infection. Inflammation leads to an increase in serum proteins such as fibrinogen, immunoglobulins, ferritin and alpha-1-antitrypsin, which are known as acute phase reactants. These proteins cause red cells to become adherent to each other and hence sediment faster. An ESR is a sensitive but not particularly specific test for inflammation. The presence of a significantly elevated ESR (>100 mm/h) should raise the suspicion of a connective tissue disorder, chronic infection such as tuberculosis or bacterial endocarditis, malignancy or a paraprotein. In the elderly with headache and an elevated ESR, giant cell (temporal) arteritis should be considered (see Ch. 1).

The CRP is a specific acute phase reactant whose hepatic synthesis is upregulated predominantly by interleukin-6 (IL-6), which in turn is upregulated in inflammation. Its half-life is only a few days. As such, the CRP tends to mirror the clinical course of inflammation more closely than an ESR.

Melanie's twin sister becomes symptomatic with fatigue and arthralgia and questions if she could also have lupus. Investigation reveals a positive ANA and the presence of antibodies against dsDNA. The development of lupus in her sister raises questions about aetiology and the role of genetic versus environmental factors in the predisposition to disease. The issues surrounding aetiology, management and clinical outcome are discussed below.

---

models of the disease. In SLE, supporting data for each of these parameters makes the case for genetic predisposition compelling. In twin studies, there is a higher concordance for disease in monozygotic (24%–60%) than in dizygotic twins (5%). Similarly, family studies have provided convincing evidence of a genetic basis in SLE by identifying an increased prevalence of disease in siblings from the same family compared with the normal population.

Numerous studies have attempted to find associations between candidate genes and patients with SLE. Of these the major histocompatibility locus genes have been the most extensively studied. The B8-DR3 haplotype is associated with SLE in Caucasian individuals. Since these genes are in linkage disequilibrium with other MHC genes, the extended haplotype associated with SLE is A1-B8-C4A0-DR3-DQW2. The DQ genes have been shown to correlate better with autoantibody formation than with clinical phenotype, for example anti-Sm has been associated with DR2, 4, 7 and DQ6; anti-Ro with DR2, 4 and DQbeta; anti-phospholipid antibodies with DR4, 7 and DQ6 and 7.

Genome wide association studies (GWAS) have identified many risk loci for SLE susceptibility, each conferring a small increased relative risk of disease. There is no one single gene defect as the cause of SLE. Interestingly, a number of these loci are concentrated in the dendritic cell/interferon alpha pathways for antigen presentation and suggest a role for this pathway in disease pathogenesis.

Interesting facts

Lupus patients are predisposed to an increased risk of heart disease, irrespective of their medications. The treating doctor should take stricter measures to control cardiac risk factors. The main cause of death in lupus is cardiovascular disease.

Interesting facts

Two out of 100 children whose mother has lupus will get lupus. No one gene will predispose to the disease. Environmental triggers are important with sunlight, drugs especially 'sulpha' antibiotics, smoking, infections and stress (mental or physical) exacerbating or triggering the disease.

Treatment

The management of SLE is largely dependent on the severity of the disease and the type and extent of organ involvement. Simpler measures such as education and psychosocial intervention can affect morbidity and mortality and should therefore not be underestimated. Infections that can mimic flares should be excluded and/or treated early and aggressively.

General principles (prevention)

Avoid the sun

This includes the use of sunscreen (at least SPF 50), a hat, long-sleeved clothing or even a change in occupation. Vitamin D supplementation is usually required.

Avoidance of infections

This includes routine vaccination (may require yearly influenza vaccines) and prompt treatment of any infection.

Tight control of cardiovascular risk factors

Attention to control of hypertension is important in minimizing damage to the renal vasculature and preventing atherosclerosis, along with smoking cessation, lipid control through diet and medication. A healthy weight and diet and exercise should be encouraged

Contraception

Healthy pregnancy is possible in the majority of women with SLE, particularly in those with good disease control for more than six months. Contraception is important in women with active disease, particularly lupus nephritis as pregnancy may cause further deterioration of already tenuous renal function along with increased foetal morbidity and mortality. It is clear from all the published data that as the degree of renal insufficiency increases, the risk that renal function will worsen during pregnancy rises sharply. The issue of contraception is also of strong relevance if cytotoxic therapy is being used as the effects of such therapy on an unborn foetus are of concern. High dose oestrogens may be contraindicated in those with active SLE or those with a history of thrombosis or APAS.

Regular follow-up

Some indicators of disease flares can only be detected by urine or blood tests. Regular follow-up with a physician to monitor for potential side-effects from medications or disease flares should be performed.

Drug therapy

Non-steroidal anti-inflammatory drugs (NSAIDs)

These are useful for symptomatic relief and are usually given as first-line treatment, either alone or in combination with the other drugs discussed below, for mild flares of inflammatory symptoms such as serositis and arthritis. The significant side-effects of gastrointestinal bleeding and renal impairment should be looked for closely. Since NSAIDs may affect renal function by decreasing renal perfusion or by causing acute interstitial nephritis, they should be discontinued in patients suspected of having renal involvement. Renal impairment is thought to arise by inhibition of the vasodilatory prostaglandins that mediate renal perfusion and is more prevalent in the elderly and in those with pre-existing renal impairment. NSAIDs may also aggravate hypertension via promoting salt and water retention in the kidney.

An unusual feature of ibuprofen (a conventional NSAID) in SLE patients is its propensity to induce an aseptic meningitis syndrome characterized by headache, fever and meningism. The symptoms resolve on cessation of the drug.

Anti-malarials

Hydroxychloroquine is useful for the dermatologic, musculoskeletal and mild constitutional manifestations of lupus, and has been shown to be a useful adjunct in managing more severe organ involvement. Its mechanism of action is uncertain but it may work by interfering with lysosomal function and thus impairing phagocytic activity, preventing dendritic cells from binding self-antigens through Toll-like receptors. It is a weak immunosuppressant that does not require regular blood monitoring and is usually used in conjunction with sunscreen and topical steroids. Side-effects include corneal deposits and retinal toxicity. These side-effects are less with hydroxychloroquine than with chloroquine. Although the risk of retinal toxicity due to hydroxychloroquine is low, formal ophthalmological review every 12 months to detect any restriction in visual fields is recommended.

Corticosteroids

These drugs, already discussed in Chapter 1, form the cornerstone of treatment for the acute active manifestations of lupus. Corticosteroids can be given intravenously for acute life-threatening presentations, intra-articularly, topically, orally and at times intralesionally for discoid lupus. Prednisone significantly increases susceptibility to infection dependent on the dose and duration, along with numerous metabolic risks. Other agents are frequently used to facilitate reduction in steroid dose where possible.

Immunosuppressive agents

These agents are often used as 'steroid-sparing' agents to provide more potent immunosuppression in those with disease unable to be controlled by the above agents alone. The commencement of potent immunosuppressive therapy such as cyclophosphamide is never undertaken lightly, especially in a female of reproductive age. Due consideration needs to be given to contraception, suppression of ovulation with gonadotropin-releasing hormone (GnRH) analogues or even the harvesting of eggs for storage prior to commencement of therapy. The effects of such medication on a foetus are obviously poorly studied and pregnancy should be avoided. This must be clearly explained to the patient.

Cyclophosphamide

This alkylating agent reduces the risk of end-stage renal disease in diffuse proliferative lupus nephritis. Its substantial side-effect profile includes bone marrow toxicity, nausea, infertility, alopecia, bladder cancer and an increased long-term risk of haemoatpoietic malignancy. One of the metabolites of cyclophosphamide (acrolein) is directly toxic to the bladder mucosa and thus the administration of cyclophosphamide should always be followed by a generous fluid intake to flush through the breakdown products of the drug. Mesna (sodium 2-mercaptoethanesulfonate) may be given to further minimize the likelihood of haemorrhagic cystitis. Cyclophosphamide is usually reserved for severe organ-threatening disease such as Class III and IV nephritis and is usually administered intravenously on a 'pulse' basis every 2–4 weeks for induction of remission.

Mycophenolate mofetil

This drug is commonly used in the treatment of lupus nephritis because of its efficacy and good tolerability. It is generally preferred over cyclophosphamide except in the setting of very severe disease. The compound is a potent, selective, uncompetitive and reversible inhibitor of inosine monophosphate dehydrogenase which inhibits the de novo pathway of guanosine nucleotide synthesis necessary for DNA synthesis. Because T and B cells have no other salvage pathways of producing guanosine, mycophenolic acid has a very specific and potent cytostatic effect on these cells.

Azathioprine

The limiting side-effects of azathioprine are bone marrow toxicity and gastrointestinal intolerance. Long-term usage increases the risk of haematopoietic malignancy. While less toxic than cyclophosphamide, it is less effective in severe renal disease. It has a role as a steroid-sparing agent or may be used to maintain remission after successful induction with mycophenolate or cyclophosphamide. Co-administration with allopurinol should be generally avoided and only undertaken with great caution due to the fact that both drugs inhibit xanthine oxidase and accumulation of high levels of either drug may manifest as profound cytopenias.

Cyclosporin and tacrolimus

These are calcineurin inhibitors that are sometimes used as a steroid-sparing agents, particularly in patients unable to tolerate one of the more 'traditional' drugs mentioned above. They suppress T cell activation and are sometimes added to mycophenolate in the setting of resistant disease. Cyclosporin has a long list of potential side-effects, including renal impairment, hypertension, hirsutism, tremor and immunosuppression. Renal toxicity is dose-dependent and predictable, occurring especially in those with pre-existing renal impairment. Another complicating factor is its potential interaction with other medications metabolized by the cytochrome P450 enzyme pathway. These include macrolide antibiotics (erythromycin) and certain calcium channel blockers which elevate serum cyclosporin levels. Tacrolimus is generally better tolerated than cyclosporin but still requires close monitoring of drug levels to prevent toxicity. Regular monitoring of renal function, blood pressure and urinalysis is mandatory.

Other agents

The role of methotrexate in the treatment of SLE is uncertain despite it having established itself as the drug of choice in the treatment of RA (see Ch. 1). It is sometimes

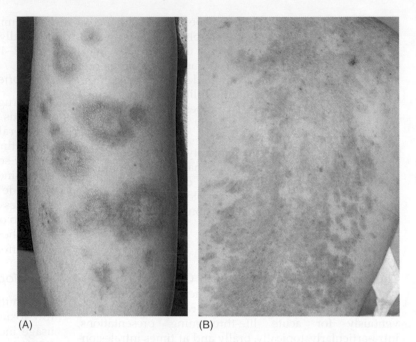

Fig. 9.7 Subacute cutaneous lupus erythematosus. (A) Annular lesions on the upper arms. (B) Erythematous papules and plaques on the back. (Source: High, W.A., 2021. Chapter 22: Autoimmune connective tissue diseases. In: High, W.A., Prok, L.D. (Eds.), Dermatology Secrets, sixth ed. Elsevier Inc.; Fig. 22.2. © 2021.)

(A)

(B)

used as a steroid-sparing agent, particularly for arthritis in SLE. Dapsone is sometimes used in the management of discoid, subacute cutaneous, bullous and profundus skin lesions due to SLE. Haematological side-effects are common and should be monitored.

Rituximab (anti-CD20 monoclonal antibody) with the ability to deplete B cells has been widely used in the management of renal and non-renal manifestations despite failing to meet its endpoint in clinical trials. Belimumab is another antibody targeting B cells (anti-BLISS) that is used as second-line therapy for moderate disease in some parts of the world, though its relatively modest efficacy and high cost have limited its use. Recent studies of anifrolumab (anti-interferon alpha) have met their primary endpoints and it is hoped it will become another treatment option for those with moderate to severe SLE.

Variants of SLE

SLE is a heterogeneous disorder that may manifest in a variety of presentations that collectively form a syndrome. These include the following:

Subacute cutaneous lupus erythematosus

This term refers to a specific group of patients distinct from SLE characterized by photosensitive skin lesions which wax and wane without residual scarring. They are usually distributed in the 'V-shaped' area of the chest and extensor surfaces of the arms. The skin lesions are usually papules or plaques with a small amount of scale and may be associated with arthralgia or arthritis

and a positive anti-Ro (SS-A) antibody in approximately 70% of cases. They may enlarge into confluent areas which may mimic psoriasis (Fig. 9.7).

Neonatal lupus

Some children born to mothers with SLE may develop a lupus dermatitis that fades over the ensuing months. They may display transiently positive ANA tests. Thrombocytopenia due to maternal antiplatelet antibodies traversing the placenta, haemolytic anaemia or leukopenia may also occur. Less commonly, the infants may develop congenital heart block which requires placement of a permanent pacemaker. Anti-Ro/La (SS-A/SS-B) antibodies are present in approximately 80% of mothers of children with congenital heart block and are thought to play a pathogenic role in this disorder through damaging the developing cardiac conduction system in utero.

Drug-induced lupus

This syndrome is seen in patients without a prior history of SLE that have recently been placed on a drug and develop fever, arthritis and serositis typical of SLE. These clinical features are usually less florid than those with 'idiopathic' lupus. Serology reveals a positive ANA with or without antibodies to dsDNA. Antibodies to histones occur in 90% of cases. The anti-histone antibodies are non-specific and can be seen in as many as 50% of idiopathic SLE. Complement levels are often normal. Unlike SLE there is usually no renal or CNS involvement. Drugs implicated include the TNF inhibitors, procainamide, hydralazine, sulphonamides, methyldopa and isoniazid. Procainamide is the drug most strongly associated with drug-induced SLE. Clinical symptoms improve when the drug is withdrawn.

Further reading

Dorner, T., Furie, R. 2019. Novel paradigms in systemic lupus erythematosus. The Lancet, 393, 2344–2358.

Firestein, G.S., Budd, R.C., Gabriel, S.E., et al. (Eds.), 2020. Firestein and Kelley's Textbook of Rheumatology, eleventh ed. Elsevier Saunders, Philadelphia.

West, S.G., Kolfenbach, J. 2020. Rheumatology Secrets, fourth ed. Philadelphia, Elsevier Saunders.

TRAUMA AND THE MUSCULOSKELETAL SYSTEM

Chapter objectives

After studying this chapter, you should be able to:

1. Understand and describe the biological processes involved in the healing of fractures.

2. Outline principles of management of fractures and understand how to initially manage injuries of the musculoskeletal system.

3. Recognize broad groupings of complications of fractures.

4. Understand the principles by which life- and limb-threatening injuries are assessed and priorities of management are assigned.

5. Understand the functional anatomy of the knee and recognize and describe the significance of ligamentous injuries of the knee.

Terence Moopanar and Andrew Ellis

Introduction

Trauma in the musculoskeletal system occurs after major or minor injury involving the soft tissues of the body (bones, joints, cartilage, ligaments, tendons, muscles etc.). Substantial energy imparted to hard and soft tissues from incidents such as motor vehicle accidents and falls from height often produce fracture to bones that require surgical intervention by orthopaedic surgeons. Blunt trauma is more common but penetrating trauma (from bullets in particular) is not uncommon in some parts of the world. High-energy trauma is potentially limb or life threatening and so immediate assessment and resuscitative measures are always prioritized in the clinical setting. Recognizing that life-threatening injury has many reversible elements, the American College of Surgeons has developed a programme that is taught worldwide to provide a system of recognition, prioritization and treatment of such injury. This system, known as advanced trauma life support (ATLS), provides a systematic approach in which life-threatening injury is first identified in a process known as primary survey. Problems with the Airway, Breathing, Circulation, neurological Disability and Exposure (ABCDE) to the environment are sought and treated while the patient is resuscitated, and then other less important injury is identified by means of secondary survey. It is beyond the scope of this chapter to deal any more with this system, except to say that it forms the backbone of modern trauma management. ATLS is a registered trademark of the American College of Surgeons Committee on Trauma, and medical practitioners working in the field of injury are strongly advised to seek this qualification.

Interesting facts

Injury deaths worldwide are estimated at more than 5 million per year. Motor vehicle crashes (road traffic accidents) cause more than 1 million deaths annually and 20–50 million significant injuries. Trauma remains the leading cause of death between 1 and 44 years of age. It is estimated that more than 1 in 10 people will die from injury. Global trauma-related deaths are estimated to cost more than US$500 billion annually.
Source: American College of Surgeons Committee on Trauma. 2008. ATLS Student Course Manual, eighth ed.

Terminology

The terminology used in the setting of trauma helps accurately describe musculoskeletal injury such that effective management can be executed without delay. Regarding injury to bones, here are some common terms used that you will commonly come across:

Fracture: a structural crack or break in the continuity of bone.

Open fracture: where the skin overlying the fracture is breached, allowing communication between the fracture and the outside. Open fractures are often referred to as compound fractures.

Closed fracture: the overlying skin is intact. It is also often referred to as a simple fracture.

Pathological fracture: a fracture caused by normal force in abnormal bone.

Stress fracture: a fracture caused by repeated mechanical stress.

Insufficiency fracture: a type of pathological stress fracture associated with osteoporotic bone, for example a compression fracture of the thoracic vertebra occurring in a postmenopausal woman (see Ch. 5).

Greenstick fracture: a type of incomplete fracture that occurs in children. Because of the relatively high moisture content and strength of collagen in children, bones tend to bend or fracture incompletely (typically one side is broken and the other side only bent).

Growth plate or physis: areas in bone consisting of cartilage until skeletal maturity.

Diaphysis: shaft of a long bone. Consists of cortical or lamellar bone. Loads well in compression but does not tolerate torque (twisting) force well.

Metaphysis: the flare of a long bone towards the joint. Consists of cancellous or trabecular bone.

Epiphysis: the part beyond the growth plate leading up to the joint surface. Blends with the growth plate scar to form the metaphysis beyond skeletal maturity.

Dislocation: disruption of a joint such that the normally opposing joint surfaces have no contact with each other.

Subluxation: disruption of a joint such that the normally opposing joint surfaces have some contact with each other but are not congruous.

Pathophysiology

Bone has a remarkable capacity to heal, far exceeding that of all other connective tissues. Unfortunately, hyaline articular cartilage has none (see Ch. 6). The inherent determination of fractures to repair is viewed as a highly efficient, primitive response to injury. Moreover, many residual deformities from fractures can remodel with time and leave no trace of the original injury.

The repair process is different in cortical and cancellous bone and this is not at all surprising when one considers the functions and biology of the two tissues (summarized in Table 10.1; return to Ch. 5 to review this in more detail).

<table>
<tr><td>Case
10.1</td><td>Trauma: 1</td></tr>
</table>

Case history

Max is a 20-year-old apprentice plumber. He is travelling home from visiting family in the country when he is involved in a high-speed motor vehicle accident. His car hits a tree near the outskirts of a large town. The police report suggests that high speed, alcohol and fatigue have all contributed to the accident. The ambulance report shows that he is conscious (Glasgow Coma Score (GCS) 14), was restrained and has signs indicative of a right knee injury, an open fracture of the right femur and a fracture of the right ankle. He has no other injuries.

He is brought to the Emergency Department where life-threatening injury is excluded and resuscitation commences along the ATLS guidelines discussed above. The GCS is a uniform system for quantifying the extent of neurological injury.

It is particularly important for monitoring change in levels of consciousness and neurological deterioration because of increasing intracranial pressure after head injury. Such a cause of change after injury might be an expanding extradural haematoma, for example. The GCS allows accurate monitoring of this change and, because of standardization, interobserver error and vagaries of description are minimized. Three main areas are assessed and the sums of the sections are combined to give a score. A GCS of 8 or below has become the generally accepted definition of coma. In this case, our patient has a GCS of 14, indicating that he is not in a coma and has a mild head injury only.

Radiographs are taken after the patient has been stabilized. These show a fracture-dislocation of the right femur through the diaphysis (Fig. 10.1), a fracture-dislocation of the right ankle (Fig. 10.2) and a swollen right knee without any obvious bony injury.

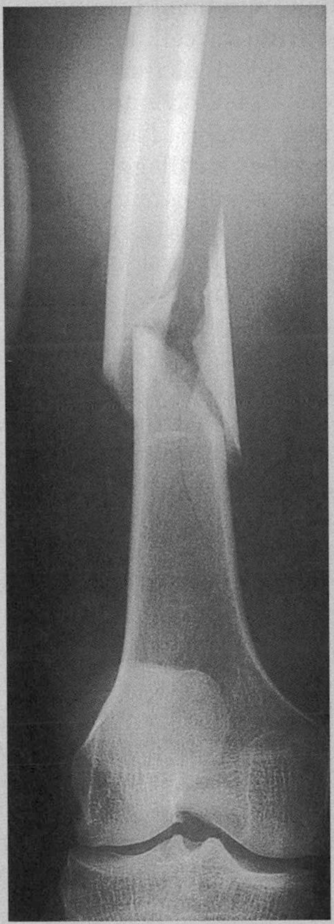

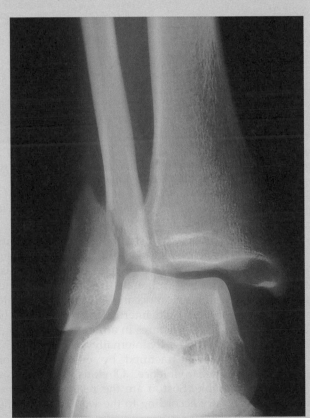

Fig. 10.1 Radiograph (AP view) showing a comminuted fracture of the shaft of the femur with a large butterfly segment.

Fig. 10.2 Radiograph (AP view) showing fracture/dislocation of the ankle.

In general terms, cancellous or trabecular bone is strong in compression and weak in tension. Most often its honeycomb, sponge-like structure fails in compression, for example a crush fracture of a vertebral body with excessive axial loading as sustained in a fall from a height. The tissue is compacted as the trabecular bone fails. Healing is directly between endosteal surfaces with no significant periosteal (indirect) contribution. The process is favoured by immobility (fixation) and the close apposition of the fracture surfaces. Hence, the very mechanism of injury produces circumstances conducive to healing. The rich blood supply is central to the reparative

Table 10.1 Features of cortical and cancellous bone

	Cortical	*Cancellous*
Location	Diaphyseal (shaft) bone	Metaphyseal (marrow) bone (carpal, tarsal, vertebral and flat bones)
Function	Mechanical	Primarily metabolic
Cortex	Thick	Thin
Periosteum	Thick	Thin
Turnover	Slow	Rapid
Blood supply	Slow	Rich

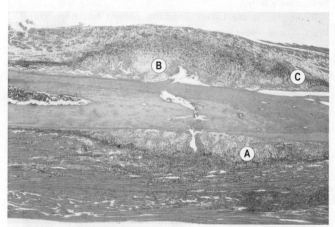

Fig. 10.3 Histology of healing fracture of diaphyseal bone. (A) Early woven bone from organization of haematoma, which is well advanced (B); (C) note that the periosteum has been lifted by trauma.

process. Non-union of a vertebral crush fracture is unknown.

According to the mechanism of certain cancellous bone fractures, there may be a gap at the fracture site. A displaced metaphyseal fracture is an example of this. Endosteal bone does not proliferate to fill the defect and delayed union or non-union occurs. This is the rationale of open reduction and rigid internal fixation of widely displaced metaphyseal fractures in adults. Fracture fragments are reduced and rigidly internally fixed.

Diaphyseal bone is fractured by either direct or indirect (transmitted) violence. Obviously, the forces involved are variable. So too are the resultant fracture patterns, which vary according to the way in which the forces are applied.

The reparative tissue has two components – one from the periosteum and the other produced by osteoinduction of primitive local mesenchymal stem cells. It is a highly efficient healing mechanism (Fig. 10.3).

The periosteal component

When the periosteum is lifted from the underlying cortical bone, whether it be by trauma, tumour or pus, it responds by laying down bone. This is an activation of the normal process of bone formation. This component is always most in evidence in a fracture on the side with the least tissue disruption. It does not entail endochondral ossification and results from activity of osteoblasts in the inner *cambium* (Latin: bark) layer of the periosteum. Periosteal new bone formation is stimulated by movement and is abolished by rigid internal fixation. In osteosarcoma (a primary tumour of bone), the periosteum is lifted by the tumour and new bone may form under the elevated periosteum giving rise to the radiological sign called Codman's triangle.

Osteoinduction

The fracture haematoma provides the tissue scaffold for the transformation into the definitive reparative tissue. This is a complex process that until recently was not well understood. Local, primitive mesenchymal cells are transformed into osteoblasts under the influence of bone morphogenetic proteins (BMPs) of humoral and platelet origins, and other undefined cytokines. This transformation sees a spectrum of cellular events in the resultant callus. The histological picture is far from homogeneous. Areas where an endochondral sequence is proceeding are seen immediately adjacent to foci of ossification without an antecedent cartilage phase as well as areas of intermediate cellular appearance. The overall picture is one of intense cellular activity. A biopsy of callus, viewed out of the context of trauma, could easily be misinterpreted as a neoplastic process.

The haematoma is rapidly invaded by blood vessels (angiogenesis) and the subsequent callus acquires its own circulation. This is essential for normal healing. It has been postulated that the local release of vascular-stimulating factors is central to this event, but the control mechanisms have not yet been identified. Further, it follows that successful vascularization will depend upon the integrity of the encompassing soft tissues. Hence, a variable degree of impairment of repair, even to the point of non-union, is not an unexpected sequel in those injuries where the surrounding soft tissues are severely crushed and traumatized.

Fracture callus is best viewed as temporary tissue. It is gradually formed into a three-dimensional mesh of relatively disorganized woven bone, which under the influence of physical forces, and especially muscle activity, is gradually transformed into highly organized lamellar bone with a cortex with central remodelling and re-establishment of the medullary canal.

Ligaments, tendons and joint capsules are designed to transmit tensile forces and are thus extremely strong in tension. They are far stronger in tension than is cancellous bone. When there is a traumatic angular deformation of a joint, the ligament may be injured (partially or completely ruptured) or it may be torn off (avulsed) from its metaphyseal attachment, taking with it a piece of bone which may be small (often erroneously called a 'chip') or quite large, according to varying circumstances. Such injuries are called avulsion fractures and,

Case 10.1 Trauma: 2

Case note: Potential damage to the knee joint

Max's left knee is observed to be swollen with obliteration of the normal contours. The swelling extends above the patella. It is important to examine the knee joint for evidence of ligamentous damage, as it is known that a significant percentage of patients with a fracture of the shaft of the femur have concomitant knee ligament injury. This is not surprising given the forces that must be applied to the limb to produce a diaphyseal fracture.

in many instances, the fragment will not unite with its bed because of the displacement and the inability of the underlying cancellous bone to bridge the gap.

Interesting facts

Internal fixation of fractures generally does not speed up time to union but will reduce rates of malunion (healing in poor position), improve function, reduce hospitalization time and cost and hasten return to work.

Describing a fracture

Fracture description plays an important part in managing musculoskeletal injury. Fractures can be described by their anatomical location (e.g. humeral shaft), joint involvement (intra- or extra-articular), comminution (simple vs multiple pieces of bone at the fracture site), involvement of the growth plate (physis), open or closed (bone communicating with the environment at the time of injury), pathological (where the bone is compromised, e.g. metastatic disease) or periprosthetic (if a prosthesis is involved at the site of injury). Clinicians may often use classification systems, such as the Garden classification system for femoral neck fractures and the Salter Harris classification system for growth plate injuries, to further describe common fracture patterns.

When beginning to learn to describe factures seen on an X-ray, it is useful to think about length (is the fracture undisplaced/translated and 'out to length' or 'off ended' and shortened), alignment (is the fracture in varus or valgus in the coronal plane; and/or in pro- or recurvatum in the sagittal plane) and rotation (is there internal or external rotation). It is therefore useful to assess an orthogonal view to ensure that the pattern of the fracture is completely appreciated.

Diagnosis of fracture

Diagnosing most fractures is usually easy. When a fracture occurs, a patient can usually give a history of a

Box 10.1 Physical signs of fracture

- Exquisite local tenderness
- Crepitus
- Deformity
- Swelling
- Loss of function

significant event, immediate and significant pain associated with loss of usefulness of the affected part and certain signs on examination (Box 10.1).

If the fracture is in a weight-bearing bone, a patient will find it very difficult to walk; if it is in the forearm, the patient might have to hold or support it with the opposite arm. To the examining doctor there may be swelling and bruising, and very marked local tenderness along the palpable part of the bone; deformity may be present and the patient will not easily use the affected limb. In some cases, the sign of crepitus will be demonstrated. This is the unique grating feeling of bone against bone and should not be actively sought in the conscious patient because of the amount of pain involved.

Most fractures occur in the way that Max's has; as the result of a single episode by a force powerful enough to fracture normal bone. An abnormal force has been applied to normal bone leaving the fracture. Cortical bone usually fails when a torque or twisting force is applied that exceeds the strength of a bone to resist a fracture. Occasionally, a normal force can be applied to abnormal bone leading to fracture, and in this case, this is known as a *pathological fracture*. Pathological fractures occur in abnormal bone and these might be bones affected by neoplastic disease (primary or secondary) or by metabolic process (e.g. rickets, osteomalacia, osteoporosis or Paget's disease). An accurate history is very important in ascertaining the exact mechanism of the fracture. Often it is the relatively minor nature of the injury that occurs that alerts the treating doctor to the presence of a pathological fracture.

Another type of fracture occurs when a normal stress is applied to normal bone but in an abnormal way. This is known as a stress fracture and occurs often when repetitive stress is applied in such a way as to cause fatigue failure of bone by means of a small crack that propagates under the repeated stress. Such a fracture might occur in athletes who over-train or in army recruits who do an excessive amount of marching.

The examining doctor should be able to localize the area very well and have a high suspicion of the presence of fracture in a conscious patient (Table 10.2) and thus be able to organize specific investigations (usually plain orthogonal X-rays will suffice).

Management of fractures

After attention to first aid and treatment of associated injuries or haemorrhage, treatment involves reduction of the fracture (if there is displacement) and holding the fracture reduced. Early stability, from the time of injury or first medical assessment, can be provided by means of external temporary splints. Such temporary splints, made of padded boards, temporary plaster half casts (backslabs) or specially made adjustable tubular frames, are an important part of the first aid of fractures.

Undisplaced fractures may be well treated by closed means without the need to align or 'reduce' the fracture. A well-moulded cast may be all that is required for many fractures. Use of such a cast usually involves splinting the joint above and below a fracture so that the muscle forces that might lead to further displacement are neutralized. In the first few hours and days, swelling must be looked for, the plaster checked to ensure that it is not too tight and the limb rested and supported. This might be done with a triangular sling in the upper limb or by means of crutches and not bearing weight in the lower limb. Healing would be expected along the lines discussed previously. Generally, a cancellous fracture of the upper limb (e.g. radius) would heal in an adult in about 6 weeks. A diaphyseal fracture takes twice as long, and a potentially weight-bearing fracture might need protection for a further period. In children, fractures often heal in about half the time of healing in adults, given their accelerated biological mechanisms.

Fractures that are displaced usually need to be aligned or reduced, to prevent the complication of malunion (healing in a non-anatomical position) and the resultant loss of function, obvious deformity or altered biomechanics that this might produce. Reduction may be closed (skin envelope intact, alignment achieved by manipulation of the limb) or open (the surgeon operates, opens the fracture and directly aligns it). Holding the fracture reduced may be by continuous traction, plaster or internal fixation. Reduction by closed manipulation usually involves traction along the line of the bone and, if further reduction is required, application of a force usually opposite to that which caused the fracture. Reduction must be confirmed by X-ray examination. Operative or open reduction is indicated if closed reduction is not possible or inadequate. Some of the indications for open reduction are listed in Table 10.3. The principles of treatment of an open fracture such as Max sustained are outlined in Box 10.2.

Fractures need careful follow-up and monitoring by an experienced practitioner. This is to ensure that the position is maintained, the adjacent joints exercised and that plasters and splints are maintained. Radiographs are used to monitor healing and position (Figs 10.4–10.6). Physiotherapy is an important adjunct to treatment, especially to regain joint motion after a period of immobility.

Complications of fractures

Fracture complications are best thought of as *early* or *late*. Early complications are those that might be considered to occur within the first few days. Hypovolaemia and infection are the two main examples of early complications.

Infection

Continuity of the fracture site with the bacteria-laden outside world is a serious complication. Infection (osteomyelitis) jeopardizes healing as well as bringing with it other complications such as excessive joint stiffness. Uncontrolled or poorly controlled sepsis may lead to limb loss. Open fractures are exposed to the outside and always result in a variable amount of dirty, devitalized and dead tissue around the fracture site, and these favour infections (Table 10.4). This is why wound debridement and lavage should be carried out as soon as possible and, ideally, in less than 6–9 hours after the injury. Prophylactic antibiotics should be given to all patients with open fractures.

Infections in open fractures include gas gangrene, which is caused by the organism *Clostridium perfringens* and associated with significant mortality and morbidity due to a toxin produced by the organism. Amputation and death are distinct outcomes when a patient contracts this infection. Tetanus, caused by *Clostridium tetani*, has been a significant problem in the past, but now is thankfully very rare (in the first world), because of a programme of immunization and the ready availability of tetanus immunoglobulin. *C. tetani* produces a neurotoxin, which causes significant contracted paralysis of muscles that may lead to failure to ventilate and thus death. In the face, the contracted paralysis produces the *risus sardonicus tetani* or violent contraction of muscles, which can be prevented by anaesthesia or by nursing the patient in a darkened quiet room. Infections of the musculoskeletal system are discussed further in Chapter 11.

More commonly, however, deep infection usually occurs with skin commensals and in up to 85% of infections associated with open fractures, *Staphylococcus aureus* from the patient's own skin is implicated.

Fat embolism syndrome

When a diaphyseal bone is fractured, fat embolism syndrome may develop. Whether this occurs through direct release of marrow fat into lacerated venules or by means of precipitation of chylomicrons within the intravascular system is subject to some controversy. The features of this

Table 10.2 Decision-making in musculoskeletal injury

Questions	Answers
What was the mechanism of injury?	Does the history fit the fracture pattern?
	Reduction is achieved by reversing the mechanism of injury (dislocation also)
What are the deforming forces?	These must be overcome to achieve reduction. Remember gravity works 24 hours a day
What are the neurovascular structures and organs (solid and hollow) at risk?	Always (in your mind's eye) paint the anatomy on the radiographs in three planes
Would further views or another form of imaging be helpful?	Anteroposterior and lateral X-rays are the minimal requirement
Is the bone normal?	Pathological fracture
Is it a fracture through cortical (diaphyseal) or cancellous bone?	Different mechanisms of healing
	Different methods of management
Is the fracture stable or unstable?	Examination under anaesthesia may be required. If deduced to be unstable, it must be made stable, or more so, by closed (plaster cast, etc.) or open means (internal fixation)

Case 10.1 — Trauma: 3

Clinical examination of the knee

The collateral ligaments

The stability of a joint is first examined in full extension. The tip of the index finger is placed over the middle of the joint line laterally and a varus stress is applied distally. If the lateral ligament is intact, there should be no opening of the joint space. The medial collateral integrity is similarly tested with a valgus stress. However, the anterior cruciate ligament (ACL) is taut in full extension, and if the medial collateral ligament (MCL) is ruptured, it may not be possible to open the joint medially. Hence, to test the MCL, the joint should be flexed 15–20 degrees, and in Max's knee the examining finger detects a slight but definite opening at the joint line in its midpart. This indicates a partial tear in the MCL. If the anterior cruciate and MCL are both ruptured, then the joint can be widely opened with a valgus stress when the knee is in full extension.

The cruciate ligaments

Both knees are flexed to approximately 90 degrees with Max supine and the feet placed together and parallel on the table. The joints are then viewed from the side. If the posterior cruciate ligament is ruptured, the tibia on the injured side will sag posteriorly on the femur. If the ACL is disrupted, common in football or skiing injuries, then the tibia can be passively drawn forward on the femur to a much greater degree than on the uninjured side (the anterior drawer sign). Slight anterior movement of the tibia on the femur is observed in normal knees. Further, with an ACL rupture, the knee can be passively hyperextended (into recurvatum). The cruciates are judged to be intact in Max's knee.

Pathology of ligament injuries

The configuration of the bundles of collagen in ligaments, and especially those that are fan-shaped, is such that for any given position of a joint, there is not equal tension on all collagen bundles. Further, the collagen is irregularly dispersed in the attachment to bone (Sharpey's fibres). When an angulatory force is applied to a joint, those bundles under maximum tension absorb the energy first, where it may be dissipated with only a small number of fibres actually rupturing. This is a safety mechanism. It explains why minor sprains are so common, moderate sprains such as Max sustained are rather infrequent and complete ruptures are unusual. In Max's case with slight opening on the medial joint line, the effective functional length of the ligament has been increased. The ligament does not shorten (contract) and some laxity will remain as a legacy to the injury. A complete rupture of the MCL is an indication for surgical repair. Moderate injuries such as Max has are not amenable to surgery. In minor sprains, the functional length of the ligament is not altered and there are no long-term consequences.

Longer-term considerations

The future of Max's knee will depend much upon maintaining the quadriceps mechanism in good condition and, as soon as pain and fracture healing permit, a regular isometric exercise programme will be instituted. Provided good muscle control is regained, Max will be able to function well from the point of view of his knee and even participate in sport. Many professional athletes have persistent laxity of the collateral ligamentous complexes and even cruciate-deficient knees, but still participate at a high level provided they have good muscle control. All sport is conducted with the knees flexed and here muscle control is vital. The player with persistent ligamentous laxity is always apprehensive about being caught off-guard, such as when he is tackled, and this is one reason why recurrent injuries in the ligamentous-deficient knee are so common.

Trauma: 4

Fracture diagnosis and treatment priorities

In Max's case, physical examination revealed marked swelling in the mid-thigh and ankle associated with quite marked pain and a tendency for abnormal movement to occur as the limb was being examined. Pain limited the examination. Palpation of the bony landmarks around the ankle and the lateral border of the right femur showed that tenderness was particularly localized to the areas of fracture. Max was unable to move his right limb and was in significant pain.

Plain radiographs proved to be all that was required to see the obvious break in cortical bone in Max's femur with significant displacement (see Fig. 10.1). The X-ray image of the ankle showed a degree of subluxation of the ankle joint that is obvious (see Fig. 10.2).

Question

Look at the X-rays of Max's fractures and attempt to describe them so that another doctor could paint an accurate picture of the fracture without looking at the X-rays.

Fractures might be described in their radiological appearance in terms of the following parameters:

- site
- extent
- configuration
- relationship of the fragments to each other (displaced, angulated, rotated, lengthened or shortened)
- whether the fractures are open to the skin or not.

Fractures can be associated with significant bleeding, and the priority of initial treatment with Max is to restore the circulatory loss associated with his hypovolaemic state. Loss of blood volume can be associated with quite marked physiological change. Initially, venous return falls leading to a decrease in the diastolic filling pressure and/or volume of the heart. This leads to a fall in cardiac output and may lead to significant failure of perfusion of end-organs, which untreated, might lead to death. The body has a number of protective measures in place to compensate for this, including the ability to sense a decrease in mean arterial pressure (by carotid and aortic baroreceptors, leading to an immediate sympathetic response). The sympathetic response leads to release of adrenaline and noradrenaline, allowing immediate constriction of arterioles, causing a rise in peripheral resistance and also helping to control bleeding. There is a reflex tachycardia in an attempt to improve output and perfusion and there is vasoconstriction of non-essential vascular beds (e.g. in the skin and abdomen). These changes often lead to a measurable alteration in signs and symptoms, including a fall in blood pressure and a rise in the heart rate; the patient may be pale, sweaty and peripherally shut down. The respiratory rate will increase in an attempt to improve oxygenation and the urinary output will fall in response to decreased renal perfusion.

Table 10.3 Fractures that require surgical stabilization

Type of fracture	Reason
Pathological fractures	Unlikely to heal spontaneously
Intra-articular fractures	To optimize joint function and to prevent secondary osteoarthritis
Open fracture	To reduce risk of infection
Unstable fracture (e.g. short oblique tibia and fibula)	Rates of malunion high by closed means
Slow-healing fracture (e.g. fractured neck of femur)	Surgical treatment leads to early mobilization and reduction in complications of prolonged bed rest (pneumonia, pressure sores, thromboembolic complications). Public health benefit from reduced hospitalization costs
Associated high levels of avascular necrosis (e.g. comminuted proximal humerus, subcapital femur)	Joint function likely to be affected. Often require artificial joint replacement (arthroplasty)

Box 10.2 Priorities of treatment of open fractures

- Identify and treat associated life-threatening injury
- Intravenous fluid resuscitation
- Intravenous antibiotics
- Splint limb and dress wound
- Tetanus prophylaxis, appropriate to immunization status
- Early surgical consultation
- Early surgical debridement and stabilization of fracture

syndrome are often associated with an acute respiratory distress and the presence of petechial haemorrhage (often best seen in the conjunctiva or axilla). The development of adult respiratory distress syndrome is strongly associated with the presence of fat embolism. The fat precipitates in the capillary system of the lung, causing impaired oxygenation and may exacerbate confusional states associated with hypovolaemia and decreased cerebral perfusion. The treatment is largely supportive by means of oxygenation of the patient, which may be achieved by simple measures such as oxygen by mask, but might lead to the need to intubate and ventilate the patient by means of an endotracheal tube in an intensive care unit.

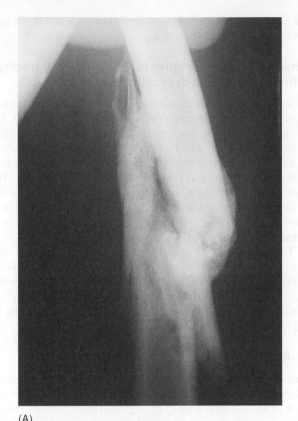

(A)

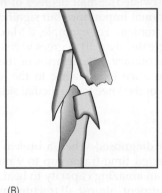

(B)

Fig. 10.4 (A) Radiograph of healing bone. Note the immature callus of early healing: although trabecular patterns are evident, the new cortex is yet to be established. At this stage, the femur would not withstand unprotected weight bearing. (B) Line drawing of original fracture fragments.

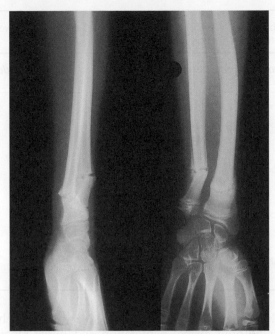

Fig. 10.5 Radiographs of fractures of the distal radius and ulna at 4 weeks post-injury in a child aged 8 years. In the ulna, periosteal new bone formation is less marked on the radial aspect where it was disrupted. There is metaphyseal osteopenia from immobilization and the open growth plate.

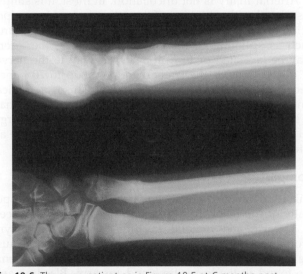

Fig. 10.6 The same patient as in Figure 10.5 at 6 months post-injury. The effect of remodelling has led to an improvement in alignment.

Injury to adjacent vessels and nerves

Nerves and vessels are intimately associated with the skeleton, and neurovascular injury must always be excluded when dealing with a fracture of the skeleton. Peripheral pulses must always be palpated and both the sensory and motor functions of individual peripheral nerves formally assessed. There are some fractures that are particularly prone to the development of neurovascular injury because of the particularities of their anatomy. For example, the common peroneal nerve passes very close to the head of the fibula, near the knee and is often injured in high fibula fractures. The radial nerve is intimately adjacent to the humerus in the radial groove in the mid-posterior portion of the humerus. Fractures of the humeral shaft in this area may cause nerve injury. Nerve injury most commonly occurs by means of stretching, occurring once the stabilizing function of bone has been lost. Such stretching injury (neuropraxia) is not uncommon and resolves for most individuals in less than 6 weeks. If, however, the stretching has been so significant that the nerve has been torn or even lacerated

Table 10.4 Classification of open fractures after Gustilo: severity of fracture is strongly linked with prognosis

Classification	Description	Deep infection rate (%)
Type I	Clean wound <1 cm	0
Type II	Laceration >1 cm, without extensive soft tissue damage	1–2.5
Type IIIA	Extensive soft tissue damage or resulting from high-energy trauma	
Type IIIB	Extensive soft tissue loss with periosteal stripping and bone exposure	10–25
Type IIIC	As above but with arterial injury requiring repair	

by the sharp bone ends, such recovery is unlikely to occur without formal exploration and nerve repair. If the neural sheath is intact, this condition is known as axonotmesis; if the nerve sheath is torn, it is known as neurotmesis. Return to Chapter 3 for a review of nerve injuries.

Arterial injury is not uncommon. In most, it is simply associated with a kinking of the artery caused by malposition of the limb and responds well to simple measures such as splinting of the fracture. However, the artery may be lacerated or torn in a similar way to the nerve. In dislocations of the knee, there is an up to 70% incidence of injury to the popliteal artery. This is a surgical emergency, as muscle ischaemia cannot last longer than 6 hours without unrecoverable damage. Early surgical opinion is warranted and the patient may require an interposition arterial graft.

Compartment syndrome

This is not an uncommon complication of fractures, especially of the tibial diaphysis. It is also occasionally seen in forearm and femoral fractures. Compartment syndrome is associated with bleeding into an area of muscle surrounded by tight fascia; commonly such systems are found in the lower limb and forearm. Bleeding and tissue damage causing swelling within the closed fascial system can lead to pressures being raised within the fascial envelope. Fascia is unyielding and has no ability to stretch. Pressures soon exceed the relatively low venous capillary emptying pressure, allowing further swelling to occur because arterial capillary filling still continues. This compounds the swelling until arterial capillary pressure is exceeded, and the muscle can become ischaemic. Note that it is still possible for a palpable distal pulse to be present as arterial capillary filling pressure is only about 35–40 mm Hg. The signs and symptoms that alert to a compartment syndrome include intense pain (unrelieved by analgesics), pain on stretching the

affected muscles and altered sensation (paraesthesia and decreased sensation); motor paralysis is a late sign.

Regional pain syndromes (CRPS, Sudeck's atrophy, reflex sympathetic dystrophy, causalgia)

This is a broad term that describes excess and prolonged pain and inflammation after injury. The syndrome has acute and chronic (when symptoms last greater than 6 months) and is associated with significant alteration of sympathetic nervous function of the limb, including altered sweating, swelling and vasomotor change. The limb often develops a severe regional osteoporosis owing to disuse. These symptoms usually resolve with treatment in most cases over time but rare severe cases may persist and be profoundly disabling.

The treatment is usually multidisciplinary and difficult, and the condition is slow to resolve. Early mobilization, physiotherapy, psychotherapy and medication (paracetamol, NSAIDs, gabapentin, topical anaesthetics, corticosteroids and opioids) have all been shown to be efficacious in treatment.

Malunion

This occurs when the fracture heals in a less than anatomical position. Malunion may result in a bone being shorter; bent in the coronal (front) or sagittal (side) plane; or even rotated axially (twisted). Small degrees of malunion may have little functional importance but significant malunion can be a major problem. For example, if Max's femur were to heal with a greater than 10 degrees varus malunion, he may develop secondary osteoarthritis of the medial compartment of the knee joint owing to the shifting of his mechanical axis of the knee to the medial side.

Non-union

A non-union is diagnosed when a broken bone fails to heal in an expected time frame (up to 9 months). Bones generally have an amazing capacity to heal, and with the appropriate treatment, almost all fractures will heal without complication.

Non-union occurs when a fracture fails to unite and radiographs show no progress to union in successive films. Non-unions are relatively rare, but Max has had a high-energy fracture of his femur with tissue stripping and loss of some local blood supply, so he has about a 5% risk of non-union of his femur. Apart from a poor blood supply, other causes of non-unions include too much movement at the fracture site (poor stability), separation of the bone ends, interposition of tissue, bone loss and infection. Risk factors for non-union include smoking, diabetes, increasing age, obesity, hormonal issues (thyroid and parathyroid endocrinopathies), vitamin D deficiency and NSAID use.

Of all fractures, the tibia in its distal third is most susceptible to non-union because of its poor blood supply. Surgical intervention by means of bone-grafting or surgical stabilization is often required.

In some circumstances, there may be a 'delayed union' which refers to progressive healing in a slower than expected time frame. This is usually due to biological factors such as a poor blood supply at the fracture site.

Avascular necrosis

Avascular necrosis refers to the death of bone due to a lack of blood supply. The term osteonecrosis is also commonly used to describe this process, which causes tiny cracks in the bone when the blood supply is severely compromised. Eventually, the structural integrity of the bone may be compromised to such an extent that the mechanical loads cause collapse, pain and eventual disability.

Avascular necrosis maybe associated with long-term use of high-dose steroid medications and excessive alcohol intake. Fractures occurring in bones with a precarious blood supply may also lead to this complication. Avascular necrosis is a significant clinical problem in subcapital fractures of the femur, and fractures of the scaphoid and the talus.

Functional anatomy of the knee joint

The key anatomical structures of the knee relevant to osteoarthritis were reviewed in Chapter 6. Here, we will review the anatomy of the knee joint with an emphasis on its functional anatomy relevant to musculoskeletal injury as per the case discussion.

General joint morphology

Inasmuch as major morphological changes were required for hominids to walk upright and to stand erect with minimal effort, these are unique to the human knee and set it apart from the knee joints of all other creatures.

In the erect position, the line of centre of gravity passes behind the hip joint and in front of the knee and ankle joints. In full extension, the hip and knee joints are said to be 'locked'. Extension of the former is restrained by the substantial iliofemoral ligament, the strongest ligament in the body. Stability of the locked knee is dependent upon the femoral condyles, which are flattened in an anteroposterior direction (a human trait), and the collateral ligaments, which become taut in extension, as does the anterior cruciate ligament (ACL). Further, the upper surface of the tibia slopes backwards, resisting hyperextension.

The locking of the hip and knee joints allows humans to stand without activity of the respective extensor mechanisms. The reader can readily confirm this. As the hip and knee flex, as they do when we walk or run, these muscle groups come into action to stabilize the joints. Standing is a very efficient mechanism. On the other hand, the ankle joint cannot be locked and the plantigrade position is maintained by the tonic activity of the calf muscles, which force the foot against the ground. The reader will recall that humans get sore and stiff in the calves on prolonged standing, but not so in the buttocks and thighs. Next, stand with the hips and knees flexed at about 20 degrees. You will soon appreciate that it takes considerable muscle effort to maintain this position. Hence, a flexion contracture of the knee joint constitutes a significant disability, particularly if the joint is painful owing to an arthropathy. A flexion contracture of up to 30 degrees in the hip joint can be accommodated by increasing lumbar lordosis.

The femur makes a coronal plane angle of 6–10 degrees with the tibia in the fully extended position. This is relatively larger in the female because of the wider pelvis. This configuration results in a tendency for the patella to move laterally when the quadriceps muscle contracts (Fig. 10.7). This is resisted by the elevated lateral femoral condyle, which is well seen in profile. The upper surfaces of the tibial plateaus are increased in an anteroposterior direction to accommodate the flattened femoral condyles (those of the chimpanzee are much rounder). Lastly, the ACL, which becomes taut in extension, helps guide the femur medially on the tibia in the last 15 degrees of extension – the screw-home movement.

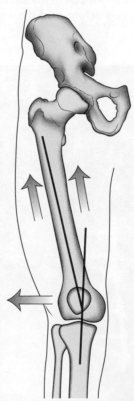

Fig. 10.7 Patella instability. The longitudinal axis of the femur makes an angle of approximately 6–10 degrees with the tibia. The angle is slightly more in females because of the wider pelvis. A strong contraction of the quadriceps muscle will tend to displace the patella laterally. This is resisted by the direct attachment of the vastus and medialis components of the quadriceps to the inner margin of the patella.

Trauma: 5

Management

Max's initial management aims to treat the pathological changes that occur with hypovolaemia and to support the physiological response. He will be given oxygen to improve his oxygen saturation and intravenous fluids to replace loss and to help maintain his cardiac output. Two large-bore intravenous lines might be inserted so that the fluid can be delivered quickly and a urinary catheter might be passed to measure his urinary output. He will be given analgesia to relieve his pain, and the leg will be splinted for this reason as well.

We know from our examination that Max has a fracture of the shaft of his femur, an injury to the medial collateral ligament (MCL) of the knee and an intra-articular fracture of the ankle. We know from basic principles that his fractures would heal if they were managed by closed (non-operative) means. However, a diaphyseal fracture of the femoral shaft might take some months to heal. A single bone fracture of cortical bone is quite likely to be unstable and there will be a degree of shortening and perhaps rotational deformity unless the fracture is accurately reduced. There are strong pulls of muscles, both quadriceps and hamstrings, which will tend to shorten the limb, and the pull of the adductors distally might lead to a varus or bow deformity of the femur.

The intra-articular fracture of the ankle has some subluxation. Articular cartilage does not bear abnormal force well as you already understand from considering the pathogenesis of osteoarthritis in Chapter 6. An intra-articular fracture, not anatomically reduced, will lead to high contact pressures and the development of premature secondary osteoarthritis within the joint in a high percentage of cases. Without restoring congruity of the ankle joint, the patient is likely to develop a painful secondary osteoarthritis within 10 years (Fig. 10.8).

For these reasons, surgery is indicated in Max. Additionally, you recall that there is an open wound over Max's femoral fracture. This makes it likely that Max's femur has become contaminated with skin organisms, or possibly with debris from the road or his clothing. Without surgical cleaning of this area, he is likely to develop a deep infection, which could lead to the development of osteomyelitis, as will be discussed in Chapter 11. For this reason, surgery is indicated to provide wound toilet (Fig. 10.9). This is the act of debridement and cleaning of a contaminated fracture that much reduces the risk of osteomyelitis. *Debridement* comes from the French – to unbridle, and means to separate the risk of infection from the better outcome expected by the patient. Surgery combined with antibiotics is the only way to do this.

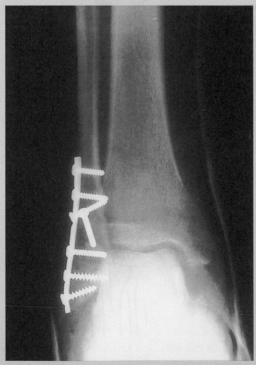

Fig. 10.8 AP radiograph of Max's ankle after internal fixation.

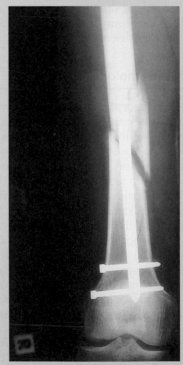

Fig. 10.9 AP radiograph of Max's knee after intramedullary nailing.

This crucial mechanism results in grooving of the antero-lateral surface of the intercondylar notch and the smooth depression can be easily seen and felt in well-preserved bones.

Muscle control

The extraordinarily powerful quadriceps group is attached distally to the readily palpable tibial tubercle. It becomes well developed and very strong in athletes, especially weightlifters – you lift with your knees. The vastus medialis controls patellar position by virtue of its fleshy attachment to the medial patella margin and it aids in the 'screw-home' movement required for full extension. It is the most specialized part of the quadriceps mechanism and atrophies quickly with disuse. Moreover, once weakened and atrophic, it is difficult for it to regain full strength and muscle bulk.

Range of motion

The normal range of movement is from 0 to 150 degrees and approximately 60 degrees of flexion is required for normal gait on flat ground. Because the cruciate and collateral ligaments become taut in full extension, no rotation is possible in this position. When the knee is flexed, there is approximately 15 degrees of internal and external rotation and these movements are produced by the medial and lateral hamstrings, respectively. This is a small degree of freedom in both directions given the enormous stresses that athletes place upon their knees, particularly when the foot is fixed to the ground by cleats or rubber soles. Little wonder then that athletes are plagued by self-induced knee injuries. Natural selection did not take the demands of soccer, basketball and the like into its deliberate, gradual determinations.

Ligaments

Ligaments, like tendons, are composed almost exclusively of type I collagen. The lateral collateral ligament can easily be felt when the knee is flexed to 90 degrees and crossed over the opposite thigh. This structure plays a relatively minor role in stability of the fully extended knee. When the knee is flexed, as it is in all human activities except standing, lateral stability is efficiently and effectively provided by the strong, wide iliotibial band. This is tensed by the action of the tensor fascia lata and gluteus maximus muscle, three-quarters of which is inserted in the fascia lata, of which the band is a specialized part. The reader can verify this by standing on tiptoe with the knee and hips slightly flexed. The band is easily felt and will be noted to become less taut in the fully upright stance.

The medial collateral ligament (MCL) is fan-shaped and distally has a wide attachment to the upper, inner aspect of the tibia, this strong structure being needed medially to combat the valgus deformity force in weight bearing, secondary to the femorotibial angle. The axis of flexion and extension passes through the condyles.

Joint capsule

This is 'redundant' anteriorly and posteriorly to allow flexion/extension by virtue of a loose criss-cross arrangement of capsular (collagen) fibres. Small amounts of elastin are so placed between bundles to assist in recoil after deformation. When a capsular injury or inflammation occurs, periarticular collagen is laid down (fibrosis) but then it is along the lines of stress and not in the preferential way described. Collagen is a virtually inextensible molecule and so too are ligaments and tendons – they have to be to serve their designated functions. Hence, capsular and periarticular fibrosis is an important cause of joint contractures and the associated disability.

Menisci – the semilunar cartilages

These structures are fibrocartilaginous notwithstanding the loose terminology. They are peculiar to joints where movements on either side of them are in different planes. They are crescentic in shape with tibial attachments at both ends (horns). The outer one-third is made up of distinct circumferential fibrous lamellae and it has a limited blood supply at the periphery. Centrally, the lamellated structure is lost and the avascular, more homogeneous tissue, is distinctly more cartilage-like. This tissue pattern indicates that the outer regions must withstand tensile forces and, more centrally, compression.

By their contour, with the upper surfaces being slightly concave, the menisci enhance joint stability. They also help in the distribution of synovial fluid essential for joint lubrication. They function as 'thrust pads', familiar to engineers. That is, they move in and out of the joint with flexion and extension. The reader can substantiate this as follows. Place the index finger immediately above the sharp anterior tibial margin adjacent to the patella tendon. Here the firm, rubbery meniscus can be palpated. With the knee flexed to 90 degrees there is a shallow depression, which is obliterated as the joint is extended. The flattened inferior surface of the femoral condyle pushes the meniscus in a centrifugal fashion. The articular surface of the femur is grooved anteriorly to articulate with the meniscus and a shallow depression for this contact is seen in lateral radiographs.

Movement in the sagittal plane largely takes place between the femur and the meniscus and rotation between the meniscus and the tibia. As stated earlier, the femur rotates medially on the tibia as the joint is fully extended. If these movements are not synchronized, the meniscus may be trapped between the ends of the two bones and tear. It may occur, for example, if the foot is firmly fixed to the ground in an internally rotated position, and the flexed knee is suddenly extended as in rising quickly from a semi-crouched position. The medial

TRAUMA AND THE MUSCULOSKELETAL SYSTEM

meniscus is more liable to injury than its lateral counterpart, because it is attached to the inner aspect of the MCL, which makes it more immobile than its lateral fellow. The popliteus muscle is a flexor of the knee joint and its tendon is attached to the posterior part of the lateral meniscus. Hence, when the joint is flexed, the lateral meniscus is retracted posteriorly out of harm's way.

When a meniscus is torn in its mid-substance, the tear will not heal spontaneously (cf. hyaline articular cartilage). Longitudinal tears in the outer vascular lamellae have the capacity to repair, as do peripheral detachments.

Further reading

Apley, A.G., Solomon, L. (2001). *A System of Orthopaedics and Fractures*, eighth ed. Arnold, London.

Bullough, P.G. (2009). *Atlas of Orthopaedic Pathology with Clinical and Radiological Correlations*, fourth ed. Mosby, Philadelphia.

McRae, R. (2006). *Pocketbook of Orthopaedics and Fractures*, second ed. Churchill Livingstone, Edinburgh.

INFECTION AND THE MUSCULOSKELETAL SYSTEM

11

Bill Walter

Chapter objectives

After studying this chapter you should be able to:

1. Understand how microorganisms reach bones or joints.

2. Understand the possible effects of microorganisms on bones, growth plates, articular cartilage and intervertebral discs.

3. Diagnose infection in musculoskeletal tissues.

4. Understand the principles of management of musculoskeletal infections.

5. Describe the possible outcomes of infection in bones, joints and intervertebral discs.

Introduction

Microorganisms abound in nature, and many find the environment and nutrients needed for growth and reproduction on or within other living organisms. Such microorganisms live in a balanced situation with their host that ensures survival of both host and parasite. Humans have developed a complex immune system that allows such co-existence to continue.

Infection is the process by which a microorganism enters into a damaging relationship with its host. If the microorganism injures the host to a sufficient degree, disturbances result in the host, which manifest as disease. Included among the microorganisms that cause disease in the musculoskeletal system are bacteria, fungi (and fungus-like organisms), protozoa, helminths and viruses. In addition, inflammation in joints (synovitis) can occur without direct invasion by microorganisms, but as a reaction to infection elsewhere in the body, perhaps as a response to circulating breakdown products.

It is the combination of the presence of microorganisms, inflammation and tissue destruction that constitutes 'clinical infection'. The case histories that follow are typical of musculoskeletal infections, and their discussion provides not only a clinical picture, but also knowledge of physiological and pathological mechanisms that are essential for the understanding of principles of management. If those principles are followed the potential adverse effects on the normal function of the host can be minimized.

General principles of musculoskeletal infection

In the musculoskeletal system there are several types of infections:

- *Septic arthritis*, in which the microorganisms infect a joint and surrounding tissues.
- *Osteomyelitis*, in which the microorganisms infect the bone. The bone may be living or dead. If the dead bone is detached from living bone, it is called a *sequestrum*. With long-term osteomyelitis of dead bone, a new layer of living bone may be formed around the infected dead bone and this is called an *involucrum*.
- *Myositis*, in which the microorganisms infect muscle. Most commonly viral, this condition is rarely caused by bacteria or fungi.
- *Infected hardware*, in which the microorganisms infect the space adjacent to orthopaedic hardware such as joint replacements (periprosthetic joint infections) or plates, screws or nails used for fracture treatment and osteotomy.

Once infection is established, it is the outcome of the host and parasite contest that determines the effect of the infection. Microorganisms may:

- be repelled and eradicated, with restitution of the tissues to their normal state

Case 11.1 — Acute osteomyelitis: 1

Case history

Simon, 4-years-old, complained to his mother that his leg was sore. That night he did not eat his evening meal with his usual enthusiasm. In the early hours of the morning, he awoke crying, and complaining that his leg still hurts. Later in the day his mother saw that he was reluctant to run around. She felt he was warm. In the afternoon, she took him to the doctor, who asked him to point to where his leg hurt, and he indicated just below the knee on the inner side of the leg. When the doctor pressed at that spot, Simon said 'Ouch!'. The skin was not discoloured. Lymph nodes in his groin were not palpable. Although he was reluctant to walk for the doctor, his knee joint range of movement was normal. His body temperature was elevated at 38.5°C. The doctor did not find any other abnormal clinical signs and made a provisional diagnosis of acute osteomyelitis of the tibia.

- be eradicated by the host but tissue destruction and inflammation lead to the formation of repair tissue that leaves a fibrous scar at the site of invasion
- remain dormant in the tissues but there is 'clinical resolution' of the disease.
- cause such tissue damage that the host is unable to survive

The 'clinical outcome' is the recovery of function in the host and is determined by the tissue responses. Those responses may be modified by effective treatment, tipping the balance between microorganism and host in favour of the host.

The mere presence of microorganisms is not sufficient to produce disease. They must invade the host tissues, to enter, multiply, spread and produce toxic substances. The body has defences against this. The ability to produce a disease is known as *pathogenicity*. The comparative pathogenicity of various organisms is known as *virulence*. Very small numbers of virulent bacteria produce disease, whereas larger numbers are required of less virulent organisms. The invasiveness of microorganisms relates not only to the toxins that they produce, but also to enzymes, which may allow them to spread by tissue dissolution and protect them from host phagocytes.

Portals of entry

In order to produce diseases of the musculoskeletal system in man, organisms must gain access to those tissues. There are several ways in which this may occur:

- haematogenous spread by bacteraemia or septicaemia from a primary site of colonization (skin, mouth, gut) if barriers to spread have been breached

- direct access by puncture of the skin and deeper tissues following injury, with organisms carried in by the penetrating instrument
- direct access at the time of elective surgery or following surgery for open injury
- local spread from infected adjacent tissues.

Biofilm

Bacteria can exist in two forms in the body: *planktonic* bacteria drift or float as individual organisms in fluid, and *sessile* bacteria are organised into groups attached together and may be fixed in one place to form a biofilm. Bacterial biofilms typically form on the surfaces of orthopaedic hardware or on a sequestrum and provide protection for the bacteria against the normal host defences. A biofilm is comprised of bacteria that are attached to these surfaces and are embedded in a matrix of extracellular material. These biofilms can exhibit sophisticated pillar or mushroom architectures with intricate channel networks providing access to environmental nutrients. The bacteria in a biofilm exhibit an altered phenotype with respect to growth, gene expression and protein production.

The biofilm lifecycle includes attachment, accumulation, maturation and dispersion. Mature biofilm is more resistant to host defences (including phagocytosis) and antibiotic treatment and therefore chronic infections are more difficult to eradicate than acute infections. The time to maturation of a biofilm varies depending in on the organism and environmental factors but laboratory studies show the beginnings of biofilm formation within a few minutes. Biofilm formation may make the removal of the infected hardware or sequestrum necessary in order to eradicate chronic infection.

Staphylococcus aureus is a common cause of bone and joint infections in all age groups and is particularly noted for its ability to form biofilm.

Host defences against infection

The host, for its part in the host–parasite relationship, has a resistance to invasion by microorganisms and the effects of their toxins that can be assessed in terms of non-specific and specific factors.

Non-specific factors are those acting against a variety of microorganisms:

- physiological, physical and chemical barriers at the portal of entry (skin or mucous membrane)
- phagocytosis (intracellular killing of microorganisms)
- the reticuloendothelial system
- the inflammatory response.

The specific factors are those that confer resistance against a specific infectious agent and come under the heading of immunity. Such immunity may be natural (not acquired through previous contact with the infect-

ing agent), or acquired (passively or actively). Passive acquired immunity is a state of relative temporary insusceptibility to an infectious agent that has been induced by the administration of antibodies that were formed in another host, rather than formed by the individual person. Monoclonal antibodies, or polyvalent antisera, are examples. Tetanus immune globulin is a product of autologous human serum that contains antibodies against tetanus toxin. Active immunity is a state of resistance built up in an individual following effective contact with the foreign antigens; that is the microorganisms or their products. Active immunization against tetanus requires injection of deactivated tetanus toxin. The antibodies are manufactured by the host. Adaptive or acquired resistance to infection requires a specific response by the host to enable it to eradicate a particular infection.

The resistance of acquired immunity is a complex subject, but as reviewed in Chapter 1, there are two major subgroups:

1. *humoral immunity*, or the active production of antibodies; and
2. *cellular immunity*, in which certain lymphoid cells recognize material as foreign and initiate a chain of responses that permit them to destroy intracellular organisms.

Humoral immunity involves the production and secretion of special protein molecules called antibodies by cells of the lymphoid system. The antibodies circulate in the blood and body fluids, having been stimulated to appear by the presence of antigens. Antibodies may induce resistance to infection because they:

- neutralize toxins or cellular enzymes
- have direct bactericidal or lytic effect
- block the infective ability of microorganisms
- agglutinate microorganisms, making them more susceptible to phagocytosis
- opsonize microorganisms and therefore aid phagocytosis.

Cell-mediated immunity depends on the ability of sensitized lymphocytes to kill foreign cells by direct contact. Lymphocytes are found in lymphoid tissue (bone marrow, thymus, spleen, lymph nodes and lymph) and in the blood. In Chapter 1 we described how humoral immunity is mediated by B lymphocytes derived from stem cells in the bone marrow. These are stimulated by antigen to divide and form plasma cells, which then secrete antibodies against the antigen concerned. The other lymphocyte population, the T lymphocytes, are responsible for cellular immunity.

The presence of antibodies, and their amount, can sometimes be used to determine whether or not a person has had contact with an antigen; this is useful in the diagnosis of some infections and in determining a person's response to treatment. Similarly, the ability of T cells to respond to challenge by some antigens can be used as a diagnostic technique.

The tissues that are regularly in contact with the external environment, such as skin, mucous membrane and cornea, have adaptations that resist invasion by microorganisms, and it is usually only at times when the continuity of the tissue surface is breached that infection occurs. The deeper tissues such as bone and joint do not have the same natural barriers to infection. Muscle is also a deeper tissue, but has a lower incidence of primary infection than bones or joints, for unknown reasons.

Also important are alterations in function of one or more organ systems in the host. The normal ecological balance of symbiotic organisms resident on the host may be upset by burns, trauma, surgery, hospitalization or antibiotic therapy. Disrupted anatomical barriers consequent on burns, trauma, bites, other infections, ischaemia or the presence of foreign materials (including implanted prostheses) alter normal relations. If the person has diabetes, renal failure, diseases of the haematopoietic system or is taking immunosuppressive drugs, the normally protective inflammatory response may be altered. Diseases of the lymphoreticular system, cancer, debilitating diseases, malnutrition and cigarette smoking have an effect on the way the body meets challenges from microorganisms.

Acute haematogenous osteomyelitis, septic arthritis and periprosthetic joint infection are all more common in males than females; however, the reason for this is unclear.

Blood supply of bone

The clinical patterns of acute osteomyelitis are different in infants, children and adults. The most likely explanation is that the blood supply and structure of bone in the three age groups is different (Fig. 11.1). The common sites of infections in infants and children are in the lower limbs, both bones and joints, whereas the spine is the bone site most commonly affected by haematogenous infection in adults. This probably reflects the larger vascular beds or the nature of blood flow in the vessels in those sites. You will recall from Chapter 5 that children have a well-defined growth plate (physis), while adults do not have a growth plate. In infants, a growth plate is present, but it is less well defined, and has some vessels that penetrate it and thereby con-

nect the epiphysis and metaphysis of the bone. The physis is cartilaginous, and therefore capable of being 'expanded' by dividing and growing cells, whereas adult bone can only grow by apposition on its surface. At the junction of metaphysis and physis, small blood vessels are open-ended, growing towards the physis. At that point, the contents of the lumen can escape and lie adjacent to physeal cartilage. If an embolus of bacteria (septicaemia or bacteraemia) escapes from such a vessel, and the size of the inoculum is sufficient to cause an infection (a measure of virulence), and there is a tropism (attraction) of the pathogenic bacteria for cartilage, then an infection may be initiated.

Once a metaphyseal infection is initiated, cell death occurs and an inflammatory process follows. Intramedullary (within the marrow cavity) inflammation in the metaphysis of a long bone further impairs the circulation to the bone and ischaemia occurs around the initial septic focus or abscess. Because the direction of flow of blood in bone is dependent on pressure differences in capillaries, the nutrition of the cortical bone of the metaphysis may be secondarily impaired. The ischaemic necrosis of bone allows pus (the consequence of infective inflammation) to spread from the initial focus within the cancellous bone of the metaphysis through the bone cortex, and through the medullary cavity.

Acute infection of bone and joints

Diagnosis of acute bone infection

The absolute diagnosis of infection in bone requires that microorganisms be detected at a site in bone. The sim-

---

Case 11.1 Acute osteomyelitis: 2

Case note: Aetiology

The doctor made a diagnosis of acute haematogenous osteomyelitis. Osteomyelitis is inflammation (-itis) of bone (osteo-) and bone marrow (myel-), and is normally due to infection. Some books call it *osteitis* but it is not possible to distinguish if bone can be infected without the marrow component. The primary infection is usually blood-borne in infants and children and the first site of lodgement of the bacterial embolus is in small blood vessels within the medullary (marrow) cavity of the bone.

Case 11.1 Acute osteomyelitis: 3

Case note: Relating clinical features to pathology

The fact that Simon pointed to the metaphyseal region of his tibia as his site of pain, and the doctor found tenderness at precisely that site links the anatomy of the region to the pathology and observed clinical picture. In adults, metaphyseal osteomyelitis is uncommon, and haematogenous osteomyelitis is less common than direct invasion of bone. When haematogenous in adults, osteomyelitis is most frequent in the vertebrae.

Had Simon been examined when he first complained of his leg being sore, the doctor may not have found tenderness at the tibial metaphysis. However, the pathological sequela of the infectious process in the intervening hours, then untreated, leads to purulent oedema fluid collecting beneath the periosteum of the bone cortex, providing a critical clinical sign – *finger-point tenderness at the metaphysis of a long bone in a child*. If this sign is found, acute osteomyelitis should be considered the most likely diagnosis until proven otherwise.

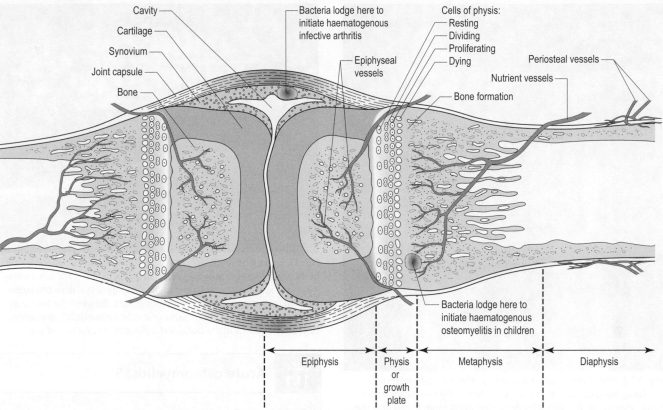

Fig. 11.1 The anatomy of bone and joint in a child. The terms used to describe the parts of the bone are shown. Note the relationship of the site of initiation of a metaphyseal abscess to the blood supply and junction of dead cartilage and forming bone adjacent to the physis.

plest way to confirm bone infection is to put a needle at the site of tenderness and to aspirate for pus. Any material collected should then be subjected to Gram staining and microbiological culture. However, this is not always possible and other investigations are usually necessary.

Although bone is an easy tissue to image, changes in bone on plain radiographs, characteristic of infection, do not appear for several days after the infection has started. When present, the most typical change is the laying down of thin layers of bone on the periosteal surface (Fig. 11.2). By the time that occurs, the infective process may be well established and difficult to abort by treatment. Nevertheless, plain radiography should always be performed as it may show an alternative diagnosis. The best investigation to perform is ultrasound imaging. It is non-invasive, not painful, and shows an image of the tissues in real time. An anechoic zone adjacent to bone (i.e. under the periosteum) means a collection of liquid and in the clinical setting confirms a diagnosis of osteomyelitis (Fig. 11.3). Furthermore, an aspirating needle can be guided by the ultrasound image to enter the liquid for the collection of a sample.

Blood cultures should also be performed, since organisms can be grown in cultures of blood taken from about half the children who have acute osteomyelitis, confirming also the septicaemic nature of the condition.

Haematological examination may show neutrophil leukocytosis or a rise in the erythrocyte sedimentation rate (ESR) or C-reactive protein (CRP) level, but they are not specific for osteomyelitis. These tests will also help to determine whether the patient has any underlying condition that has affected the immune system, thereby permitting the infection to be initiated.

In typical cases of acute osteomyelitis, no other investigations are required for diagnosis. A management scheme for a patient with pain, fever and loss of joint function in which a provisional diagnosis of osteomyelitis is considered is shown in Figure 11.4. Sometimes the condition is *atypical*, affecting an unusual bone (e.g. clavicle, calcaneus), a site that is concealed (e.g. vertebra, pelvis) or due to an uncommon pathogen (fungus, *Salmonella*). Then it may be appropriate to determine whether or not it is bone that harbours the pathology, and which bone. The most sensitive test for determining altered bone metabolism is a radioisotope bone scan. Bone scans usually employ ^{99m}technetium as the γ-emitter and a bisphosphonate as the molecule that binds to bone. Very small increases in bone formation, such as a response to infection (although not specific for infection) can be detected. Bone scans may thus locate a site, but not necessarily the pathological process. If tests locate the bone site, then it may be necessary to biopsy that site by needle or trephine aspiration to confirm an infection and identify the causative organism. Magnetic resonance imaging (MRI) can also provide valuable information about bone and the soft tissues adjacent to bone, including the presence of pus.

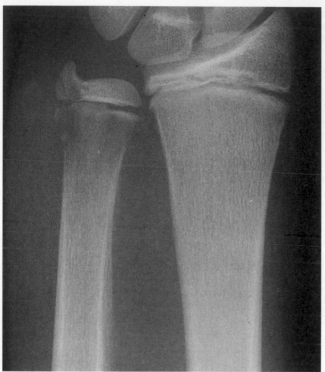

Fig. 11.2 Plain radiograph showing the effects of osteomyelitis involving the distal end of the ulna. Note the thickness of the soft tissue shadow of the skin adjacent to the distal ulna. It indicates the swelling that should be clinically obvious. Note the loss of bone that has occurred in the metaphysis of the ulna, which follows the site of initial abscess formation. Note the layers of bone that have been laid down by periosteal activity just proximal to the focus of the intramedullary osteomyelitis. In this radiograph you have evidence of bone destruction, bone formation and inflammation. These findings would be typical about 10 days after the osteomyelitis started.

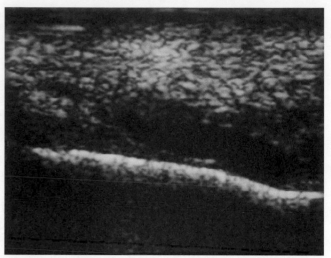

Fig. 11.3 Diagnostic ultrasound image from a child with osteomyelitis of the tibia. The cortex of the tibia is depicted by the continuous white line in the lower part of the figure. Overlying muscle is depicted by the dappled grey and black lines in the upper part. Between the two is an area from which there are no ultrasonic echoes (anechoic), appearing black. It is adjacent to the bone and represents a collection of pus.

| Case 11.1 | **Acute osteomyelitis: 4** |

Case note: Investigations

In Simon's case, the diagnosis of acute haematogenous osteomyelitis of the proximal tibia was almost certain, as he had classical clinical features. Plain radiography was normal. Ultrasound imaging showed that there was a liquid collection adjacent to his proximal tibia on its medial side. His haemoglobin level was 142 g/L, his white blood cell count was 14×10^9 cells/L with 79% neutrophils, and his ESR was 45 mm in 1 h and CRP 100 mg/L.

Treatment of acute bone infections

The appropriate treatment depends on knowledge of the causative microorganism. Treatment demands that the use of antibiotic drugs, surgery, or both, be considered. Most of the infants and children who have acute haematogenous osteomyelitis are infected with *S. aureus*. The sooner the treatment commences after making the provisional diagnosis of acute osteomyelitis, the more likely the condition is to be cured and the amount of tissue destroyed by the infection to be minimized (Fig. 11.5).

| Case 11.1 | **Acute osteomyelitis: 5** |

Case note: Treatment

Simon was treated with the intravenous administration of flucloxacillin in a dose of 100 mg/kg body weight per day, given 6-hourly, after checking that he did not have an intolerance to penicillin. As his condition improved quickly, assessed by his general wellbeing, loss of pain, decrease in tenderness and improved appetite, the intravenous line was removed 60 h after his admission to the hospital and the same dose of the antibiotic continued orally. It was given between meals and he was *not* given ice cream 'to help the medicine go down!'.

In contrast, chronic osteomyelitis, discussed below, requires that the causative organism be determined before treatment starts, as the likely organisms are much more diverse and, therefore, selection of an antibiotic on a 'best-guess' principle is more likely to be wrong. In chronic osteomyelitis, the urgency of intervention is much less, as the level of pain is less, the risk of septicaemia is less and the structural alteration of the tissues has already occurred.

Interesting facts

In the case of suspected ACUTE osteomyelitis attempts should be made to confirm the diagnosis and identify the infecting organism but antibiotic treatment of the suspected organism should not be delayed while waiting for the results of culture and other tests. Treatment can be altered when the results become known. In CHRONIC osteomyelitis it is more common to identify the causative organism before treatment begins.

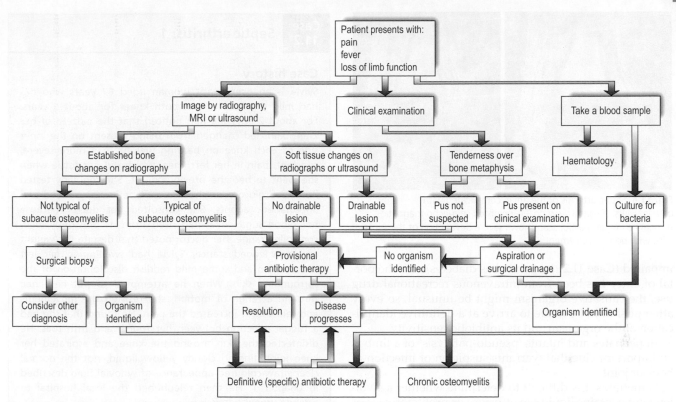

Fig. 11.4 Algorithm for management of a patient with pain, fever and loss of function in a limb when a diagnosis of osteomyelitis is considered. Note that the three important tasks are: (1) take a history; (2) take a blood sample; (3) image by ultrasound and plain radiography.

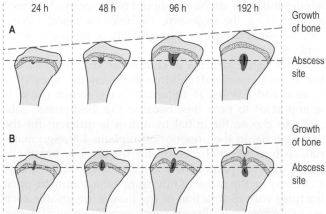

Fig. 11.5 Effects of infection of growing bone. (A) The growing end of a bone at four successive time periods demonstrating how the bone growth moves relative to the initial site of abscess formation. As a consequence of growth, the growth plate (physis) moves away from the site of the abscess, leaving behind a sequestrum of dead unresorbed cartilage (depicted by a vertical line), which harbours masses of bacteria. (B) What may happen to the shape of the articular surface of the joint and the physis, if the site of lodgement of the initial embolus is within a vessel that crosses the growth plate. Growth adjacent to that site is prevented because the dividing cells within the physis are destroyed by the infection.

Diagnosis of acute joint infections

Any non-traumatic acute condition affecting a joint should be assumed as being an infection until proved otherwise. The best way to confirm the diagnosis is to aspirate the joint and examine its contents by Gram stain, cell count, crystal examination and culture. Infection initiates an inflammatory response and neutrophils enter the joint cavity. A cell count of greater than 10^5 cells/mm^3 is consistent with an infection, while half that value or more is suggestive. The analysis of synovial fluid and the information that can be gained from it was addressed in Chapter 1. It will be the next day before any bacterial colony growth may be seen but treatment should start before then. If the Gram stain demonstrates bacteria, it can also guide the choice of the correct antibiotic, as the organisms that commonly cause septic arthritis are limited in number. *S. aureus* and streptococci are Gram-positive cocci, while *Haemophilus influenzae* are Gram-negative rods.

Interesting facts

Since immunization against *Haemophilus influenzae type b* has been introduced, the incidence of that organism as a cause of septic arthritis in children has decreased markedly.

The larger joints of the body are those most commonly infected. If an unusual joint is involved or if the infection has followed an inadvertent joint puncture (e.g. tooth, thorn or fishbone), then it is likely that an unusual organism will be the cause. If the immune state of the patient is

INFECTION AND THE MUSCULOSKELETAL SYSTEM

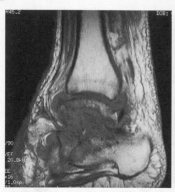
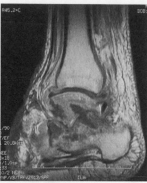

Fig. 11.6 Septic arthritis of the ankle complicated with osteomyelitis. Sagittal view on T1-weighted spin-echo magnetic resonance imaging (MRI) scan shows severe destruction of the subtalar joint with bone involvement.

impaired (Case 11.2: 1 – Sylvia has diabetes) or if the portal of entry has been from intravenous recreational drug use, the causative organism might be unusual, so every attempt should be made to arrive at a definitive identification of the organism and its antibiotic sensitivity.

In neonates and infants 'pseudo-paralysis' of a limb is an important clue that warrants suspicion of infection of bone or joint.

Sometimes it is difficult to determine whether a swollen joint contains liquid (an effusion) or proliferative synovium, or both. Moreover, in deeper joints such as the hip or shoulder, the joint cannot be palpated. If uncertainty exists as to whether a joint contains an effusion, the best tool to confirm it is MRI (Fig. 11.6). Alternatively, ultrasound, which is a quicker and easier examination than MRI, which will also delineate a joint effusion.

Interesting facts

In any joint in which there has been rapid onset of pain, in the absence of trauma, infection must be suspected, and assumed to be present until proved otherwise.

Treatment of acute joint infections

An algorithm for the management of suspected septic arthritis is shown in Figure 11.7. The important principles of management of bone and joint infections are shown in Box 11.1.

Location of the site of infection

Locating the site of infection involves clinical examination and usually imaging procedures. Confirmation should be by identifying microorganisms there; however, it is not always necessary to do that before starting treatment.

Identification of the causative organism

This should always be pursued, although it may not always be successful, and if an organism is strongly suspected, the

---

Case 11.2 — Septic arthritis: 1

Case history

Sylvia is an overweight woman aged 67 years who has had mild discomfort from both knees for about 5 years. For about 2 days she had noticed that the pattern of her knee pain had changed from being present on the inner side of each knee on bearing weight to a more severe, constant, pain in her left knee, which did not settle when she went to bed the previous night. She regularly tested her blood glucose, as she was a diabetic who needed oral anti-diabetic agents. She consulted her doctor because her blood sugar level had risen from its previously well-controlled range. Her doctor noted that despite her weight and bow-legged stance, Sylvia had swelling in her left knee region and some mild reddish discolouration of the surrounding skin. When he attempted to put her knee through a range of motion, she resisted the movements and said that it increased the pain. He found that she had a fungal infection between her fourth and fifth toes. He disinfected the skin around the knee and aspirated her knee joint, finding cloudy yellow liquid, not the normal clear straw-coloured appearance of synovial fluid described in Chapter 1. He then telephoned the local hospital to arrange urgent admission.

administration of antibiotics should not be delayed. As well as identifying the organism, the microbiological laboratory is able to determine susceptibility of the organism to antibiotics.

Acute septic arthritis is commonly due to *S. aureus*, but in unimmunized children between the ages of 6 months and 2 years, *H. influenzae* is a common cause. It is important to note this, because the 'best-guess' antibiotic to choose for initial treatment is different for the two bacteria. In the presence of implanted foreign material, such as internal fixation for fractures or prosthetic joints, unusual pathogens such as *Staphylococcus epidermidis* may be the cause of infection. After traumatic open fractures with destruction of the tissues, organisms such as *Escherichia coli*, *Pseudomonas aeruginosa*, *Bacteroides*, streptococci and clostridia may be found. In sexually active young people, aged between 15 and 30 years, gonorrhoea may be a cause of acute arthritis. Recreational drug takers, and immunosuppressed people may also have bone and joint infections with unusual organisms, including fungi, and therefore every attempt should be made to obtain a tissue specimen for identification early in the diagnostic process.

In chronic osteomyelitis there is no urgency to commence treatment and in all cases, identification of causative organisms should precede the starting of antibiotics. In spinal infections, aspiration biopsy should be performed, as *Mycobacterium tuberculosis* is a frequent cause, particularly in the patient originating from an area of endemic tuberculosis.

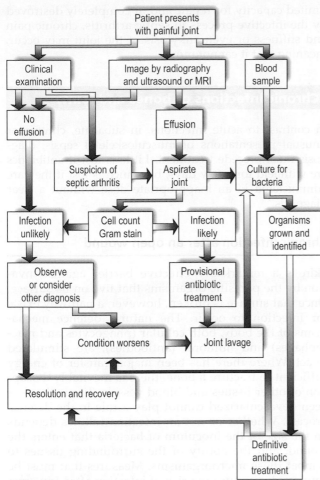

Fig. 11.7 Algorithm for management of a child with septic arthritis. Note that the three important tasks are: (1) take a history; (2) take a blood sample; (3) image by ultrasound or magnetic resonance imaging (MRI) and plain radiography.

Box 11.1 Principles of management of infection in bones and joints

- Locate the site of infection
- Identify the causative organism
- Sterilize the infected region
- Remove pus, necrotic tissue and foreign material and restore blood supply
- Monitor progress of the patient

Sterilizing the infected region

The effective way to sterilize the infected region is to use antibiotic drugs. In order to be effective, antibiotics must be able to reach the bacteria. This requires patent blood vessels sufficiently close to the periphery of the infective focus for the antibiotic to diffuse in sufficient concentration to inhibit bacterial division. The microbiological laboratory can determine the sensitivity of organisms to various antibiotics and, if necessary, determine

blood levels of antibiotics. By their presence in the tissues peripheral to an infected focus (abscess), antibiotics control the spread of invading bacteria to surrounding tissues. Bactericidal antibiotics are more effective than bacteriostatic drugs but antibiotics do not remove pus.

Surgery

The principal role of surgery is to remove pus and necrotic tissue. It should be performed in all patients with septic arthritis as soon as possible after diagnosis. Thorough and copious lavage is necessary. Lavage of joints can be performed using an arthroscope, being minimally invasive, or by open arthrotomy. In acute osteomyelitis, all patients should be prepared for surgery, although it may not be required in those who have a prompt clinical response to antibiotics alone. The indications for surgery are:

- the presence of pus as assessed on clinical grounds (and probably if detected by ultrasound imaging)
- failure of the patient to improve between two examinations by the clinician, 4–6 hours apart, after the administration of an adequate dose of provisional antibiotic and rehydration.

Antibiotic therapy

Initially, an appropriate dose of provisional ('best guess') antibiotic is given. In infants and children this should be on a body weight basis. Currently, it is appropriate to give an anti-staphylococcal bactericidal antibiotic in four daily divided doses to all children suspected of having acute osteomyelitis or septic arthritis. The precise selection of antibiotic depends on keeping local records about the causative organisms that have previously been found, and their antibiotic sensitivities. Change to a specific antibiotic, if necessary, will be guided by the results of microbiological cultures. In chronic osteomyelitis a mixed growth is often obtained. If an operative procedure is performed as part of the diagnostic process in chronic osteomyelitis to obtain a specimen for culture, the risk of bacteraemia or septicaemia at the time of surgery should be minimized by giving a single dose of an anti-staphylococcal antibiotic at that time.

The route and duration of antibiotics administration

The route and duration of treatment with antibiotics often excite debate, but current evidence does not support the prolonged use of intravenous administration. When the patient is feeling better and tolerating food, antibiotics can be given by mouth. It is important to ensure that the dose is administered regularly and that it is swallowed. Antibiotic absorption can be inhibited by food in the stomach; therefore it is advisable to administer oral antibiotics between meals. Recall that Simon was given his antibiotics between meals and his mother was told to avoid concomitant ice cream (Case 11.1: 4). Oral administration can usually be started within 3 days of the initiation of treatment. The total duration need not be prolonged.

- In the uncomplicated case of acute osteomyelitis or septic arthritis, when clinical recovery is prompt, pain disappears and function returns, a total duration of 3 weeks is probably adequate to minimize the risk of recurrence.
- In chronic osteomyelitis, the duration relates more to the type and number of surgical procedures performed than to any other indicator.

Where antibiotics are used to suppress, but not cure, chronic osteomyelitis the requirement for antibiotics can be tested by suspending the medication after a reasonable period and watching for the clinical effect. Should symptoms recur then antibiotic medication can be recommenced, without deleterious effect on the patient. It is usual to offer such a therapeutic challenge after 6 weeks of initial treatment for chronic osteomyelitis.

Monitoring progress

Clinical examination should be based on the temperature chart, the appearance of the patient, the degree of tenderness and the restriction of movement. CRP monitoring may be a useful guide, especially if not falling promptly.

The ideal outcome is to eradicate the infection and restore normal function, without structural deformity of the affected skeletal tissue, or other long-term sequel. As acute haematogenous osteomyelitis usually affects infants and children, there is an enormous capacity for repair as the child grows. In normal growth, infants' bones are completely replaced as their size increases by new bone laid down adjacent to the growth plate for length, and circumferentially under the periosteum for width. If acute osteomyelitis, which commences in the metaphysis, involves the growth plate by local spread, future growth in length may be affected, leading to a short or curved bone (see Fig. 11.5). Once destroyed by infection, growth plates cannot repair or be replaced. Articular cartilage also has a

limited capacity for repair and, if completely destroyed by the infective process in septic arthritis, chronic pain and stiffness or even ankylosis of the joint may occur, meaning that it cannot move.

Chronic infections of bones and joints

In contrast to acute infections, in subacute, chronic or unusual presentations of musculoskeletal sepsis, diagnosis must precede treatment. Little is lost if antibiotics are withheld for a few days, but much is lost if they are administered in an inappropriate dose without a clear diagnosis.

Chronic infection after an open wound

Skin is a remarkably effective barrier against invasion by the parasitic organisms that live on its surface. Once that surface is broken, however, a pathway exists for infection to occur. The natural defence mechanisms of the body, both cellular (phagocytes and macrophages) and humoral (antibodies), are stimulated to act. Where there has been major transfer of energy sufficient to fracture a bone, there is inevitably disruption of other tissues and blood vessels. Tissue that has been devascularized cannot play a role in the defence process. Whether or not an infection follows depends on the size of the inoculum of bacteria that enters the wound, and the ability of the surrounding tissues to combat those microorganisms. Measures that must be employed to reduce the risk of infection after any open wound are:

- surgical washout, meaning copious lavage with large volumes of water to wash out and dilute the inoculum

---

Case 11.2 — Septic arthritis: 2

Case note: The causative organism

The liquid aspirated from Sylvia's knee was examined and a Gram stain revealed clumps of Gram-positive cocci consistent with a diagnosis of septic arthritis. The next day there were colonies of bacteria on the culture plate, which were identified as *S. aureus*.

Case 11.2 — Septic arthritis: 3

Case note: Treatment

Following her admission to hospital, Sylvia had an intravenous line inserted. Fluid was administered via the line because she was nauseated, has diabetes and had not drunk much that day, and an antistaphylococcal, bactericidal antibiotic was given intravenously by a bolus dose every 6 h. Her blood sugar level was measured and found to be 14 mmol/L. When Sylvia was rehydrated and her blood sugar level had been reduced to normal by administration of insulin, she had lavage (washout) of her knee joint with sterile water, using an arthroscope to view the inside of the joint under spinal anaesthesia. The surgeon had warned her that if a satisfactory washout of the joint could not be achieved by that technique, the joint would have to be opened (open arthrotomy) to achieve the same result.

and any other foreign material, together with excision of any devitalized tissue; and

- inhibition of bacterial cell division by the use of antibiotics. The principle of prophylaxis is to give large doses of appropriate antibiotics as soon after the injury as possible, and to continue them for only a short period.

The organisms that are most likely to cause infection after open wounds are *S. aureus*, *P. aeruginosa*, clostridia and anaerobes, such as *Bacteroides*.

If fractures are treated by internal fixation, bacteria may adhere to the foreign surface and form a biofilm which can prevent the penetration of antibiotics in to the bacterial colonies. Such colonies may remain dormant for long periods and emerge as acute infections when the general state of the patient alters, nutritionally or by disease or change in immunity. Bone death may also occur at the site of fracture, because of the disruption of blood supply. Removal of such dead bone in the evolution of fracture healing requires considerable osteoclast activity over a long period. Some of the dead bone (sequestrum) may become incorporated into the fracture repair callus and new living bone, but act as a nidus for infection at a future date.

Joint replacement surgery has been a great advance in treatment for arthritis during the last 50 years. The surgery of joint replacement requires the excision of considerable amounts of bone adjacent to the joint in order to insert a prosthesis. The prostheses used are manufactured from several different materials – metals, high-density polyethylene, ceramics and polymethyl methacrylate as a bone cement. Such foreign material can act as a repository for bacterial colonies inevitably introduced during the surgical operation. Furthermore, wear particles from the articulating surfaces may affect the way phagocytic cells function. Infection may occur in up to 2% of patients who have joint replacement. The effect is chronic periprosthetic joint infection for which the prosthesis may have to be removed (Fig. 11.9). Antibiotic prophylaxis should be given for joint replacement surgery, using the same principles as for open fractures.

Case 11.1   Acute osteomyelitis: 6

Case note: Progress

Simon became free from pain 3 days after treatment commenced. He was discharged from hospital and his mother was told that the antibiotic treatment with flucloxacillin must continue, with regular dosage, between meals, for the next 2 weeks. He has not had any further problems. In view of his good progress, assessed clinically, no further investigations were performed, as they were unlikely to influence any therapeutic or prognostic decisions.

Case 11.2   Septic arthritis: 4

Case note: Progress

Sylvia did not fare as well as Simon. She continued to have some pain in her knee, and the swelling persisted. She had a further arthroscopic lavage, and it was found that there was very little articular cartilage remaining on her medial femoral and tibial condyles (from her osteoarthritis, although more may have been lost because of the infection). The surgeon told her that she could not have total knee replacement surgery for at least 1 year as the risk of a prosthesis becoming infected was high, in view of her recent acute septic arthritis. Remember that the presence of a foreign body decreases the local tissue defences against infecting organisms, and a small inoculum of bacteria may then cause an infection, even with organisms of low virulence or pathogenicity.

Chronic osteomyelitis

Chronic osteomyelitis is a significant health problem with substantial morbidity but low mortality. Whether it arises from acute haematogenous infection, after trauma, or following an implant, the general principles of management are identical. There is no guarantee that cure can ever be achieved, so suppression is sometimes a better concept. Recurrences can occur a very long time after the initial infection.

S. aureus remains the most common isolate, reflecting the acute infection that initiated the process. In many parts of the world, particularly where there is malnutrition, overcrowding or poverty, tuberculosis is endemic. *M. tuberculosis* reaches bones and joints by haematogenous spread, stimulating chronic inflammation, which has a different pathological pattern from that of acute inflammation but a similar association of destruction and repair of tissues. In chronic inflammation, the onset of pain is gradual rather than sudden and its severity is less intense. However, the inflammation has frequently been present for a long period before treatment is sought and irreversible structural changes may have occurred in the bones and joints involved.

The fundamental problem is the persistence of organisms. The pathological anatomy reflects the consequences of continuing necrosis and repair. Dead bone that has become detached from surrounding living bone is called *sequestrum*. The accumulation of pus in the tissues is an abscess, and a sinus is a track from the depths of a tissue to the exterior, usually made by the passage of pus. Reactive new bone is called an *involucrum*. The balance between necrosis and repair determines the outcome; the aim of management is to tip the balance in favour of the host.

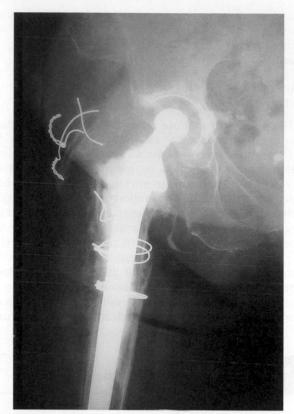
Fig. 11.9 Plain radiograph of infected hip prosthesis.

Case 11.3 Chronic infection: 1

Case history

Stewart loved his motorcycle. When he was 18 he crashed it at high speed and sustained a comminuted open fracture of his right tibia. He was taken to the nearest district hospital where he was treated without delay by the administration of an antibiotic, surgical lavage of the open wound and insertion of an intramedullary nail to internally fix the fracture after it had been realigned to an almost anatomical position. Some 10 days after his accident, his temperature rose to 39°C and there was a serous discharge from the wound. A specimen of the discharge was taken for culture, and antibiotic medication was recommenced; 10 days later he was allowed to go home, as he was feeling well. He is now 20 and has not been able to return to work as an apprentice plumber. He has continuing mild discomfort from his right leg, particularly when bearing weight. He had to use crutches for 9 months, as plain radiography did not show healing of the fracture. Every 2 or 3 months he has an acute exacerbation of pain in his tibia, a feeling of being unwell, and discharge of a small amount of pus from his shin. After taking antibiotics for a few days, he generally feels better and the pain decreases. He is now concerned that his orthopaedic surgeon might suggest that his leg be amputated below the knee (Fig. 11.8).

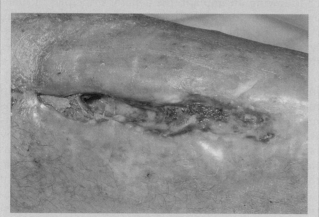

Fig. 11.8 The state of Stewart's leg on one of the occasions when he had an exacerbation of pain and purulent discharge. Note the redness and swelling of acute inflammation of the skin, the ulceration of the skin because of necrosis, and in the base of the ulcer the coagulated slough of dead tissue and pus lying on exposed bone. When bone is allowed to dry like that, it dies and acts as a reservoir for bacteria. Such dead bone is called sequestrum, and it is essential that it be removed before healing can occur. Dead bone cannot contribute to the fracture-healing process.

Case 11.3 Chronic infection: 2

Case note: Prognosis

Until all dead and foreign tissue has been removed, the risk of such exacerbations of infection always remains in cases of chronic osteomyelitis. This is the most likely reason why Stewart has had a 'flare-up' of infection in his leg. If Stewart is left with an ununited fracture of his tibia and an intermittent or continually discharging sinus, he may never regain normal function of his limb. The potential for chronic infection was caused by his open fracture in the first instance. The severity of disruption of the tissues at the time of the initial trauma is a major determinant of outcome. The incidence of chronic osteomyelitis after open fracture may be as high as 10%.

Diagnosis of chronic bone and joint infections

If the mouth of a discharging sinus is sampled to obtain a specimen, a diverse mixture of organisms may be cultured. Most of them are likely to be commensals which have colonized the superficial tissue; only tissue specimens from the depths of a sinus, or blood cultures, are useful in identifying the true causative organism in chronic osteomyelitis. Vertebral osteomyelitis is not usually associated with a sinus, so a biopsy, which can be done by a trephine or needle using radiological monitoring, is an important part of the diagnostic process. Plain radiography is usually sufficient to make a diagnosis of chronic osteomyelitis (Table 11.1).

Table 11.1 Relation of radiological signs to pathology in chronic infections

Pathological process	Radiological sign
Oedema	Soft tissue swelling; obliteration of tissue planes
Medullary infection	Osteopenia and lysis of cortical bone
Cortical infection	Cortical lucency and lysis
Subperiosteal abscess	Periosteal new bone, involucrum
Soft tissue abscess	Soft tissue swelling; obliteration of tissue planes
Localized cortical and medullary abscess	Single or multiple radiolucent cortical or medullary lytic lesions with surrounding sclerosis
Cortical necrosis	Sequestration of bone
Fistula	Migration of cortical fragments

If further detail is required, computerized tomography and sometimes magnetic resonance imaging may be helpful. A sinus can be delineated by injection of a radiological contrast agent along its track, or at the time of surgery by injecting a coloured dye, such as gentian violet. Any tissue sample removed should be subjected to histological examination to seek features of infection. That may be the only direct evidence.

Management of chronic infection

The principles of management of chronic infection of bones and joints, regardless of aetiology or the site of infection, are:

- correct and complete microbiological diagnosis
- assessment and modification of host defence mechanisms
- anatomical definition of the extent of local disease in bone and soft tissues
- correct antibiotic therapy
- surgical removal of necrotic and poorly vascularized tissue and all infected granulation
- obliteration of dead spaces left by the surgical debridement
- restoration of stability of the skeleton to allow function
- rehabilitation.

There are limited indications for surgery:

- significant disability for the patient's lifestyle or general health

Case 11.4 **Tuberculous osteomyelitis: 1**

Case history

Sachin was born in Cambodia and had grown up during the civil war in that country. At the age of 36 she had been granted emigration rights. As part of the immigration process she had undergone a medical examination, and had a chest X-ray examination. She was found to be healthy. Two years after re-establishing her family life in another country she had consulted a medical practitioner, who spoke her native language, because of pain in her back. She had not sustained any injury that she could recall. The pain was not related to her menstrual periods. It was a constant dull ache that was progressively becoming more severe. She had not experienced a fever. She had lost a little weight. Examination showed her to stand with a slight scoliosis of her thoracolumbar region, and she had lost the normally expected rhythmic pattern of movement of her back when she was asked to bend forwards. She had an area of impaired light touch sensation on the anterior aspect of her left thigh. Her left knee jerk reflex was slightly less prominent than the right. You will recall from Chapter 4 that these neurological abnormalities would constitute a so-called 'red flag'. Moreover, the report of the X-ray examination of her back stated 'infection should be excluded'.

Case 11.4 **Tuberculous osteomyelitis: 2**

Case note: Diagnosis

The spine is a more frequent site for tuberculous osteomyelitis than acute osteomyelitis. The destructive effects are on intervertebral discs as well as bone, leading to potential impairment of spinal cord function because of structural and mechanical deformity of the spine. In Sachin's case, it was the characteristic loss of the intervertebral disc height between two vertebrae that alerted the radiologist to make the comment about the possibility of infection. Regardless of the infecting organism, the structural changes in bones and joints are similar. It is essential to identify the causative organisms before commencing treatment.

- appropriate patient expectations and commitment to multiple surgeries and prolonged treatment
- prior stabilization of systemic disease (including cessation of cigarette smoking)
- adequate local conditions (skin, blood supply) in the affected limb
- technical feasibility of any planned reconstruction.

Case 11.4 Tuberculous osteomyelitis: 3

Case note: Pathology

Osteomyelitis of the spine destroys intervertebral discs and parts of the adjacent vertebrae so that an angular deformity, or kyphus, results. The hunchback of Notre-Dame probably had tuberculosis. The vertebrae usually fuse together when the infection is controlled. The level of the spine infected determines whether spinal cord dysfunction may follow as a result of the cord being stretched over the kyphus. In the lumbar region, nerve roots occupy the spinal canal and are less vulnerable to stretch. Pus from the infection may, however, enter the spinal canal and produce an extradural abscess with nerve root or spinal cord dysfunction. This may explain the abnormal neurological findings in Sachin's case.

If a vertebral body is affected, the pus may track forwards causing a paravertebral abscess. In the lumbar region such an abscess frequently enters the substance of the psoas muscle(s) and tracks down to the groin within the psoas sheath, leading to a 'cold abscess' in the groin when the sinus breaks through the skin. Chronic osteomyelitis in a long bone may lead to pathological fracture of that bone – if that occurs, the fracture may not unite.

The use of antibiotics may be an alternative to suppress the disease. Usually a prolonged course is not necessary, although short courses (6 weeks) may have to be repeated from time to time. However, in tuberculosis, antituberculous antibiotics, given as multiple drug combinations, are usually effective in controlling and eradicating the disease after about 9 months' administration.

Acknowledgements

We acknowledge Professor Sydney Nade, author of the earlier edition of this chapter, for his contribution.

alopecia – excessive loss of hair.

ankylosis – when the joint becomes stiff or fused in a particular position.

arthropathy – pathology in a joint, but sometimes used as a generic term for arthritis.

arthroplasty – surgery to a joint to modify its surface or structure including joint replacement.

arthrotomy – surgical incision of a joint capsule.

autoantibody – an antibody directed against self-components.

biological treatment – a medication derived from living sources such as cell culture.

biopsychosocial – considers biological, pscyhological and social factors and their interactions in understanding symptoms.

bursa – a 'cushioning' sac, lined by synovium and normally containing a small amount of synovial fluid, lying between areas of friction to allow opposing surfaces to slide smoothly against each other.

capsulitis – inflammation of the outer lining of the joint, i.e. the joint capsule.

chondrocyte – principal cartilage cell responsible for synthesis of extracellular matrix.

condyle – a rounded protuberance that occurs at the ends of some bones.

crepitus – grating sound elicited on moving a joint.

cyclooxygenase – an enzyme responsible for synthesis of prostaglandins and thromboxanes.

cytokine – polypeptides which act non-enzymatically and regulate host cell function.

denervation – interruption of the nerve supply to muscles or skin.

depolarization – the sudden surge of charged particles across the membrane of a nerve or muscle cell.

dermatome – the skin segment of the body supplied by a given spinal nerve.

diaphysis – the shaft of a long bone.

dislocation – disruption of a joint such that the normally opposing joint surfaces have no contact with each other.

effusion – excessive synovial fluid accumulation within the joint cavity.

enthesitis / enthesopathy – inflammation at site of tendinous insertion into bone.

epicondyle – the protuberance above a condyle.

epiphysis – the end of the long bone beyond the growth plate leading up to the joint surface.

erosion – localized loss of integrity of the articular surface, usually due to invasion by inflamed synovium.

fracture – a structural break in the continuity of bone.

glomerulonephritis – inflammation of the glomerulus of the kidney.

glycosaminoglycan – complex polysaccharides consisting of long chains of sugar molecules attached to an amino group.

haemarthrosis – blood within synovial cavity.

haplotype – the particular combination in any individual of specific HLA (human leukocyte antigen) gene alleles.

histocompatibility antigen – a white blood cell marker determined by certain genes important in transplant graft acceptance or rejection; sometimes called HLA (human leukocyte antigen).

humoral – refers to the 'fluid' component of blood, as opposed to circulating cells.

immunosuppression – suppression of immune system, usually by drugs.

intima – the inner layer of the wall of a tissue such as the synovium.

labrum – a lip like structure around the margins of joint.

malar – a rash over the facial cheeks typically seen in systemic lupus erythematosus.

meniscus – fibrocartilaginous discs that divide the cavity of certain synovial joints.

mesangium – the part of the glomerulus comprised of phagocytic cells and extracellular matrix.

metalloproteinases – a family of enzymes which contain a metal atom in their structure and can degrade cartilage and other connective tissues.

metaphysis – the flare of a long bone towards the joint.

monarthritis – joint inflammation involving only one joint.

myopathy – a disorder of skeletal muscle.

nociception – the sensation of pain.

oligoarthritis – joint inflammation involving less than six joints.

open fracture – a fracture where the overlying skin is breached, allowing communication between the fracture and the outside.

osteoblast – the cell responsible for bone formation.

osteoclast – the cell responsible for bone resorption.

pathogenicity – ability to cause pathology (disease).

pathological fracture – a fracture caused by normal force in abnormal bone.

periarticular – occurring 'near the joint'.

physis – the growth plate in a long bone.

polyarthritis – joint inflammation involving six or more joints.

proteoglycan – large molecules made up of glycosaminoglycans linked to the proteins.

radiculopathy – pathology involving a spinal nerve root.

serositis – inflammation of the lining surface of the heart (pericarditis), lungs (pleuritis) or abdomen (peritonitis).

spondyloarthritis – inflammation involving spinal joints.

spondylosis – degeneration affecting the intervertebral discs.

stress fracture – a fracture caused by repetitive 'normal' forces.

subluxation – disruption of a joint such that the normally opposing joint surfaces have some partial contact with each other.

synovectomy – removal of synovium either by surgery or by treatment with radioactive isotopes.

synovium – a normal thin layer of tissue within the joint that produces synovial fluid.

tendonitis – inflammation of a tendon.

tophus – collection of sodium urate crystals in tissues.

valgus – a deformity that displaces the distal part of a joint away from midline.

varus – a deformity that displaces the distal part of a joint towards the midline.

vasculitis – inflammation of blood vessels.

Index

Note: Page numbers followed by 'f' indicate figures, 't' indicate tables and 'b' indicate boxes.